Progress in Drug Research
Fortschritte der Arzneimittelforschung
Progrès des recherches pharmeceutiques
Vol. 43

Progress in Drug Research
Fortschritte der Arzneimittelforschung
Progrès des recherches pharmaceutiques
Vol. 43

Edited by / Herausgegeben von / Rédigé par
Ernst Jucker, Basel

Authors / Autoren/ Auteurs
Harold E. Bays and Carlos Dujovne · Eric J. Lien, Hua Gao and
Linda L. Lien · N. Seiler and C. L. Atanassov · Shradha Sinha and
Mukta Srivastava · Mark P. Hayes and Kathryn C. Zoon.

1994   Birkhäuser Verlag
                   Basel · Boston · Berlin

Editor:

Dr. E. Jucker
Steinweg 28
CH-4107 Ettingen
Switzerland

© 1994 Birkhäuser Verlag, P.O. Box 133, CH-4010 Basel, Switzerland
Softcover reprint of the hardcover 1st edition 1994

Printed on acid-free paper produced from chlorine-free pulp

ISBN-13:978-3-0348-7158-7   e-ISBN-13:978-3-0348-7156-3
DOI: 10.1007/978-3-0348-7156-3

Contents · Inhalt · Sommaire

Foreword

Volume 43 of «Progress in Drug Research» contains five reviews and the various indexes which facilitate its use and establish the connection with the previous volumes. The articles in this volume deal with high cholesterol blood levels and other dyslipidemias; search of ideal antihypertensive drugs; the natural polyamines and the immune system; biologically active quinazolones and with production and action of interferons.

In the 35 years the PDR has existed, the Editor has enjoyed the valuable help and advice of many colleagues. Readers, the authors of the reviews, and last but not least, the reviewers have all contributed greatly to the success of this series. Although the comments received so far have generally been favorable, it is nevertheless necessary to analyze and to reassess the current position and the future direction of such a review series.

So far, it has been the Editors intention to help disseminate information on the vast domain of drug research, and to provide the reader with a tool with which to keep abreast of the latest developments and trends. The reviews in PDR are useful to the non-specialist, who can obtain an overview of a particular field of drug research in a relatively short time.

The specialist readers of PDR will appreciate the reviews' comprehensive bibliographies, and, in addition, they may even get fresh impulses for their own research. Finally, the readers can use the 43 volumes of PDR as an encyclopedic source of information.

It gives me great pleasure to present this new volume to our readers. At the same time I would like to express my gratitude to the authors who willingly accepted the task of preparing extensive reviews. My sincere thanks also go to the Birkhäuser Verlag, and, in particular to Mrs. L. Koechlin and Mssrs. H.-P. Thür, E. Mazenauer and G. Messmer. Without their personal committment and assistance, editing PDR would be a nearly impossible task.

Basel, September 1994   DR. E. JUCKER

Vorwort

Der vorliegende 43. Band der Reihe «Fortschritte der Arzneimittelforschung» enthält fünf Übersichtsartikel sowie die verschiedenen Register, welche das Arbeiten mit diesem Band erleichtern und den Zugriff auf die vorhergehenden Bände ermöglichen.

Die Artikel des 43. Bandes behandeln – wie das Inhaltsverzeichnis zeigt – verschiedene aktuelle Gebiete der Arzneimittelforschung und ermöglichen es dem Leser, sich rasch einen guten Überblick über diese Gebiete zu verschaffen.

Seit der Gründung der Reihe sind 35 Jahre vergangen. In dieser langen Zeitspanne konnte der Herausgeber immer auf den Rat der Fachkollegen, der Leser und der Autoren zählen. Ihnen allen möchte ich meinen Dank abstatten. In diesem Dank sind auch die Rezensenten eingeschlossen, denn sie haben wesentlich zum guten Gedeihen der Reihe beigetragen. Viele Kommentare und Besprechungen waren lobend. Trotzdem ist es angebracht, die Frage nach dem Sinn und Zweck der «Fortschritte» zu stellen und zu überüprüfen.

Nach wie vor ist es unser Ziel, neueste Forschungsergebnisse in Form von Übersichten darzustellen und dem Leser auf diese Weise zu ermöglichen, sich verhältnismässig rasch und mühelos über bestimmte aktuelle Richtungen der Arzneimittelforschung zu informieren. Es wird ihm die Möglichkeit geboten, sich im komplexen und sich rasant entwickelnden Fachgebiet auf dem laufenden zu halten und den Kontakt zur aktuellen Forschung aufrechtzuerhalten.

Die Übersichten der «Fortschritte» bieten dem Spezialisten eine wertvolle Quelle der Originalliteratur dar, erlauben ihm nützliche Vergleichsmöglichkeiten, und sie können u.a. seine eigene Forschung befruchten. Für alle Leser der «Fortschritte» stellt die Reihe mit ihren ausführlichen Verzeichnissen eine nützliche Quelle von enzyklopädischem Wissen dar, so dass das gesamte Werk auch als Nachschlagewerk dienen kann.

Zum Gedeihen der Reihe haben die Autoren massgebend beigetragen; ihnen allen sei hier gedankt. Dank gebührt auch dem Birkhäuser Verlag, insbesondere Frau L. Koechlin und den Herren H.-P. Thür, E. Mazenauer und G. Messmer.

Basel, September 1994   DR. E. JUCKER

Progress in Drug Research, Vol. 43 (E. Jucker, Ed.)
© 1994 Birkhäuser Verlag, Basel (Switzerland)

Drugs for treatment of patients with high cholesterol blood levels and other dyslipidemias

By Harold E. Bays[1] and Carlos A. Dujovne[2]

[1] The Lipid Center, Advanced Cardiovascular Institute, Audubon Regional Medical Center, One Audubon Plaza Drive, University of Louisville School of Medicine, Department of Endocrinology and Metabolism, Louisville, Kentucky 40127, USA; and
[2] The Lipid and Arteriosclerosis Prevention Clinic, Division of Clinical Pharmacology, Department of Medicine, University of Kansas, Kansas City, Kansas, USA

Correspondence to:
Harold E. Bays, M.D., Medical Director, The Lipid Center, Advanced Cardiovascular Institute, Audubon Regional Medical Center, One Audubon Plaza Drive, Louisville, Kentucky 40217, USA

1   Introduction

Atherosclerotic coronary artery disease (ASCAD) is the most common cause of morbidity and mortality in most developed nations. Dyslipidemia increases the risk of ASCAD. Diet, lifestyle habits, and/or lipid-acting drugs that favorably affect lipid blood levels have been shown to decrease progression, or in some cases induce regression of ASCAD. Therefore, lipid-acting drugs have been recommended for dyslipidemic patients with ASCAD, or at high risk for ASCAD, who do not correct their lipid blood levels after diet and lifestyle recommendations. The choice of the type of lipid-acting drug/s should be based on the blood lipid profile, as well as the potential effectiveness, tolerance, and toxicity anticipated in the individual patient.

2   Results of clinical trials of lipid-acting treatments: Peripheral vascular disease

One of the most accessible vascular beds to monitor the progression of atherosclerosis is the peripheral circulation. It is presumed, though not definitively established, that similar risk factors and similar mechanisms promote atherosclerotic lesions in the peripheral circulation as in the coronary arteries. Decreased progression, and increased regression of peripheral atherosclerotic disease of the lower extremities has been shown to be directly proportional to level of correction of dyslipidemia by various lipid-acting drugs [1–4]. Lipid-acting drugs have been shown to decrease the progression, and increase regression of asymptomatic carotid atherosclerotic lesions [5].

3   Results of clinical trials of lipid-acting treatments: Atherosclerotic coronary artery disease (ASCAD)

3.1   Primary ASCAD prevention trials

Primary prevention trials (Table 1) have shown that treatment of dyslipidemia is associated with a decrease in the onset of ASCAD, despite significant differences in the mechanism of action and differences in the various types of treatments. This suggests that correcting dyslipidemia is

Table 1.
Examples of primary ASCAD prevention trials in the treatment of dyslipidemia*

Author (Study/year)	Duration (years)	Treatment	Summary of major findings	Reference
Dayton S. et al. (VA Diet Trial, 1969)	5–8	Diet	A 13% reduction in total cholesterol blood levels in treated patients was associated with a 30% reduction in coronary/peripheral vascular disease and a 20% reduction in myocardial infarction and sudden death.	[71, 72]
Miettinen M. et al. (Finnish Study 1972)	6+6	Diet	An approximate 15% reduction in total cholesterol blood levels in treated patients was associated with a 53% reduction in ASCAD deaths in men and a 34% reduction in ASCAD deaths in women.	[72, 73]
Coronary Drug Project (CDP, 1975/1986)	6/15	Niacin	A 10% reduction in total cholesterol blood levels in treated patients was associated with a 27% reduction in nonfatal myocardial infarction and a 3.1% reduction in ASCAD deaths. After 15 years, treated patients had an 11% reduction in overall mortality.	[8, 9]
WHO Clofibrate Study (1978)	5	Clofibrate	A 9% reduction in total cholesterol blood levels in treated patients was associated with a 20% reduction in ASCAD events, no change in fatal ASCAD events, an increased rate of cholecystitis and 28% increase of cancer – particularly gastrointestinal cancer.	[11]
Hjermann I. et al. (Oslo Diet-Heart Trial 1981)	5	Diet, Antismoking advice	A 13% reduction in total cholesterol blood levels in treated patients was associated with a 47% reduction in fatal and nonfatal myocardial infarction and sudden death.	[74]
LRC-CPPT (1984)	7	Cholestyramine	A 13% reduction in total cholesterol and 20% reduction in LDL-C blood levels in treated patients was associated with a 19% reduction in fatal and nonfatal myocardial infarction.	[12–14]
MRFIT (1982)	7	Special** intervention	A 7% reduction in total cholesterol in treated patients compared to a 3% reduction in total cholesterol blood levels in controls was associated with no statistical difference in ASCAD deaths. However, among a subset of patients with hypercholesterolemia at entry into the study, the "special intervention" group had a 32% reduction in ASCAD deaths.	[75, 76]
Frick MH et al. (Helsinki Study 1987)	5	Gemfibrozil	An 11% reduction in total and LDL cholesterol, a 35% decrease in triglyceride, and a 11% increase in HDL-C blood levels in treated patients was associated with a 34% reduction in coronary artery disease.	[15, 16]

* The trials listed are at least 5 years in duration.
** "Special intervention" in the MRFIT included recommendations towards dietary treatment of hypercholesterolemia, regular physical exercise, antihypertensive treatment, attaining ideal body weight, and cessation of cigarette smoking. The lack of benefit may have been related to the fact that 1/3 of participants did not receive cholesterol lowering dietary instruction because they were not hypercholesterolemic, some antihypertensive drugs worsened cholesterol blood levels, and the reduction in total cholesterol between the diet treated and control group was only about 3%.

an effective intervention in decreasing the onset and progression of ASCAD – whether by diet, lifestyle intervention and/or by lipid-acting drugs [6–16]. Compared to secondary ASCAD prevention trials that have often demonstrated beneficial results in as early as 2 years, primary ASCAD prevention trials typically require up to 15 years to demonstrate statistical significance. Lipid-acting drugs that have thusfar been shown to decrease the onset, morbidity and/or mortality of ASCAD in primary prevention trials include resins, niacin, and fibrates.

One of the first primary prevention trials was the Coronary Drug Project (CDP) [8, 9]. The CDP was designed to study the effects of different lipid-acting treatments on the onset of ASCAD. Treatments that had to be discontinued due to adverse events included high dose estrogen (which increased thrombotic ASCAD events) and dextrothyroxine (which increased cardiac dysrhythmias). Clofibrate was found to result in a mild reduction in total cholesterol and modest reduction in ASCAD events and ASCAD deaths. However, clofibrate was associated with worsening of other vascular morbidities (e.g. angina, pulmonary embolism, and thrombophlebitis), as well as a marked increase in gall bladder disease.

Niacin treatment was found to be effective in improving lipid blood levels and reducing ASCAD events. Furthermore, a 15-year follow up of patients in the CDP treated with niacin demonstrated a 11% reduction in cardiac as well as overall mortality [9].

The WHO primary prevention trial [11] demonstrated that a mild reduction in total cholesterol blood levels with clofibrate was associated with a mild reduction in ASCAD events, but no change in fatal ASCAD events. However, due to the increased rate of cholecystitis and the increase in the rate of cancer – particularly gastrointestinal cancer – the authors concluded that clofibrate should not be recommended as a lipid-acting drug for primary prevention of ASCAD.

In 1984, the Lipid Research Clinics Coronary Primary Prevention Trial (LRC-CPPT) [12, 13] demonstrated a clear reduction in ASCAD events and ASCAD deaths with resin lipid-acting drug treatment. The results of this landmark trial supported a "1:2 rule of primary prevention" in that every 1% reduction in total cholesterol blood level decreased the risk of ASCAD by 2%. A 6-year post trial follow-up of this 7-year trial demonstrated that although the beneficial effect of cholestyramine treatment in the prevention of ASCAD did not persist beyond the cessation of treatment, cholestyramine was found to be safe and efficacious treatment for hypercholesterolemia, with only a nonsignificant increase in cancer and cholecystitis [14].

Finally, the Helsinki Heart Trial [15] was a primary prevention trial in which treatment of dyslipidemic men with gemfibrozil resulted in a decrease in low density lipoprotein cholesterol (LDL-C), decrease in triglyceride, and an increase in high density lipoprotein cholesterol (HDL-C) blood levels with an overall reduction in onset of ASCAD. A reexamination of this trial revealed that patients with an elevated triglyceride blood level and/or elevated LDL-C/HDL-C ratio had the greatest risk for ASCAD [16]. In fact, the LDL-C/HDL-C ratio was more prognostic than LDL-C and HDL-C alone in predicting the onset of ASCAD in dyslipidemic men. Furthermore, over 70% of the reduction in ASCAD risk in gemfibrozil treatment group occurred in the subset of men with triglyceride blood levels greater than 2.3 mm/liter (< 200 mg/dl) and LDL/HDL ratio greater than 5.0. The authors concluded that the subset of men with elevated triglyceride blood levels and elevated LDL/HDL cholesterol ratios (which constituted only about 10% of the trial population) benefitted most from gemfibrozil treatment.

3.2   Secondary ASCAD prevention trials

Secondary prevention trials have shown that improvement in dyslipidemia with diet, ileal by-pass surgery, exercise, and/or lipid-acting drugs may decrease the progression of atherosclerotic lesions in patients with pre-existing ASCAD. This is clinically relevant in that patients with ASCAD are most likely to benefit from aggressive treatment to correct dyslipidemia and reduce other ASCAD risk factors because of their marked increased risk for future ASCAD, regardless of cholesterol blood levels [7].

For example, a meta-analysis of primary ASCAD prevention trials demonstrated only 6 fewer myocardial infarctions (MI's) than expected per 1000 patients after 5–10 years of treatment of dyslipidemia. Conversely, a similar meta-analysis of secondary ASCAD prevention trials demonstrated 27 fewer MI's than expected per 1000 patients after 1–5 years of treatment of dyslipidemia [7]. Clearly, patients with ASCAD denote a subset of patients who are most at risk for ASCAD progression and are most likely to benefit from aggressive treatment to correct dyslipidemia. Lipid-acting drugs that have been shown to decrease the progression, induce regression, and/or otherwise reduce the recurrence of ASCAD in trials of secondary prevention include resins, niacin, statins [17] and fibrates.

Secondary ASCAD prevention trials have provided information regarding

Table 2.
Angiographic secondary prevention trials in the treatment of dyslipidemia

Author (Study/year)	Duration (years)	Treatment	LDL-C	HDL-C	TG	ASCAD Progression Treated/Control	ASCAD Regression Treated/Control	Reference
Nikkila E.A. et al. (1984)	7	Clofibrate, niacin or both	−19%	+10%	−38%	17% / 38%	? / ?	[77]
Brensike J.F. et al. (NHLBI 1984)	5	Cholestyramine	−26%	+ 8		32% / 49%	7% / 7%	[18] [78]
Blankenhorn D.H. et al. (CLAS 1987)	2	Colestipol/Niacin	−43%	+37%	−22%	39% / 61%	16% / 2%	[18] [79]
Cashin-Hemphill L. et al. (CLAS II 1990)	4	Colestipol/Niacin	−40%	+37%	−18%	48% / 85%	18% / 6%	[18] [80]
Ornish D. et al. (Lifestyle Heart Trial 1990)	1	Diet/lifestyle	−37%	+ 0	+18%	14% / 32%	41% / 32%	[18] [81]
Kane J.P. et al. (UCSF Familial Hypercholesterolemic Trial 1990)	2	Combination of colestipol, niacin, and/or lovastatin	−38%	+28%	−19%	20% / 41%	33% / 13%	[82]
Brown B.G. et al. (FATS 1990)	2.5	Colestipol/Niacin or Colestipol/Lovastatin	−34% −48%	+41% +14%	−29% − 9%	25% / 46% 22% / 46%	39% / 11% 32% / 11%	[83]
Buchwald R. et al. (POSCH 1990)	5	Ileol by-pass	−38%	+ 4%	+20%	37% / 65%	14% / 6%	[84]
Watts G.F. et al. (STARS 1992)	3	Diet Diet and cholestyramine	−16% −35%	NC NC	−20% NC	15% / 46% 12% / 46%	38% / 4% 33% / 4%	[85]
Schuler G. et al. (1992)	?	Diet, exercise	− 8	+ 3	−24%	23% / 48%	32% / 17%	[86]
Blankenhorn D.H. et al. (MARS 1993)	2	Lovastatin	−38%	+ 8%	−21%	29% / 41%	23% / 12%	[87]

the quantitative angiographic changes in coronary artery lumen, as well as the onset of ASCAD events with various lipid-acting treatments. The study design and entry criteria of various angiographic secondary ASCAD prevention trials listed in Table 2 differ substantially from trial to trial. Some of these trials have reported the percentage change in arterial lumen, while as others have reported the percentage of patients who have progression or regression in coronary artery lesions. Therefore, the results of the various secondary ASCAD prevention trials listed in Table 2 are not necessarily comparable. However, in general, these studies support a "2:1:1 rule of secondary prevention", in that every 2% reduction in LDL-C blood level decreases the risk of ASCAD progression by about 1% and induces regression by about 1%.

With regard to onset of ASCAD events, a meta-analysis of 8 secondary ASCAD prevention trials of diet and lipid-acting drugs demonstrated that a 10% reduction in the total cholesterol blood level was associated with a 19% decreased risk of nonfatal MI's, 12% decreased risk of fatal MI's, and a 15% decrease risk of overall MI's [7]. Furthermore, a review of many of the angiographic secondary ASCAD prevention trials listed in Table 2 demonstrated a 25–89% reduction in all ASCAD events in treated versus control groups [18]. Finally, at least two of the secondary ASCAD prevention trials have demonstrated that treatment of dyslipidemia is associated with a decrease in overall mortality compared to controls [9, 18, 19]. Although regression of atherosclerotic lesions with aggressive treatment of dyslipidemia has become a potential treatment goal for many patients with ASCAD, several points should be understood. Firstly, the angiographic finding of widening of coronary artery lumen ("regression") found in angiographic ASCAD secondary prevention trials may involve mechanisms independent of alterations in blood lipid levels including lysis of fully occlusive thrombi, healing of acutely disrupted plaque, remodeling of the underlying vascular architecture, and relaxation of arterial vasomotor tone [18].

Secondly, the potential for regression may be largely dependent on the stage of the atherosclerotic lesion. For example, "early" or minimal lesions composed predominantly of lipid-laden macrophages (and possibly smooth muscle cells), typically maintain an intact intimal structure. These asymptomatic lesions, that are often found early in life, may be reversible with treatments of dyslipidemia (Tables 1 and 2). Alternatively, "mature" or advanced lesions such as the atheroma, are typically composed of extracellular lipid debris, proliferated smooth muscle, hemorrhagic and thrombotic material, fibrotic scar tissue, and typically have a disrupted intima. These lesions are thought to be less susceptible to significant regression despite aggressive treatment of dyslipidemia.

Finally, while as the "regression" in secondary prevention ASCAD trials in Table 2 has been shown to occur much more frequently in treated patients compared to controls, the absolute widening of individual arterial lumen is modest [18]. Nevertheless, the risk of ASCAD progression and ASCAD events is markedly reduced. It is proposed that treatment of dyslipidemia reduces the lipid/foam cell content and thus reduces the risk that the plaque will fissure, disrupt, thrombose and otherwise progress [18]. Hence, although treatment of dyslipidemia may be associated with only a modest improvement in arterial lumen, the reduction in the risk of subsequent ASCAD events may be substantial.

Therefore, optimal treatment of patients at high risk for onset or recurrence of ASCAD should begin before the development of the irreversible atheromatous lesion. One important treatment is aggressive reduction of LDL-C blood levels in patients with, or at high risk for ASCAD. The National Cholesterol Education Program (NCEP) Expert Panel [20] has recently reduced the desired goal of treatment of LDL-C blood levels in patients with ASCAD who are candidates for secondary prevention. This reflects the theory that potential reversibility of atherosclerotic lesions is more likely to occur with LDL-C blood levels below, and perhaps substantially below 100 mg/dl. However, even if this optimal goal is not reached, clinical trials have shown that any substantial reduction in LDL-C blood levels below pre-treatment levels may reduce atherosclerotic progression. This has been demonstrated in many of the secondary ASCAD prevention trials that selected patients on the basis of the presence of ASCAD, and not the degree of dyslipidemia. Improvement in even mild to moderate dyslipidemia was associated with a decreased risk of progression and an increased rate of regression compared to untreated controls [18].

4   Dietary treatment

The National Cholesterol Education Program (NCEP) Expert Panel has recently reaffirmed the importance of dietary modifications as the first-line treatment for patients with dyslipidemia [20]. As noted in Tables 1 and 2, primary and secondary trials have shown dietary intervention to be effective in decreasing progression, or possibly increasing regression of ASCAD. A low fat diet may improve many ASCAD risk factors including improvement in dyslipidemia in many patients, as well as weight loss in overweight patients, decrease in blood pressure, increase in glucose sensitivity, and decrease in risk of thrombosis. In addition, if saturated fats are replaced by an increase in foods high in antioxidants such as vitamins A, E, and C, the progression of atherosclerosis may also be reduced [21].

If dietary fats are to be used, saturated fats should be avoided. Dietary intake of saturated fats increase LDL-C blood levels while as both poly- and monounsaturated fats decrease LDL-C blood levels. But, while as dietary monounsaturated fatty acid consumption may preserve or possibly increase HDL-C blood levels, polyunsaturated fatty acids may decrease HDL-C blood levels. Furthermore, diets high in monounsaturated fats have been shown to generate LDL-C that are resistant to oxidation [22–24]. Conversely, diets high in polyunsaturated fatty acids may be associated with increased LDL-C oxidative modification and degradation by macrophages [22, 25]. If these findings are confirmed and found to be clinically relevant, it may be best to recommend monounsaturated fatty acids (e.g. olive oil or canola oil) as the oils/fats of choice. However, because the use of either poly or monounsaturated has not as yet been confirmed to decrease ASCAD by clinical trials, and because the intake of total fat, regardless of saturation status, has been associated with the increased likelihood of new ASCAD lesions [26], patients with, or at high risk for ASCAD should adhere to the NCEP guidelines of low total fat intake.

5   Lipid-acting drug treatment

If dietary treatment is unsuccessful in correcting lipid blood levels, the NCEP guidelines recommend lipid-acting drug treatment based on LDL-C blood levels and ASCVD risk factors [20]. The National Institutes of Health have also provided suggestions regarding the need for treatment of HDL-C and triglyceride blood levels. These recommendations are outlined in Table 3.

5.1   Choice of lipid-acting drugs

Although considerable variability exists in the recommendations of lipid-acting drugs based on lipid blood level profiles, Table 4 outlines our recommendations as to the choice of single-agent, lipid-acting drug treat-

Table 3.
Recommendations for treatment of dyslipidemia (Adapted from Bays HE, Dujovne CA) [88]

A. NCEP recommendations for treatment of adult cholesterol values based on LDL-C blood levels and cardiovascular risk[1]			
	Low-risk patients	High-risk patients	Secondary prevention[2]
Desirable LDL-C blood levels	<160 mg/dl (<4.13 mm/l)	<130 mg/dl (<3.35 mm/l)	<100 mg/dl (<2.58 mm/l)
High LDL-C blood levels that may require drug therapy	>190 mg/dl (>4.9 mm/l)	>160 mg/dl (>4.13 mm/l)	>130 mg/dl (>3.35 mm/l)

B. Draft NIH recommendations[3] for adult HDL-C and/or trigylceride blood level measurement[4]
Two or three fasting HDL-C and triglyceride blood levels, at least 1 week apart, should be measured before lipid-acting drug therapy is started. Fasting HDL-C blood levels should be measured in patients with two or more risk factors for ASCVD.[5]
Fasting triglyceride blood levels should be measured in patients with lipemic serum, lipemia retinalis, xanthomas, or acute pancreatitis.
Both fasting HDL-C and triglycerides should be measured whenever serum total and LDL-C blood levels are evaluated, particularly in patients with the following.

History of ASCVD
Two or more risk factors for ASCVD[2]
Previously diagnosed hypercholesterolemia
Family history of dyslipidemia
Disorders associated with ASCVD risk and dyslipidemia (e.g., diabetes, peripheral vascular disease, obesity, renal failure)

C. Authors' criteria for lipid-acting drug therapy and treatment goals of fasting adult blood lipid values based on cardiovascular risk			
	Low-risk patients	High-risk patients	Secondary prevention[2]
LDL-C			
High LDL-C blood levels that may require drug therapy	>190 mg/dl (>4.90 mm/l)	>160 mg/dl (>4.13 mm/l)	>130 mg/dl (>3.35 mm/l)
Desirable LDL-C blood levels	<160 mg/dl (<4.13 mm/l)	<130 mg/dl (<3.35 mm/l)	<100 mg/dl (<2.58 mm/l)
HDL-C[5]			
Low HDL-C blood levels that may require drug therapy	<30 mg/dl (<0.77 mm/l)	<35 mg/dl (<0.90 mm/l)	<40 mg/dl (<1.03 mm/l)
Desirable HDL-C blood levels	>35 mg/dl (>0.90 mm/l)	>40 mg/dl (>1.03 mm/l)	>45 mg/dl (1.16 mm/l)
Triglycerides[5]			
High triglyceride blood levels that may require drug therapy to prevent ASCVD or pancreatitis/xanthomas	>500 mg/dl (>5.65 mm/l)	>200 mg/dl (>2.26 mm/l)	>200 mg/dl (>2.26 mm/l)
Desirable triglyceride blood levels	<200 mg/dl (<2.26 mm/l)	<200 mg/dl (<2.26 mm/l)	<150 mg/dl (<1.70 mm/l)
LDL/HDL ratio Desirable LDL/HDL ratio[6]	<4.0	<3.0	<3.0

[1] NCEP, National Cholesterol Education Program; NIH, National Institutes of Health; LDL-C, low density lipoprotein cholesterol; HDL-C, high density lipoprotein cholesterol; ASCVD, atherosclerotic cardiovascular disease.
[2] Secondary prevention includes patients with personal history of ASCVD disease. High risk includes patients with two or more of the following: men > 45 years old, women > 55 years old (or with premature menopause without estrogen replacement therapy), family member of premature ASCVD, current cigarette smoking, hypertension, low HDL-C, diabetes mellitus, presence of peripheral vascular disease, obesity with body weight > 30% above ideal body weight.

[3] These are proposed guidelines from the 1992 National Institute of Health Consensus Development Conference statement "Triglycerides, High Density Lipoprotein and Coronary Heart Disease". Publication of the official recommendations is pending.
[4] Blood lipoprotein levels should be obtained only if accurate measurement, counseling, follow-up, and appropriate treatment (if needed) can be ensured.
[5] The NCEP has not yet made recommendations on isolated low levels of HDL-C or isolated elevated triglyceride blood levels.
[6] The LDL/HDL cholesterol ratio may be useful for assessing ASCVD risk, but the need for drug therapy should be based on lipoprotein blood levels.

Table 4.
Choices of lipid-acting drugs according to blood lipid abnormalities (Adapted from Bays HE, Dujovne CA) [89]

LDL-C	HDL-C	Triglycerides	Drugs of Choice*
↑	normal	normal	Resins, niacin, statins
↑	normal/↑	↑	Niacin, statins, fibrate
normal	normal/↓	↑	Fibrates, niacin, fish oils, statins**
normal	↓	normal	Niacin, statins, fibrates**

LDL-C, low density lipoprotein cholesterol; HDL-C, high density lipoprotein cholesterol
* Drugs are listed in general order of preference. However, ultimate choice should be based on anticipated benefits, tolerance, and toxicity for the individual patient
** Treatment for isolated elevation in triglyceride and/or HDL-C blood levels has not yet been shown to decrease progression of ASCVD

ment for selected lipoprotein disorders. However, the ultimate choice should be made on the anticipated benefit and potential toxicity to the individual patient.

5.2   Postmenopausal estrogen replacement treatment (ERT)

The same ASCVD risk in women occurs approximately 10–15 years later in life compared to men. Because the risk of ASCVD gradually increases after the menopause, by 75 years of age, the ASCVD risk of women is equal to that of men. The ASCVD risk may be particularly accelerated if menopause is prematurely induced by bilateral oophorectomy [27, 28]. The premenopausal endogenous estrogen may account for reduced ASCAD risk in women that may extend many years into the menopause [29].
Although yet to be proven by controlled, prospective clinical trials, most retrospective/population studies (and re-evaluation of earlier studies) now support an overall 40–50% reduction in atherosclerotic myocardial disease with estrogen replacement treatment (ERT) doses equivalent or less than

Table 5.
Blood lipid level effects of postmenopausal estrogen replacement therapy (ERT) compared
to pretreatment values

Oral Estrogen Replacement (ERT)	TC	LDL-C	HDL-C	TG
Unopposed ERT	↓	↓↓	↑↑	↑↑
With MPA	↓	↓↓	–	–/↑
With C-19 NTD	↓	↓	↓	–/↑
Unopposed Parenteral ERT**	–/↑	–/↓	–/↑	–/↑

Total cholesterol, LDL-C = Low density lipoprotein cholesterol, HDL = High density lipo-
protein cholesterol, TG = Triglycerides, MPA = Medroxyprogesterone acetate, NTD = Nor-
testosterone derivatives (e.g. norgestrel, norethindrone, and norethindrone acetate)
Arrows represent changes from pretreatment blood lipid levels:
↓   = Decreased by 5–10%,   ↑   = Increased by 5–10%
↓↓ = Decreased by 10–25%,   ↑↑ = Increased by 10–15%
–   = No change
* The estrogen component is considered to be "low dose" estrogen such as 0.625–1.25mg/day
oral conjugated equine estrogen or estrone sulfate, and 1–2 mg/day micronized estradiol. The
percentage change listed is a generalization based on results of several studies [10, 33, 35].
Lipid blood levels responses to postmenopausal estrogen replacement treatment are depend-
ent on many factors and may significantly vary between individuals.
** Parenteral estrogen replacement includes 0.05 mg twice a week of transdermal estradiol,
or 1.25 mg at bedtime intravaginal conjugated equine estrogen.

1.25 mg of conjugated estrogen daily [30, 31]. The impact on the risk of stroke is probably minimal [32].

Although the benefit of ERT in reducing ASCVD is probably multifactorial, one of the main effects of ERT may be on blood lipid levels. Unopposed ERT may improve blood lipids by increasing HDL-C and decreasing LDL-C blood levels. However, triglyceride blood levels may be adversely increased by ERT in a dose-dependent manner, particularly in women with pretreatment elevations in triglyceride blood levels [33–35].

Concurrent progestin treatment may be necessary in women with uteri to reduce the increased risk of uterine cancer that may occur with ERT alone. However, progestins may diminish estrogen's favorable effects upon LDL-C and HDL-C blood levels. Triglyceride blood levels may be favorably decreased. Overall, if estrogen is given with a progestin with minimal androgenic properties such as medroxyprogesterone, most studies have shown an overall mild to moderate decrease in LDL-C, mild increase in triglyceride, and unpredictable effect on HDL-C blood levels [33, 34].

Table 6.
Contraindications to estrogen replacement treatment

Absolute contraindications	Relative contraindications
Thromboembolic disease	Cigarette smoking
Acute cerebral/coronary artery disease	Strong family history of thrombo-embolism
Breast or endometrial cancer	Vascular or migraine headaches
Undiagnosed uterine bleeding	Major depression
Acute liver disease	Liver, gall bladder, pancreatic or kidney disease
Pregnancy	Hypertension
Immobilization of an extremity	Diabetes mellitus
	Immediate family history of breast cancer
	Seizure disorder
	Morbid obesity
	Ulcerative colitis
	Sickle cell trait or disease
	Varicose veins

Hence, the overall effect of ERT on lipid blood levels depends on the dose of estrogen, method of estrogen delivery, pre-treatment lipid blood levels and presence or absence of concurrent progestin treatment (Table 5).

Providing no contraindications exist (Table 6), ERT may be a first treatment of choice for some menopausal women to improve dyslipidemia and reduce ASCAD risk. However, ERT may provide benefits in reducing ASCVD risk beyond simply the favorable effects on lipid blood levels. In fact, the improvement in ASCVD risk by estrogens may be only 50% due to the favorable effects on blood lipid levels alone [28]. ERT has been suggested to have favorable influences on other ASCVD risk factors, such as beneficial effects on arterial endothelia [36]. Of particular interest is the clinical suggestion and experimental evidence that ERT may help prevent LDL-C oxidation [37, 38].

5.3   Resins (Bile acid sequestrants)

Included in this category of lipid-lowering agents are cholestyramine and colestipol (Table 7). Resins bind to bile acids and decrease their reabsorption in the intestine, thereby decreasing an important substrate for cholesterol synthesis. LDL-C receptor activity is subsequently increased. The decreased hepatic cholesterol production as the result of sequestration of bile acids is largely blunted by a "compensatory" increase in the hepatic

Table 7.
Bile acid resins (cholestyramine/colestipol). (Adapted from Bays HE, Dujovne CA) [89]

Doses: – Starting dose of resins is 4–5 grams (scoops) before the main meal, and advanced to. 8–10 grams before meals.
Common Side Effects: – Indigestion, abdominal pain, nausea, constipation, hemorrhoids, and increase in triglyceride blood levels.
Rare Side Effects: – Weight loss, skin rash, petechiae, transient increase in liver enzyme blood levels, and malabsorption of fat-soluble vitamins (vitamins A, D, E, and K)
Laboratory Monitoring: – Triglyceride blood levels should be routinely monitored.
Drug Interactions: – Concurrent drugs (such as thiazide diuretics, propranolol, thyroxine, warfarin, cardiac glycosides, folic acid, fat-soluble vitamins and statins) may have decreased gastro-intestinal absorption; therefore, blood levels, as well as the effects of all concurrent drugs should be regularly monitored. To minimize the decreased absorption, all drugs should be taken 1–2 hours before or 4 hours after resin dose.

production of cholesterol from other substrates. In addition, the compensatory increase in hepatic cholesterol may also result in an increase in VLDL-C production that may often increase triglyceride blood levels [39, 40]. Nevertheless, the increased activity of hepatic LDL-C receptors significantly increases the clearance of LDL-C from the blood and is thought to be the major mechanism accounting for the net reduction in LDL-C blood levels with resin drug treatment.

Resins are often a first drug of choice for patients with hypercholesterolemia because they are not absorbed and have minimal to no systemic side effects. Because of well-documented trials 'of long-term safety, resins are the only lipid-acting drugs currently recommended for use in children with severe hypercholesterolemia. They have also been shown by both primary and secondary prevention trials to be safe and effective in decreasing LDL-C blood levels and decreasing ASCAD progression (Tables 1 and 2).

Resins have a relatively high incidence of gastrointestinal adverse effects such as nausea, heartburn, abdominal pain, bloating, belching, and constipation. Furthermore, because resins may decrease the absorption of many drugs [40, 41] it is recommended that concurrent medications should be taken at least 1 hour before or at least 4 hours after treatment with resins

[39]. This dosing restriction may be difficult in patients on numerous medications, especially if resins are recommended more than once a day.

In order to increase palatability, resins may be mixed with fluids such as water or juices or food. Resins should not be cooked or heated however, because the drug may become inactive.

To reduce the risk of constipation, an increase in dietary fiber and possibly the addition of psyllium may not only provide a laxative effect, but may also contribute to a reduction in cholesterol blood levels.

High dose resins may be efficacious and well tolerated by many patients. However, perhaps the best-tolerated use of resins is low dose 8–10 grams (2 scoops, packets, or flavored bars) of cholestyramine or colestipol before the main meal alone or in combination treatment with other lipid-acting drugs such as niacin, statins, or fibrates. This combined lipid-acting drug regimen may result in a synergistic and substantial reduction in LDL-C blood levels and may be the most cost-effective treatment for severely dyslipidemic patients, or patients resistent or intolerant to higher dose single lipid-acting drug treatment [42].

5.4   Nicotinic acid (Niacin)

Niacin is a B vitamin that decreases both LDL-C and triglyceride, as well as increases HDL-C blood levels [39, 43] (Table 8). Niacin is possibly the only lipid-acting drug that consistently reduces lipoprotein (a) blood levels [Lp(a)]. Elevated Lp(a) may be an important single or additive ASCAD risk factor in some patients [44, 45].

Niacin has been shown by both primary and secondary prevention trials to be safe and effective in decreasing ASCAD progression, decrease ASCAD mortality, as well as a decrease in overall mortality [9] (Tables 1 and 2).

Niacin often causes poorly tolerated side effects, such as flushing and gastritis, that may limit patient compliance. The occurrence of these adverse effects are widely variable among patients and often unpredictable, even after years of use. Regular clinical evaluation for side effects, and regular laboratory monitoring of liver enzymes, uric acid, and glucose blood levels is indicated, particularly in patients treated with more than 1.5 grams of niacin a day.

A major side effect that limits the treatment with niacin is flushing. Several measures can be taken to increase tolerance to this common problem. These include:

(1) Patient education. If patients are warned of these common reactions, and reassured of the lack of adverse health consequences, they may be willing to tolerate adverse flushing until it diminishes with continued use.

(2) Ingestion of niacin with or after meals. Niacin is often better tolerated if taken with food.

(3) Ingestion of a 325-mg aspirin 30–60 minutes before niacin.

(4) Starting with low dose and gradually increasing the dose of niacin. A key to increasing the tolerance of niacin treatment is to slowly advance the dosage, allowing for the patient to become tolerant to the flushing.

(5) Use sustained-release niacin preparations. Slow-release preparations are associated with a decreased severity of flushing. However, hepatotoxicity is increased with doses of the sustained release niacin (i.e. greater than 1.5 grams per day) compared to the regular release crystalline niacin preparation [46, 47]. Furthermore, the sustained-release preparations may have less effect on lowering LDL-C and increasing HDL-C blood levels than the equivalent doses of regular niacin [48].

Table 8.
Nicotinic acid (Niacin) (Adapted from Bays HE, Dujovne CA) [89]

Doses: – Starting dose of niacin is 100–250 mg twice a day after meals, then advanced to 1–2 grams two to three times a day after meals preferably not to exceed 4 grams per day
Common Side Effects: – Skin flushing, nausea, pruritus, gastritis, and elevations in glucose liver enzyme, and/or uric acid blood levels
Rare Side Effects: – Worsening of peptic ulcer disease or gout, cardiac dysrhythmias, headaches – Severe liver disease with extreme rare potential for irreversible hepatic failure
Laboratory Monitoring: – During dosing adjustment, liver enzymes, glucose, and uric acid blood levels should be monitored every 6 weeks. Once dosage has stabilized, laboratory should be monitored every 3–6 months
Drug Interactions: – Concurrent diet, oral hypoglycemic drug, or insulin doses may need to be adjusted due to increases in blood sugar – Concurrent alpha-adrenergic blocking antihypertensive drugs may result in hypotension – Concurrent drugs known to have hepatic toxicity may have an additive effect on elevation in liver enzymes – Concurrent statins may increase the risk for muscle toxicity [90]

In addition to its favorable effects on blood lipid levels, it has also been suggested that niacin may have other benefits in reducing ASCAD risk such as short-term activation of fibrinolysis, reduced plasma fibrinogen, inhibition of platelet aggregation, stimulation of prostaglandin I2 production and reduction in thromboxane A2 synthesis [49, 50].

5.5   Statins [3-Hydroxy-3-methylglutaryl coenzyme A (HMG-CoA) reductase inhibitors]

Currently marketed lipid-acting drugs in this category include lovastatin, pravastatin, simvastatin, and fluvastatin (Table 9). Statins inhibit the rate-limiting enzyme in the hepatic production of cholesterol and therefore decrease total cholesterol, LDL-C, and VLDL-C (triglyceride) blood levels. HDL-C blood levels may be slightly to moderately increased. Although the results of primary prevention trials are lacking, statins have been shown by secondary prevention trials to be safe and effective in decreasing LDL-C blood levels and decreasing ASCAD progression (Table 2).
Statins are generally well tolerated. Side effects of statins in doses relative to 20 mg or less of lovastatin has been shown to not significantly differ from that of placebo [51]. Pravastatin appears to have greater hydrophilicity than statins such as lovastatin and simvastatin. This may result in lower rates of uptake in peripheral tissues and decreased diffusion across the blood brain barrier with, theoretically, less central nervous system effects. Conversely, decreased peripheral tissue uptake may limit possible antioxidant effects of statins, such as reduction in LDL-C oxidation, that occurs in the lipophilic subendothelial space [52].
From a practical standpoint, hydrophilicity concerns have not as yet shown to be clinically relevant [53]. All current statins are adequately taken up by the liver and are effective in improving dyslipidemia with relatively few side effects. Definitive and confirmatory comparative trials demonstrating an efficacy or toxicity difference among the currently marketed statins are lacking. However, the difference in chemical properties among statins may account for the clinical finding that some patients who experience adverse side effects to one statin may tolerate a switch to a different statin.
Because cholesterol synthesis is typically increased at night, statins, with their inhibition of the rate-limiting step of cholesterol synthesis, have been shown to be more effective when given in the evening compared to in the morning [49, 54, 55].

Table 9.
Statins (Adapted from Bays HE, Dujovne CA) [89]

Doses:
– Lovastatin 20 mg daily to maximum dose of 80 mg a day
– Pravastatin 20 mg daily to maximum dose of 40 mg a day
– Simvastatin 10 mg daily to maximum dose of 40 mg a day
– Fluvastatin 20 mg daily to maximum dose of 40 mg a day
Common Side Effects:
– None
Rare Side Effects:
– Gastrointestinal complaints (Indigestion)
– Neurologic complaints (headache, fatigue, sleep disorders, dizziness)
– Increase in liver enzymes
– Increase in muscle enzymes with or without myalgias
– Myalgias with or without increase in muscle enzymes
– Antibody (lupus-like) antibody response with or without symptoms
– Skin rash
Laboratory Monitoring:
– Liver and muscle enzymes should be monitored every 6–8 weeks for the first 3 months, then every 2–3 months for the remaining first year. If no laboratory symptoms occur, then enzymes may be monitored every 3–6 months.
Drug Interactions:
– Concurrent erythromycin may increase the risk for liver toxicity
– Concurrent cyclosporin may increase the risk for muscle toxicity [92–94]
– Concurrent gemfibrozil may increase the risk for muscle toxicity
– Concurrent niacin may increase the risk for muscle toxicity [90]
– Concurrent warfarin's effect may be increased with prolongation of prothrombin time

5.6   Fibrates

Included in this category of lipid-lowering agents are gemfibrozil, fenofi-
brate, bezafibrate, and clofibrate (Table 10). The NCEP chose not to identify
fibric acid derivatives as major treatments for hypercholesterolemia because of their limited effect on LDL-C blood levels [20]. However, they do
effectively reduce triglycerides and increase HDL-C blood levels and are
therefore useful for the treatment of patients with very high triglyceride
blood levels that might predispose to pancreatitis, or symptomatic eruptive
xanthomas. Furthermore, they may be useful for patients with dysbetalipo-
proteinemia and combined hyperlipidemia.
Primary [11, 15, 16] and secondary ASCAD prevention trials [9, 56–58]
have shown fibrates to be effective in reducing the progression of ASCAD,
particularly in patients with hypertriglyceridemia and high LDL/HDL ra-

Table 10.
Fibrates (Adapted from Bays HE, Dujovne CA) [89]

Doses: – Gemfibrozil 600 mg once or twice a day to maxium dose of 1200 mg a day   – Clofibrate 100 mg a day to maxium dose of 200 mg a day   – Bezafibrate 200 mg twice or three times a day to maxium dose of 600 mg a day   – Fenofibrate 100 mg three times a day to maxium dose of 400 mg a day   – Ciprofibrate 100 mg once a day to maxium dose of 200 mg a day
Common Side Effects: – Indigestion, nausea, abdominal pain, flatulence
Rare Side Effects: – Myalgias, headaches, drowsiness, insomnia, gallstone formation, gastrointestinal bleeding, hypokalemia, anemia, leukopenia   – Rash, urticaria   – Elevation in liver and muscle enzymes   – Clofibrate may increase the risk of gastrointestinal cancers, particularly cancer of the gall bladder
Laboratory Monitoring: – Liver and muscle enzymes should be monitored every 2 months for the first 4 months. If no laboratory symptoms occur, then enzymes should be monitored every 6 months.
Drug Interactions: – Concurrent oral hypoglycemic drugs may be displaced from blood carriers and therefore dose may have to be adjusted   – Concurrent statins may increase the risk of myopathy   – Concurrent warfarin's effect may be increased with prolongation of prothrombin time

tios. Due to the higher all-cause mortality (mainly due to gastrointestinal cancers), and due to the increased risk of gall bladder disease, the use of clofibrate has declined as the fibrate of choice [11].

Finally, fibrates may have other physiologic actions that may decrease ASCAD progression. For example, fibrates may decrease the platelet-derived growth factor effect on smooth muscles and reduce platelet aggregation [49], reduce fibrinogen blood levels, and cone fibrates have been suggested to possibly decrease Lp(a) blood levels.

5.7   Probucol (Table 11)

Probucol, originally developed to delay the oxidation of airplane tires, was incidentally found to lower cholesterol blood levels in animals. It was then marketed as a cholesterol lowering agent in humans. LDL-C blood levels, as well as HDL-C blood levels are reduced. Probucol has also been shown to be the most potent, and consistent antioxidant drug available.

Table 11.
Probucol (Adapted from Bays HE, Dujovne CA) [89]

Doses: – Starting dose of probucol is 250 mg twice a day to maximum dose of 500 mg twice a day
Common Side Effects: – Prolongation of QT interval on electrocardiogram – Decrease in HDL-C blood levels
Rare Side Effects: – Diarrhea, nausea, abdominal pain
Laboratory Monitoring: – Electrocardiogram should be obtained before, and at least once more 6–12 weeks after start of drug. If cardiac dysrhythmia occurs, or symptoms of dysrhythmia occurs, the drug should be stopped and heart monitoring performed. – Electrolyte, including magnesium, blood levels should be monitored regularly during drug treatment.
Drug Interactions: – Concurrent medications that prolong the QT interval on electrocardiogram (such as tricyclic antidepressants, phenothiazines, as well as antidysrhythmic such as procainamide and quinidine) or medications that impair electrical myocardial conduction may increase the risk of dysrhythmias. – Concurrent medications with intrinsic dysrhythmic potential or the effects of medications that may cause electrolyte imbalances should routinely monitored

Hypercholesterolemic patients treated with probucol in doses as low as 500 mg/day consistently results in preventing the oxidation of LDL-C. In fact, probucol doses of 250–500 mg/day may be equal to the usual dose of one gram/day in the consistent reduction in LDL oxidation [59, 60]. The dose of other antioxidants such as vitamin E may require doses as high as 800 to 1600 mg a day for similar, but less consistent reduction in LDL-C oxidation. Adverse side effects of probucol include a prolongation of the QT interval on electrocardiogram that may theoretically predispose to dysrhythmia. Probucol also decreases HDL-C blood levels that may theoretically increase ASCVD risk. However, because other treatments that decrease HDL-C blood levels (such as vegetarian diet) are not thought to increase ASCVD risk, the clinical significance of this laboratory finding is unclear.

Treatment of rabbits with high cholesterol blood levels with probucol has been shown to decrease atherosclerotic progression [61, 62]. In humans, probucol has been shown to decrease xanthomas in patients with familial hypercholesterolemia [63]. Because of the only modest effects in improving dyslipidemia, the beneficial effects found in animals and humans are thought to be predominantly through the antioxidant properties of probucol. Probucol may have other favorable effects with respect to decreasing ASCAD progression as well. These effects include a reduction in insulin-dependent diabetes in animals and inhibition of interleukin-1 release [49]. Probucol has yet to be shown by primary or secondary ASCAD prevention trials to decrease ASCAD progression, or be superior to high dose antioxidant vitamin treatment such as with vitamins E, A, and C [21]. The final analysis of the Probucol Quantitative Regression Swedish Trial (PQRST) on the use of diet plus cholestyramine compared to diet, cholestyramine, and probucol is pending. Analysis of the results of this study should help clarify the efficacy, if any, of probucol in reducing the progression of ASCVD in hypercholesterolemic patients. Until a clear benefit has been shown by clinical trials, the use of probucol should be considered only as a possible adjunct to other lipid-acting drugs.

5.8   Fish oils (Table 12)

Omega-3 fatty acids are polyunsaturated fatty acids abundant in cold-water marine fish oils such as mackerel, herring, sardines, and salmon. The omega-3 fatty acids eicosapentanoic acid (EPA) and docosahexanoic acid (DHA) found in these marine fish oils have been shown to reduce very-low-density lipoprotein (VLDL) synthesis in the liver with a reduction in triglyceride blood levels [64]. A concomitant rise in low-density lipoprotein (LDL) cholesterol and HDL cholesterol blood levels is often noted. Although some investigators believe the increase in LDL cholesterol may not be clinically adverse because of favorable altered lipoprotein configuration produced by these fatty acids [64] this has yet to be confirmed by clinical trials.

Triglyceride blood levels which exceed 1000–2000 mg/dl may benefit from treatments such as fish oils to prevent triglyceride-induced acute pancreatitis and symptomatic eruptive xanthomas.

"Cholesterol-free" fish oil preparations are available. But, because cholesterol-containing fish oil preparations contribute little to overall dietary cholesterol, and because dietary cholesterol often has limited effect on blood cholesterol levels, it is questionable as to whether cholesterol-free preparations provide any major advantages.

Because omega-3 fatty acids are precursors to prostaglandins, fish oil consumption decreases platelet aggregation and theoretically increase the risk of hemorrhage. However, it should be noted that significant bleeding

Table 12.
Fish oils (Adapted from Bays HE, Dujovne CA) [89]

Doses:
– Starting dose of 1–2 gel capsules* with meals three times a day and advanced to up to 6 gel capsules three times a day
Common Side Effects: – Indigestion, gastritis, diarrhea, fishy after-taste – Laboratory evidence of increased bleeding time with decreased platelet aggregation – Increase in LDL-C blood levels
Rare Side Effects: – Elevations in glucose blood levels – Hematomas – Toxic fat soluble hypervitaminosis with some fish oil concentrates such as cod liver oil – Weight gain (each fish oil gel capsule has 1 gram of fat)
Laboratory Monitoring: – Blood glucose levels should be monitored during the first few months of treatment – If bleeding is a risk, then bleeding time should be monitored.
Drug Interactions: – Concurrent diet, oral hypoglycemic drug, or insulin doses may need to be adjusted in patients with increase in blood sugar – Concurrent aspirin, or other drugs that decrease platelet aggregation or with warfarin anticoagulants may increase bleeding tendency

* Fish oils are generally available in 1000 mg lipid concentrates with approximately 300–600 mg of eicosapentanoic acid and/or docosahexanoic acid.

has not been reported in numerous clinical trials of fish oil therapy and, in fact, the decrease in platelet aggregation may be advantageous in decreasing the risk of acute thrombotic myocardial infarction. Also, a transient increase in glucose blood levels in patients with diabetes mellitus or glucose intolerance has also been described as an adverse effect of fish oil treatment [65]. Population studies have demonstrated that Eskimos in Greenland and Alaska, who ingest marine fish oils as much as 7 g/day (compared with an average of 0.06 g/day in modern Western diets), had a surprisingly low incidence of atherosclerotic heart disease, despite the cultural prevalence of a high-fat diet and obesity. Some studies have demonstrated a diminished rate of restenosis after percutaneous transluminal coronary angioplasty [64], while as others have shown a reduced mortality from sudden death resulting from arrhythmia in patients taking fish oil concentrate for treatment of dyslipidemia [66]. However, not all trials have shown such favorable results.

6   Cost considerations

Because ASCAD is the most common cause of morbidity and mortality of populations of developed nations, much emphasis has been placed on ASCAD prevention. However, lifetime lipid-acting drug of all dyslipidemic patients based on lipid blood levels alone could result in enormous cost. It has been suggested that 29% of the United States population 20 years of age and older, or approximately 52 million people, should currently practice dietary modifications according to NCEP guidelines. As many as 7%, or approximately 12.7 million might require lipid-acting drugs [67].

From an individual standpoint, the cost of some lipid-acting drugs may be unaffordable and prohibitive for some patients. Therefore, before consideration of lipid-acting drugs, the most cost-effective approach towards treatment of dyslipidemia includes the following:

(1)   *Begin with evaluation and treatment for underlying conditions that may contribute to dyslipidemia.* Conditions such as hypothyroidism, uncontrolled diabetes mellitus, estrogen-deficient menopausal status in women, Cushing's syndrome, obstructive liver disease, nephrotic syndrome and other rarer disorders may worsen blood lipid levels. Evaluation and treatment of these conditions can often substantially improve, if not correct dyslipidemia.

(2)   *Avoid other drugs that may contribute to dyslipidemia.* Drugs such as corticosteroids, isoretinoin, thiazides, anabolic steroids, some b-blockers, cyclosporin and progestins can often worsen blood lipid levels. When possible, these drugs should be discontinued or replaced by drugs with less dyslipidemic potential.

(3)   *Encourage the patient to adopt and maintain healthy lifestyle habits.* In addition to many other favorable effects on atherosclerotic progression, stopping smoking can often substantially improve HDL-C blood levels. Substantial reduction or abstention of alcohol intake may often dramatically improve, or sometimes normalize triglyceride blood levels in patients with moderate to severe hypertriglyceridemia. A regular physical exercise program may decrease LDL-C and triglyceride, and increase HDL-C blood levels.

(4)   *Encourage that patients follow an appropriate diet and maintain ideal body weight.* Dietary treatment may often result in substantial improvement in lipid blood levels. However, extreme variability exists and some patients may have only a modest to no favorable response,

despite dietary compliance [68]. Nevertheless, dietary treatment is still the first treatment of choice before consideration of lipid-acting drugs. Several reasons exist for this recommendation. Firstly, diets low in total, and particularly low in saturated fats have been shown by primary and secondary prevention trials to reduce the progression, and sometimes induce progression of ASCAD (Tables 1 and 2). Secondly, low fat diets often help reduce body fat and therefore may reduce ASCAD risk factors such as hypertension, insulin resistance, and propensity to thrombosis. In patients with adult onset or Type II diabetes mellitus, reduction in body weight with low fat diet can substantially improve, if not "cure" the diabetes state with substantial improvement in blood lipid levels. Finally, individual responses to dietary recommendations are widely variable. It is not uncommon to see individuals with moderate to severe dyslipidemia who have correction, or marked improvement in blood lipid levels with diet treatment alone.

(5) *Recommend lipid-acting drug treatment only to patients whose potential benefit in reducing the progression of ASCAD outweighs the potential risks and excessive costs.* The NCEP [20] has recently emphasized the need to concentrate treatment to patients with, or at high risk for ASCAD. For example, lipid-acting drug treatment of most young adults and pre-menopausal women who may have moderate dyslipidemia, but otherwise no other ASCAD risk factors is de-emphasized. Conversely, recommendations regarding the goals of treatment of patients with existing ASCAD are more aggressive [69] (Table 3).

(6) *If lipid-acting drugs are indicated, the drug regimen most likely to improve the dyslipidemia and most likely to be tolerated by the individual patient should be recommended.* Table 4 outlines some general guidelines to recommendations concerning specific lipid disorders. It is cost-effective to choose lipid-acting drugs that are most likely to improve the dyslipidemia of the individual patient. For example, although resins may be effective in lowering total and LDL-C blood levels, they may often worsen triglyceride blood levels and therefore should be used with caution in patients with pre-treatment hypertriglyceridemia. Alternatively, although statins may have mild triglyceride lowering effects, they are not the initial lipid-acting drug of choice for patients with profound hypertriglyceridemia at risk for pancreatitis or symptomatic eruptive xanthomas.

With respect to tolerance and compliance, the most cost-effective use of specific lipid-acting drug treatment depends on the anticipated benefit and potential toxicity for the individual patient.

For example, due to the poor tolerance in many patients, single lipid-acting drug treatment with high dose resins may not be as cost-effective as other regimens [70]. Conversely, lower doses may be well tolerated. Furthermore, resins have the least risk for systemic side effects compared to other lipid-acting drugs. This may result in less frequent office visits and laboratory monitoring and therefore may reduce overall cost compared to other lipid-acting drugs.

Generic niacin has been suggested as the most cost-effective for dyslipidemia because of its low cost and efficacy in improving LDL-C, HDL-C and triglyceride blood levels [70]. Unfortunately, niacin may have potential toxicity (particularly hepatotoxicity) that requires routine laboratory surveillance. Furthermore, the high degree of side effects may prompt medical office visits that might increase overall costs [70]. However, due to the low cost, generic niacin may be a cost-effective choice for patients who have adequate lipid blood level response and who tolerate the side effects. For many patients with fixed incomes, the ability to afford the cost of medicine may be the single most important consideration with regard to compliance.

In hypercholesterolemic patients, statins compared favorably with that of niacin in reduction of LDL-C blood levels. Furthermore, due to the excellent tolerability profile of statins compared to lipid-acting drugs such as resins and niacin, they may require less medical office visits, and therefore may be a cost effective choice for many hypercholesterolemic patients.

Fibrates, used primarily to treat hypertriglyceridemia, are not as cost-effective as other lipid-acting drugs in reducing LDL-C blood levels. But fibrates may be secondary only to niacin in cost-effectiveness in decreasing triglyceride and increasing HDL-C blood levels in hypertriglyceridemic patients [70]. However, fish oil treatment may be the most cost-effective triglyceride blood level lowering agent for many hypertriglyceridemic patients. Probucol, due to the modest improvement in LDL-C and the worsening of HDL-C blood levels, as well as due to the lack of human primary or secondary prevention trials demonstrating a clinical reduction in the progression in ASCAD, is not as cost-effective as other single lipid-acting drugs in lowering lipid blood levels.

Table 13.
Combination lipid-acting drug treatment [41, 89, 98]*

Dual lipid-acting drug treatment of elevated LDL-C blood levels
Resin and niacin Resin and statin Niacin and statin
Low dose combination may reduce LDL-C blood levels as much, if not more than higher doses of either agent alone. The lower dose of each may result in decreased adverse effects that may occur with high doses of single lipid-acting drug treatment. Both niacin and statin may potentially cause liver and muscle toxicity [90].
Dual lipid-acting drug treatment of elevated triglyceride blood levels
Niacin and fibrate Fish oil and fibrate Niacin and fish oil
Lowering severe elevations in triglyceride blood levels may reduce the risk of acute pancreatitis and symptomatic eruptive xanthomas, but definitive clinical trials have yet to show a reduction in ASCAD. Both niacin and fibrates may potentially cause liver and muscle toxicity.
Dual lipid-acting drug treatment of combined hyperlipidemia
Resin and niacin Resin and fibrate Statin and niacin Statin and fibrate Statin and fish oil Resin and fish oil
Niacin, fish oil, and fibrates may blunt the increase in trigylceride blood levels that may occur with resins. Statins and niacin may both cause liver and muscle toxicity [90]. Statins and fibrates may cause liver toxicity. Furthermore, statins and fibrates have been described in uncontrolled case reports to rarely cause severe myopathy with rhabdomyolysis. Some authors recommend that this combination only be used by lipid specialists, or at least with precaution [95–97].
Triple lipid-acting drug treatment [98–101]
Resin, niacin and statin
Some patients with, or at high risk for ASCAD are very resistant, even to dual drug treatment. Some of these patients may respond to 3 drug lipid-acting drug treatment. Both niacin and statins can cause liver and muscle toxicity.

* These combinations do not include drugs such as estrogen or antioxidants such as probucol.

7   Combination lipid-acting drug treatment

The most efficacious, and sometimes most cost-effective, treatment for many patients with dyslipidemia is combination lipid-acting drug treatment. The use of resins alone in doses greater than 2 scoops once or twice a day may result in an increase in side effects that may limit compliance. Conversely, low dose resins, such as 5 grams of colestipol per day, has been shown to achieve approximately 50% of the reduction of LDL-C blood levels compared with 15 grams of colestipol per day [42]. Therefore, incremental increases in resin doses may have diminishing benefit in reducing LDL-C blood levels, but have an associated increase in adverse side effects and decrease compliance.

Similarly, the adverse side effects of niacin may increase markedly with doses greater than 2–3 grams per day. And while as the bulk of the LDL-C blood level lowering effect of statins occurs at doses at or below the equivalent of 40 mg of lovastatin per day, higher doses have only modest additional blood lipid level lowering effects with an increase in potential toxicity, side effects, and monetary cost.

Therefore, the most efficacious treatment for many patients with moderate or severe dyslipidemia is combination lipid-acting drug treatment that may not only be better tolerated, but in many cases have additive or perhaps synergistic effects in improving lipid blood levels in some patients. Some combination lipid-acting drug regimens are included in Table 13.

8   Conclusion

The treatment of dyslipidemic patients with, or at high risk for ASCAD has been shown by primary and secondary clinical trials to decrease progression, and sometimes induce regression of atherosclerotic disease. Recommendations should begin with evaluation and treatment of underlying conditions that contribute to dyslipidemia, use of possible alternatives to drugs that may worsen dyslipidemia, encouragement of healthy lifestyle habits, and attaining appropriate diet and physical exercise. If dyslipidemia persists, then the most cost-effective approach towards recommending the most appropriate lipid-acting drug treatment is to reserve treatment to patients with, or at high risk for ASCAD whose expected benefit outweighs the potential risks and excessive costs.

References

1   Bilheimer D.W.: Therapeutic Control of Hyperlipidemia in the Prevention of Coronary Atherosclerosis: A Review of Results from recent Clinical Trials. Am J Cardiol, *62*, 1J–9J, 1988.

2   Barndt R. Jr., Blankenhorn D.H., Crawford D.W., Brooks S.H.: Regression and progression of early femoral atherosclerosis in treated hyperlipoproteinemic patients. Ann Int med, *86*, 139–146, 1977.

3   Zelis R., Mason D.T., Braunwald E., Levy R.I.: Effects of Hyperlipoproteinemias and their treatment on the peripheral circulation. J Clin Invest, *49*, 1007–1015, 1970.

4   Duffield R.G.M., Lewis B., Miller N.E., Jamieson C.W., Brunt J.N.H., Colchestero A.C.F.: Treatment of hyperlipidemia retard progression of symptomatic femoral atherosclerosis. A randomized controlled trial Lancet, *2*, 639–642, 1983.

5   Furberg C.D., Byinton R.P.: ACAPS Group. ACAPS: Effects of Lovastatin on Progression of Carotid Atherosclerosis and Clinical Events. Abstract from 1993 Scientific Session of the American Heart Association – Circulation section *88*, 2073, 1993.

6   The Multiple Risk Factor Trial research Group: Mortality rates after 10.5 years for participants in the Multiple Risk Factor Intervention Trial. JAMA *263*, 1795–801, 1990.

7   Rossouw J.E., Lewis B., Rifkind B.M.: The Value of Lowering Cholesterol After Myocardial Infarction. NEJM *323*, 1112–1119, 1990.

8   The Coronary Drug Project Research Group: Clofibrate and niacin in coronary heart disease, JAMA *231* (4), 360–381, 1975.

9   Canner P.L., Berge K.G., Wenger N.K., et al.: Fifteen year mortality in coronary drug project patients: long-term benefit with niacin. J Am Coll Cardiol *8*, 1245–1255, 1986.

10   Haarbo J., Hassager C., Jensen S.B., Riis B.J., Christiansen C.: Serum Lipids, Lipoproteins, and Apolipoproteins During Postmenopausal Estrogen Replacement Therapy Combined with Either 19-Nortestosterone Derivatives or 17-Hydroxyprogesterone Derivatives. Am J Med. *90*, 584–589, 1991.

11   Report from the Committee of Principal Investigators: A cooperative trial in the primary prevention of ischemic heart disease using clofibrate, Br. Heart J. *40*, 1069–1118, 1978.

12   Lipid Research Clinics Program. The Lipid Research Clinics Coronary Primary Prevention Trial results: I. Reduction in incidence of coronary heart disease. JAMA *251*, 351–364, 1984.

13   Lipid Research Clinics Program. The Lipid Research Clinics Coronary Primary Prevention Trial results: II. The relationship of reduction in incidence of coronary heart disease to cholesterol lowering. JAMA *251*, 365–374, 1984.

14   The Lipid Research Clinics Investigators. The Lipid Research Clinics Coronary Primary Prevention Trial. Arch Intern Med *152*, 1399–1410, 1992.

15   Frick, M.H. et al: Helsinki Heart Study: Primary-prevention trial with gemfibrozil in middle-aged men with dyslipidemia: Safety of treatment, changes in risk factors, and incidence of coronary heart disease. N. Engl. J. Med. *317* (20), 1237–1245,1987.

16   Manninen V., MSci L.T., Koskinen P., et. al.: Joint Effects of Serum Triglyceride and LDL Cholesterol and HDL Cholesterol Concentrations on Coronary Heart Disease risk in the Helsinki Heart Study. Circulation *85*, 37–45, 1992.

17   Pravastain Multinational Study Group: Effects of Pravastatin in Patients with Serum

Total Cholesterol Levels from 5.2 to 7.8 mmol/liter (200 to 300 mg/dl) Plus Two Additional Atheroscerotic Risk Factors. Am J Cardiol. 72, 1031–1037, 1993.

18   Brown B.G., Zhao X.Q., Sacco D.E., Albers J.J.: Lipid lowering and plaque regression. Circulation 87, 1781–91, 1993.

19   Hjermann I., Holme I., Leren P.: Oslo Diet and Antismoking Trial: Results after 102 months. Am J Med 80, 7–11, 1986.

20   Expert panel on Detection, Evaluation, and Treatment of High Blood Cholesterol in Adults. Summary of the second report of the national cholesterol education program (NCEP) expert panel on detection, evaluation, and treatment of high blood cholesterol in adults (adult treatment panel II). JAMA 269 (23), 3015–3023, 1993.

21   Bays H.E., Dujovne C.A.: Antioxidants in the treatment and prevention of atherosclerotic cardiovascular disease. Clin. Invest. Artheriosclerosis 1994; 5: 166–175.

22   Parthasarathy S., Khoo J.C., Miller E., Barnett J., Witzum J.L., Steinberg D.: Low density lipoprotein rich in oleic acid is protected against oxidative modification: implications for dietary prevention of atherosclerosis. Proc Natl Acad Sci USA 87, 3894–98, 1990.

23   Kinter M.T., Roberts R.J.: Effects of Oleic Acid on Lipoxygenase Activity and 4-Hydroxy-2-Nonenal Formation. Am. Heart Assoc. Abstract to the Council on Arteriosclerosis. Lipoprotein Modification. Page 5, 1993.

24   Carr T.P., Sawyer J.K., Rudel L.L.: Dietary Monounsaturated Fat Protects Against Coronary Artery Atherosclerosis in African Green Monkeys. Am. Heart Assoc. Abstract to the Council on Arteriosclerosis Diet and Oxidation of Lipoprotein. Page 48, 1993.

25   Nicolosi R.J., Courtemanche K.V., Behr S.R.: Increased LDL Oxidation Susceptibility and Enhanced Aortic Atherogenesis in Hamsters Fed High Polyunsaturated vs. Monounsaturated Vegetable Oils. Am. Heart Assoc. Abstract to the Council on Arteriosclerosis Diet and Oxidation of Lipoprotein. Page 48, 1993.

26   Blankenhorn D.H., Johnson R.L., Mack W.J., Il Zein H.A., Vailas L.I.: The Influence of Diet on the Appearance of New Lesions in Human Coronary Arteries. JAMA 263, 1646–1652, 1990.

27   Colditz G.A., Willett W.C., Stampfer M.J., Rosner B., Speizer F.E., Hennekens C.H.: Menopause and the Risk of Coronary Heart Disease in Women; NEJM 316, 1105–1110, 1987.

28   Connor E.B., Bush T.S.: Estrogen and Coronary Heart Disease in Women. JAMA 265, 1861–1867, 1991.

29   Isles C.G., Hole D.J., Hawthorne V.M., Lever A.F.: Relation between coronary risk and coronary mortality in women of the Renfrew and Paisley survey: comparison with men. Lancet 339, 702–705, 1992.

30   Goldman L., Tobsteson A.N.A.: Uncertainty About Postmenopausal Estrogen. NEJM 325, 800–802, 1991.

31   Stampfer M.J., Graham A.C., Willett W.C., Manson J.A., Rosner B., Speizer F.E., Hennekens C.H.: Postmenopausal Estrogen Therapy and Cardiovascular Disease. NEJM 325, 756–62, 1991.

32   Stampfer M.J.: Smoking, Estrogen, and Prevention of Heart Disease in Women. Mayo Clin Proc. 64, 1553–1557, 1989.

33   Rijpkema A.H.M., et al.: Effects of Post-menopausal Oestrogen-Progestogen Replace-

ment Therapy on Serum Lipids and Lipoprotein: A Review; Maturitas *12*, 259–285, 1990.

34   Miller V.T.: Postmenopausal Estrogen Replacement; Drug Therapy, 76–79, June 1990.

35   Walsh B.W., Schiff I., Rosner B., Greenberg L., Ravnikar V., Sacks F.M.: Effects of Postmenopausal Estrogen Replacement on the Concentrations and Metabolism of Plasma Lipoproteins. NEJM *325*, 1196–204, 1991.

36   Chang W.C., Nakao J., Orimo H., Murota S.I.: Stimulation of Prostaglandin Cyclooxygenase and Prostacyclin Synthetase Activities by Estradiol in Rat Aortic Smooth Muscle Cells. Biochim et Biophy Acta *620*, 472–482, 1980.

37   Zhu X.D., Knopp R.H.: Effect of Sex Hormones on Oxidative Modification of Low Density Lipoproteins by Placental Macrophages and Trophoblast and Their Susceptibility to Cytotoxicity. Am. Heart Assoc. Abstract to the Council on Arteriosclerosis Lipoprotein Metabolism. Page 5, 1993.

38   Shwaery G.T., Sacchiero R.J., Judd S.G., Nicolosi R.J., Foxall T.L.: Effects of Estrogen on Oxidation Ex Vivo of Low Density Lipoprotein From Hyypercholesterolemic Swine. Am. Heart Assoc. Abstract to the Council on Arteriosclerosis Diet and Oxidation of Lipoproteins. Page 48, 1993.

39   Illingworth D.R.: Management of hyperlipidemia: goals for the prevention of atherosclerosis. Clin Invest Med *14*, 211–218, 1990.

40   Steiner A., Weisser B., Vetter W.: A comparative review of the adverse effects of treatments for hyperlipidemia. Drug Safety *6*, 118–130, 1991.

41   Prihoda J.S., Illingworth D.R.: Drug Therapy of Hyperlipidemia. Current Problems in Cardiology. Mosby Year Book *17*, 551–605, 1992.

42   Superko R.H., Greenland P., et al.: Effectiveness of Low-Dose Colestipol Therapy in Patients with Moderate Hypercholesterolemia. Am J Card *70*, 135–140, 1992.

43   Henkin Y., Oberman A., Hurst D.C., et al.: Niacin revisited: clinical observations on an important but underutilized drug. Am J Med *91*, 239–246, 1991.

44   Bays H.E., Dujovne C.A., Mays B.: Elevated Lipoprotein (a) Blood Levels as the Single Treatable Risk Factor in Patients with Coronary Artery Disease. Journal of Ky. Med. Assoc. *91*, 498–500, 1993.

45   Ridker P.M., Hennekens C.H., Stampfer M.J.: A Prospective Study of Lipoprotein(a) and the Risk of Myocardial Infarction. JAMA *270*, 2195–2199, 1993.

46   Mullin G.E., Greenson J.K., Mitchell M.C.: Fulminant hepatic failure after ingestion of sustained-release nicotinic acid. Ann Intern Med *111* (3), 253–255, 1989.

47   Etchason J.A., Miller T.D., Squires R.W., et al.: Niacin-induced hepatitis: a potential side effect with low-dose time-release niacin. Mayo Clin Proc *66*, 23–28, 1991.

48   Knopp R.H., Ginsberg J., Albers J.J., et al.: Contrasting effects of unmodified and time release forms of niacin on lipoproteins in hyperlipidemic subjects. Clues to mechanism of action of niacin. Metabolism *34*, 642–650, 1985.

49   Superko R.H.: Drug Therapy and the Prevention of Atherosclerosis in Humans. Am J of Cardiol *64*, 31G–38G, 1989.

50   Hotz W.: Nicotinic acid and its derivatives: a short survey. Adv Lipid Res *20*, 195–217, 1983.

51   Dujovne C.A., Chremos A.N., Pool J.L., et al.: Expanded Clinical Evaluation of Lovastatin (EXCEL) study results: IV. additional perspectives on the tolerability of lovastatin. Am J Med *91* (suppl. 1B), 25S–30S, 1991.

52   Giroux L.M., Pare E., Davignon J., Naruszewicz M.: Simvastatin inhibits the oxidation

of low density lipoprotein by activated human monoxyte-derived macrophages. Abst of the AHA Council on Atheroscl 23, 1992.

53   Raasch R.H.: Pravastatin sodium, a new HMG-CoA reductase inhibitor. DICP 25, 388–394, 1991.

54   Hunninghake D.B., Knopp R.H., Schonfeld G., et al.: Efficacy and safety of pravastatin in patients with primary hypercholesterolemia. Atherosclerosis 85, 81–89, 1990.

55   Todd P.A., Goa K.L.: Simvastatin. A review of its pharmacological properties and therapeutic potential in hypercholesterolaemia. Drugs 40, 583–607, 1990.

56   Trial of clofibrate in the treatment of ischaemic heart disease: Five-year study by a group of physicians of the Newcastle upon Tyne region. BMJ 14, 767–75, 1971.

57   Ischaemic heart disease: a secondary prevention trial using clofibrate: report by a research committee of the Scottish Society of Physicians. BMJ 4, 775–84, 1971.

58   Carlson L.A., Rosenhamer G.: Reduction of mortality in the Stockholm Ischaemic Heart Disease Secondary Prevention Study by combined treatment with clofibrate and nicotinic acid. Acta Med Scand 223, 405–18, 1988.

59   Dujovne C.A., Harris, Gerrond L.L.C., Fan J., Muzio F.: Comparative Effects of Probucol on Lipoprotein Oxidation Susceptibility. Am J Card (In Press)

60   Jiala I., Grundy S.M.: Effect of Dietary Supplementation With Alpha-Tocopherol in the Oxidative Modification of Low Density Lipoprotein. J Lipid Research 33, 899–906, 1992.

61   Kita T., Nagano Y., Kokode M., et al.: Probucol prevents the progression of atherosclerosis in Watanabe heritable hyperlipidemic rabbit, and animal model for familial hypercholesterolemia. Proc Natl Acad Sci U.S.A. 84, 5928–5931, 1987.

62   Carew T.E., Schwenke D.C., Steinberg D.: Antiatherogenic effect of probucol unrelated to its hypocholesterolemic effect. Proc Natl Acad Sci USA 84, 7725–7729, 1987.

63   Yamamoto A., Matsuzawa Y., Yokoyama S., et al.: Effects of Probucol on xanthoma regression in familial hypercholesterolaemia. Am J Cardiol 57, 29–35, 1986.

64   Harris W.S.: Fish oils and plasma lipid and lipoprotein metabolism in humans; a critical review. J Lipid Res 30, 785–807, 1989.

65   Glauber H., Wallace P., Griver K., Brechtel G.: Adverse metabolic effect of omega-3 fatty acids in non-insulin-dependent diabetes mellitus. Ann Intern Med 108, 663–8, 1988.

66   Simopoulos A.P.: Omega-3 fatty acids in health and disease and in growth and development. Am J Clin Nutr 54, 438–63, 1991.

67   Sempos C.T., Cleeman J.I., Carroll M.D., et al.: Prevalence of high blood cholesterol among US adults: an update based on guidelines from the second report of the national cholesterol education program adult treatment panel. JAMA 269 (23), 3009–3014, 1993.

68   Hunninghake D.B., Stein E.A., Dujovne C.A., Harris W.S., et al.: The Efficacy of Intensive Dietary Therapy Alone or Combined with Lovastatin in Outpatients with Hypercholesterolemia. NEJM 328, 1213–1219, 1993.

69   Martin M.J., Browner W.S., Wentworth D., et al.: Serum cholesterol, blood pressure, and mortality: Implications from a cohort of 361, 662 men. Lancet 2, 933–936, 1986.

70   Schulman K.A., Kinosian B., Jacobson T.A., et al.: Reducing high blood cholesterol level with drugs: cost-effectiveness of pharmacologic management. JAMA 264 (23), 3025–3033, 1990.

71   Dayton S. et al.: A controlled clinical trial of a diet high in unsaturated fat in preventing complications of atherosclerosis, Circulation *40* (1, Suppl. 2),. II-1–II-63, 1969.
72   Steiner G., Shafrir E.: Primary Hyperlipoproteinemia. McGrawHill 1991.
73   Miettinen M. et al.: Effect of cholesterol-lowering diet on mortality from coronary heart-disease and other causes: A twelve-year clinical trial in men and women, Lancet *II*, 835–838, 1972.
74   Hjermann I., et al: Effect of diet and smoking intervention on the incidence of coronary heart disease: Report from the Oslo Study Group of a randomized trial in healthy men, Lancet *2*, 1303–1310, 1981.
75   Multiple Risk Factor Intervention Trial Research Group. Multiple Risk Factor Intervention Trial. JAMA *248*, 1465–1477, 1982.
76   Stamler, J., Wentworth, D., and Neaton, J.D. for the MRFIT Research Group: Is relationship between cholesterol and risk of premature death from coronary heart disease continuous and graded? Findings in 356 222 primary screenees of the Multiple Risk Factor Intervention Trial (MRFIT),JAMA *256* (20), 2823–2828, 1986.
77   Nikkila E.A., Viikinkoski P., Valle M., Frick M.H.: Prevention of progression of coronary atherosclerosis by treatment of hyperlipidaemia: a seven-year prospective angiographic study. BMJ. (Clin Res Ed). *289*, 220–3, 1984.
78   Brensike J.F., Levy R.I., Kelsey S.F., et al.: Effects of therapy with cholestyramine on progression of coronary arteriosclerosis: results of the NHLBI type II coronary intervention study. Circulation *69*, 313–324, 1984.
79   Blankenhorn D.H., Nessim S.A., Johnson R.L., Sanmarco M.E., Azen S.P., Cashin-Hemphill L.: Beneficial effects of combined colestipol-niacin therapy on coronary atherosclerosis and coronary venous bypass grafts. JAMA *257*, 3233–3240, 1987.
80   Cashin-Hemphill L., Mack W.J., Pogoda J.M., et al.: Beneficial effects of colestipol-niacin on coronary atherosclerosis: a 4-year follow-up. JAMA *264*, 3013–3017, 1990.
81   Ornish D., Brown S.E., Scherwitz L.W., Billings J.H., Armstrong W.T., Ports T.A., McLanahan S.M., Kirkeeide R.L., Brand R.J., Bould K.L.: Can lifestyle changes reverse coronary heart disease? Lancet *336*, 129–133, 1990.
82   Kane J.P., Malloy M.J., Ports T.A., et al.: Regression of coronary atherosclerosis during treatment of familial hypercholesterolemia with combined drug regimens. JAMA *264*, 3007–3012, 1990.
83   Brown G., Albers J.J., Fisher L.D., et al.: Regression of coronary artery disease as a result of intensive lipid-lowering therapy in men with high levels of apolipoprotein B. N Engl J Med *323*, 1289–1298, 1990.
84   Buchwald H., Varco R.L., Matts J.P., Long J.M., Fitch L.L., Campbell G.S., et al.: Effect of partial ileal bypass surgery on mortality and morbidity from coronary heart disease in patients with hypercholesterolemia. Report of the Program on the Surgical Control of the Hyperlipidemias (POSCH). N Engl J Med. *323*, 946–55, 1990.
85   Watts G.F., Lewis B., Brunt J.N.H., et al.: Effects on coronary artery disease of lipid-lowering diet, or diet plus cholestyramine in the St. Thomas Atherosclerosis Regression Study (STARS), Lancet *339*, 563–569, 1992.
86   Schuler G., Hambrecht R., Schlierf G., Niebauer J., Hauer K., Neumann J., Hoberg E., Drinkmann A., Bacher F., Grunze M., Kubler W.: Regular physical exercise and low-fat diet: Effects on progression on coronary artery disease. Cirulation *86*, 1–11, 1992.
87   Blankenhorn D.H., Azen S.P., Kramsch D.M., et al.: Coronary Angiographic Changes

with Lovastatin Therapy. The monitored atherosclerosis regression study. Ann Intern Med, 969–976, 1993.

88   Bays H.E., Dujovne C.A.: Cardiovascular Risk Factor Management in Primary Care. Resident and Staff Physician. 1994 (In Press).

89   Bays H.E., Dujovne C.A.: Drug Treatment of Dyslipidemias: Practical Guidelines for the Primary Care Physician. Heart Disease and Stroke *1*, 357–365, 1992.

90   Reaven P., Witztum J.L.: Lovastatin, nicotinic acid, and rhabdomyolysis. Ann Intern Med 109, 597–598, 1988. Letter.

91   Ayanian J.Z., Fuchs C.S., Stone R.M.: Lovastatin and rhabdomyolysis. Ann Intern Med *109*, 682–683, 1988.

92   Corpier C.L., Jones P.H., Suki W.N., et al.: Rhabdomyolysis and renal injury with lovastatin use: report of two cases in cardiac transplant recipients. JAMA *260*, 239–241, 1988.

93   Norman D.J., Illingworth D.R., Munson J., et al.: Myolysis and acute renal failure in a heart-transplant recipient receiving lovastatin. N. Engl J Med *318*, 45–47, 1988. Letter.

94   Smith P.F., Eydelloth R.S., Grossman S.J., et al.: HMG-CoA-reductase inhibitor-induced myopathy in the rat: cyclosporin A interaction and mechanism studies. J Pharmacol Exp Ther *257*(3), 1225–1235, 1991.

95   Pierce L.R., Wysowski D.K., Gross T.P.: Myopathy and rhabdomyolysis associated with lovastatin-gemfibrozil combination therapy. JAMA *264* (1), 71–75, 1990.

96   Duell B.P., Illingworth D.R.: Combination Therapy With HMG CoA Reductase Inhibitors and Gemfibrozil: Practical or Perilous. Heart Disease and Stroke, 260–261, May/June 1993.

97   Bays H.E., Dujovne C.A.: Combination Therapy With HMG CoA Reductase Inhibitors and Gemfibrozil: Practical or Perilous Author's Reply. Heart Disease and Stroke, 261–262, May/June 1993.

98   Stein E.A.: Management of Hypercholesterolemia. Am J. Med. *87*, 4A-20S–4A-27S, 1989.

99   Malloy M.J., Kane J.P., Kunitaka S.T., Tun P.: Complementarity of colestipol, niacin, and lovastatin in treatment of severe familial hypercholesterolemia. Ann Intern Med *107*, 616–623, 1987.

100   Stein E.A., Lamkin G.E., Bewley D.Z., Henschen S.: Treatment of severe familal hypercholesterolemia with lovastatin , resin, and niacin (abstr). Arteriosclerosis *7* (5), 517a, 1987.

101   Stein E.A., Turner T., Mellies M.T.: Triple drug therapy for heterozygous familial hypercholesterolemia. Arteriosclerosis *3* (5), 485a, 1983.

Progress in Drug Research, Vol. 43 (E. Jucker, Ed.)
© 1994 Birkhäuser Verlag, Basel (Switzerland)

In search of ideal antihypertensive drugs: Progress in five decades

By Eric J. Lien[1*], Hua Gao[1] and Linda L. Lien[2]

[1] Department of Pharmaceutical Sciences, School of Pharmacy, University of Southern California, Los Angeles, CA 90033, USA; [2] R.Ph. 10728 Kelmore St, Culver City, CA 90230, USA
* To whom correspondence should be addressed.

1   Introduction

Among the three major causes of death in developed countries, namely, cardiovascular diseases including heart attack, stroke, and all forms of cancer, the first two are associated with hypertension. Because of the important health impact, many antihypertensive agents have been introduced in the last 50 years. In this review, we shall focus our attention on the following groups: (1) renin inhibitors, (2) calcium channel blockers, (3) α- and β-adrenergic blockers, and (4) angiotensin converting enzyme (ACE) inhibitors.
Theoretically, to serve as an effective drug, an ideal antihypertensive agent should possess the characteristics listed in Table 1.

Table 1.
Characteristics of an ideal antihypertensive agent (adapted and expanded from [1, 2]).

1.	Orally, or transdermally active.
2.	Good duration of action 12–24 hrs, or longer.
3.	Slow onset, induces a decrease in blood pressure, not too pronounced and similar in supine and standing positions (no orthostatic hypotension).
4.	No negative inotropic effect or chronotropic effect (tachycardia) on the heart.
5.	No tolerance (no tachyphylaxis).
6.	No severe adverse reaction (e.g. nephrotoxicity, hepatotoxicity or idiosyncrasy), no reduction of physical capacity or mental alertness.
7.	Suitable for long-term therapy (months or years).
8.	Of reasonable cost, and with no significant interactions with other drugs.
9.	No severe rebound in blood pressure upon discontinuation.

Figure 1 shows the slow improvement of the therapeutic efficacy of various types of antihypertensive drugs introduced during 1940–1990.
Various biochemical and pharmacological sites of action of different antihyptertensive agents are depicted in Figure 2. These target sites include adrenergic α_2 receptors in the central nervous system for clonidine type of drugs, sympathetic nervous system for α- and β-blockers, key enzymes involved in the renin-angiotensin cascade, and calcium channels in the heart and the vessels.

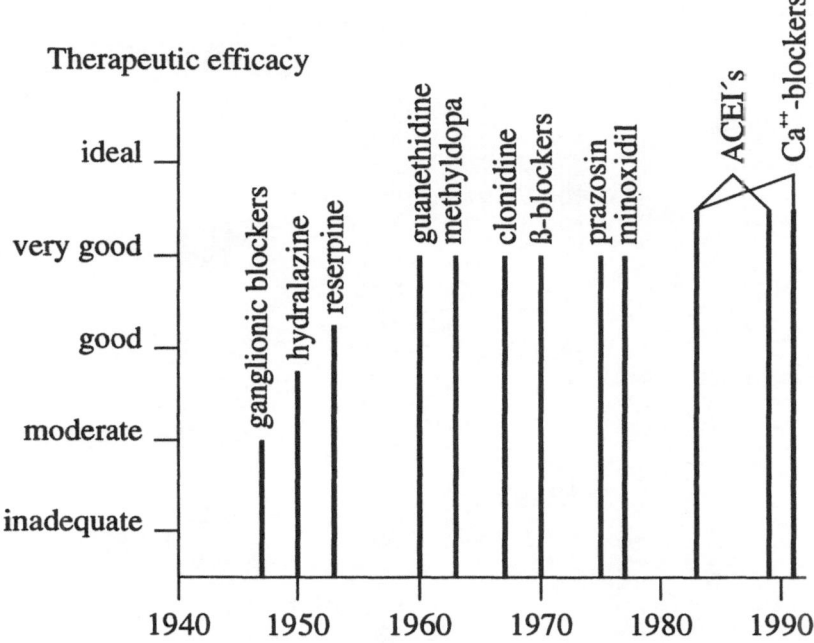

Fig. 1.
Introduction of various antihypertensive drugs with different therapeutic efficacies during 1940–1990.

1.1   Renin inhibitors

A wide range of effects caused by angiotensin II is shown at the bottom of Figure 2. Since renin inhibitors act at the upper stream of the cascade, it is generally believed that specific renin inhibitors should have fewer side effects as compared to ACE inhibitors. Intensive effort is being focused on the search of non-peptide, orally available renin inhibitors [3–7]. Several promising compounds still undergoing clinical trials are summarized in Table 2, together with the amino acid sequences of renin and some proto-types of inhibitors.

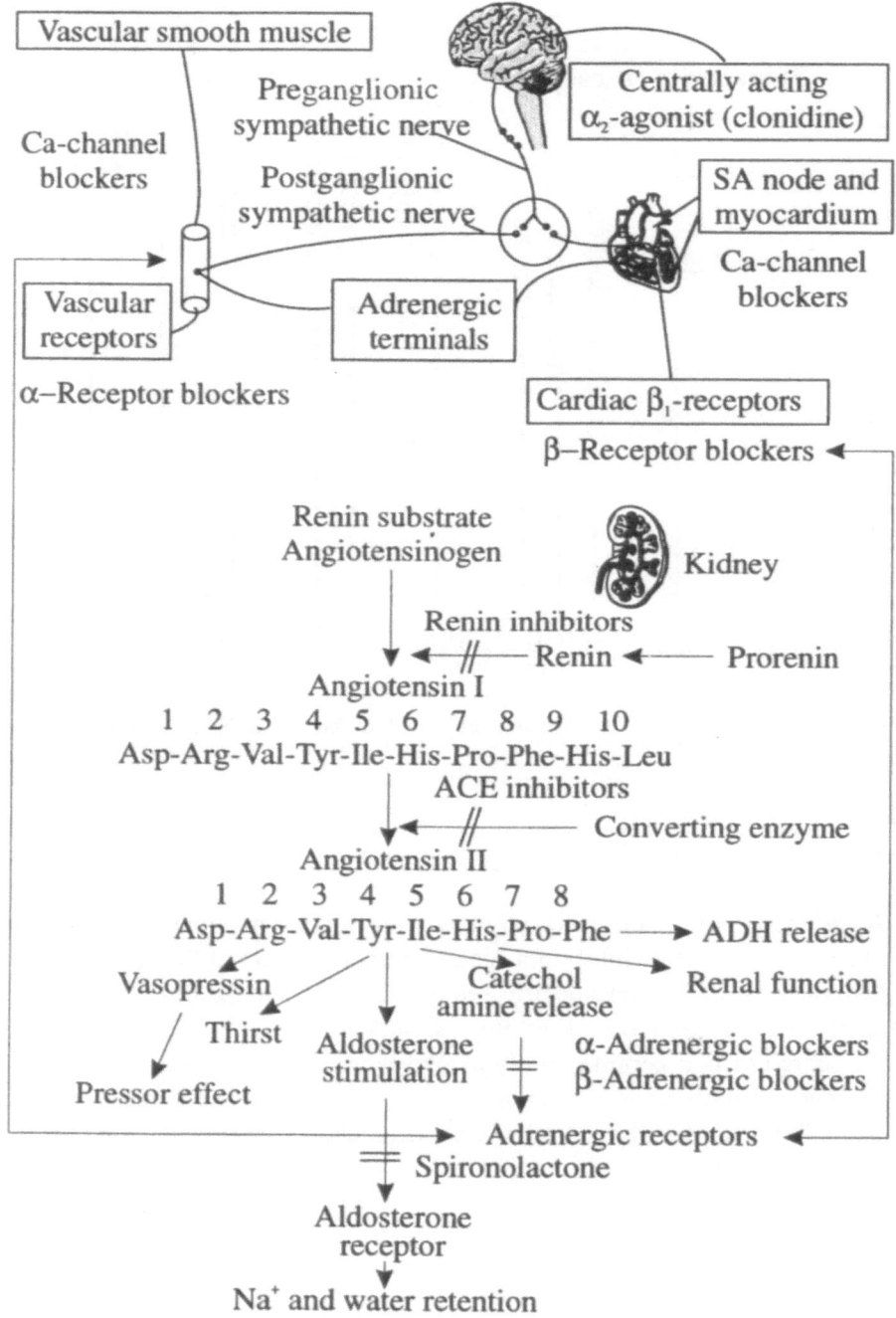

Fig. 2
Different biochemical and pharmacological target sites for various antihypertensive agents.

1.2   FDA rating and classification

The system for rating new drugs used until the end of 1991 is as the following:

Class 1 = New molecular entity
         A = Important therapeutic gain
         B = Modest therapeutic gain
         C = Little or no therapeutic gain

The classification system used beginning in 1992 is shown below:

         P = Priority review, therapeutic gain
         S = Standard review, substantially equivalent
         E = Used to treat life-threatening or severely debilitating illness
         V = A designated orphan drug

Currently the most commonly prescribed antihypertensive agents are calcium channel blockers, angiotensin converting enzyme inhibitors (ACEI's), and to a lesser extent β-adrenergic blockers and α-adrenergic blockers.

2   Calcium channel blockers

Table 3 summarizes the structures and indications of calcium channel blockers developed between 1962 and 1993. These calcium channel blockers or antagonists for calcium ion are generally divided into three major groups: verapamil type, diltiazem type and 1,4-dihydropyridine derivatives [8, 9]. Detailed descriptions of the structure-activity relationship and pharmacological profiles of the specific drugs marketed between 1986 and 1993 are given under generic names. The beta adrenergic blockers with the same essential pharmacophore but different auxopharmacophore [10, 11] are shown in Table 4, while the α-adrenergic blockers used clinically are given in Table 5.
Besides their use as antihypertensive agents some calcium channel blockers have indications as antiarrhythmic, antianginal and for neurological defects due to spasm following subarachnoid hemorrhage (See Table 3).

Table 2.
Human renin binding sites with angiotensinogen and various inhibitors [3–7].

Compound	Structures* RENIN		IC$_{50}$ (nM)	Clinical study

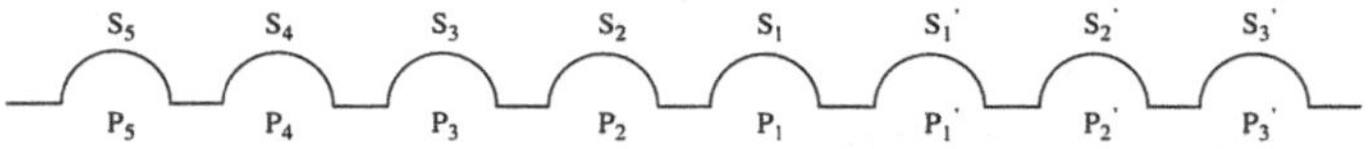

S_5 S_4 S_3 S_2 S_1 $S_1{'}$ $S_2{'}$ $S_3{'}$

P_5 P_4 P_3 P_2 P_1 $P_1{'}$ $P_2{'}$ $P_3{'}$

HUMAN ANGIOTENSINOGEN

Asp$_1$ - Arg$_2$ - Val$_3$ - Tyr$_4$ - Ile$_5$ - His$_6$ - Pro$_7$ - Phe$_8$ - His$_9$ - Leu$_{10}$ ▼ Val$_{11}$ - Ile$_{12}$ - His$_{13}$ ... Protein

Renin Inhibitors

Compound	Structures	IC$_{50}$ (nM)	Clinical study
Substrate analog (RIP)	Pro - His - - - - Pro - - - Phe - - - His Lys - - - Tyr - - - - - Val - - - - Phe - - - - Phe	2000	
Reduced peptide isostere (H-142)	R Pro - His - - - - Pro - - - Phe - - - His - - - - Leu - - - - Val - - - - - Ile - - -- His - - - Lys	10	
Pepstatin A	Iva - - - Val - - - Val - - - - - --- - - Sta - - - ------- Ala - - -- Sta	20,000	

Inhibitors containing statine or modified statine

Compound	Structures	IC$_{50}$ (nM)	Clinical study
Scrip	Iva - His - - - - Pro - - - Phe - - - His - - - - - - - - Sta - - - - - - - - Leu - - - - Phe - NH$_2$	20	
CGP 2928	Z - Arg - Arg - - - - Pro - - - Phe - - - His - - - -┐ H$_3$CO(BOC)Lys - His - - - - - Ile - - - - - - - - Sta -┘	10	
SR 43845	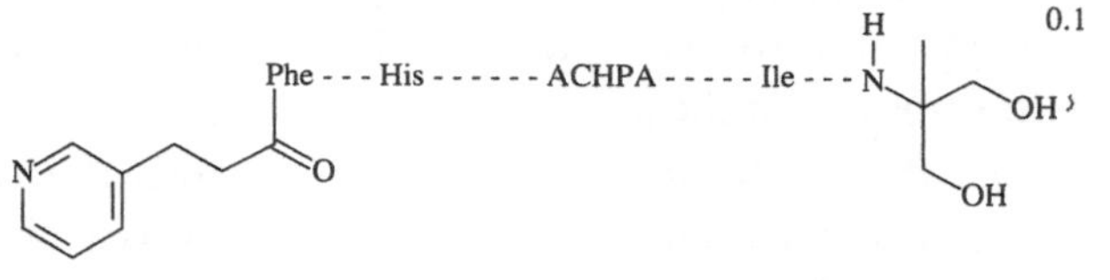 Phe - - - His - - - - - - ACHPA - - - - - Ile - - - N(H)... OH ... OH (with pyridine-propanoyl group)	0.1	
A 64662	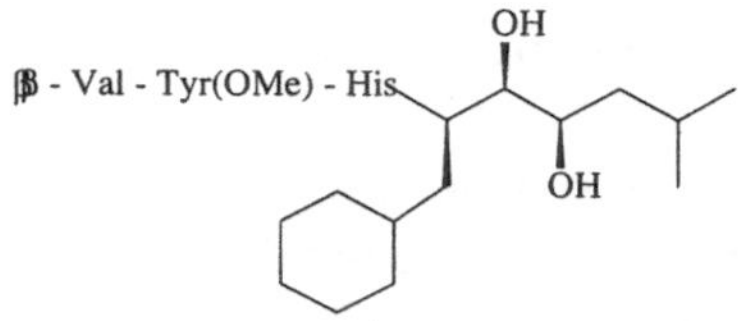 β - Val - Tyr(OMe) - His... (OH, OH, cyclohexyl group)	0.6	

Table 2. (continued)

Compound	Structures* RENIN	IC$_{50}$ (nM)	Clinical study
Enalkirin	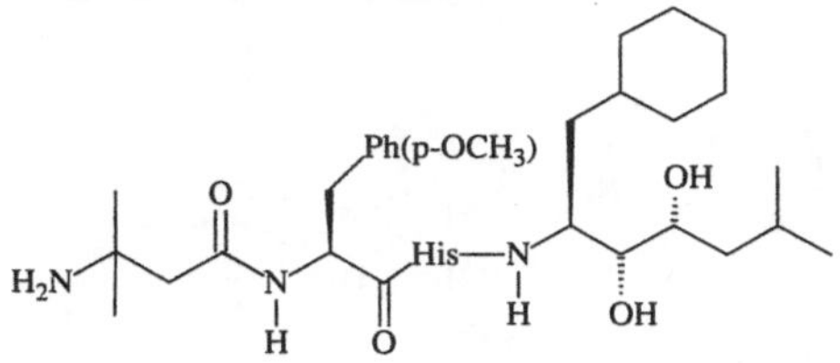	0.8	Yes
Ditekirin	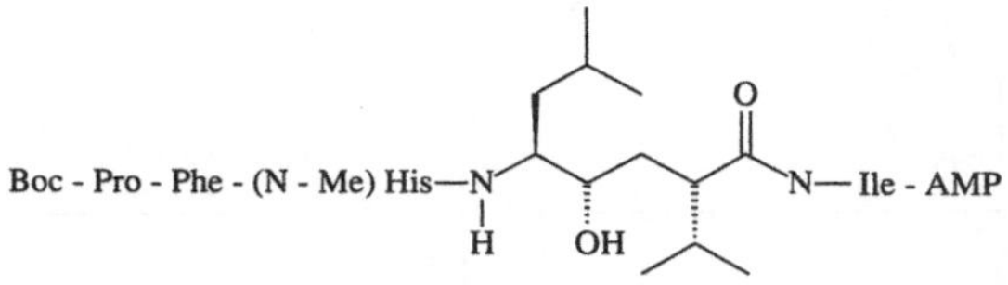		Yes
CGP 38, 560A	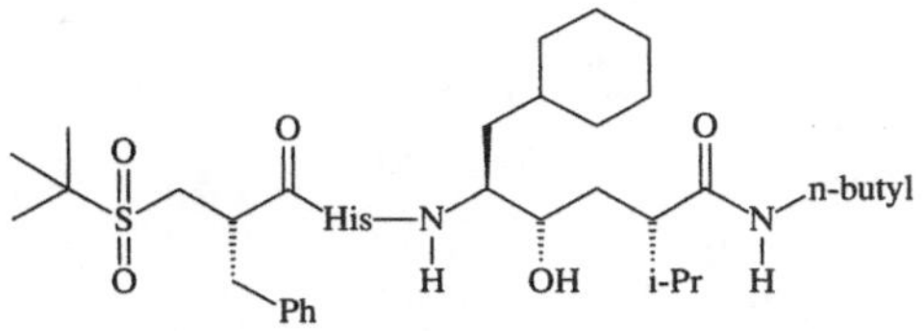	1 0.7	Yes
Ro-42, 5892	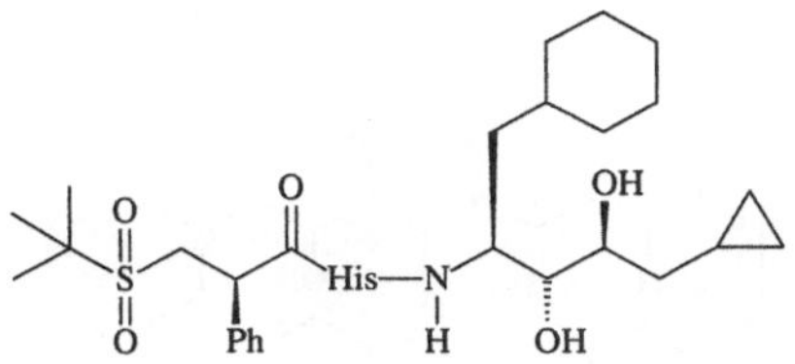		Yes (promising)
ES-8891	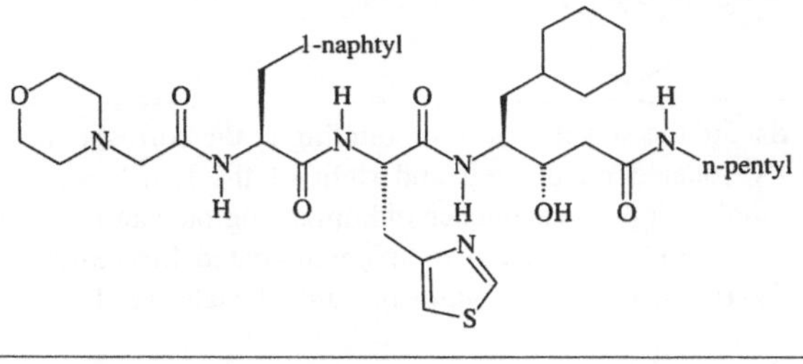	1.1	Yes
FK-744	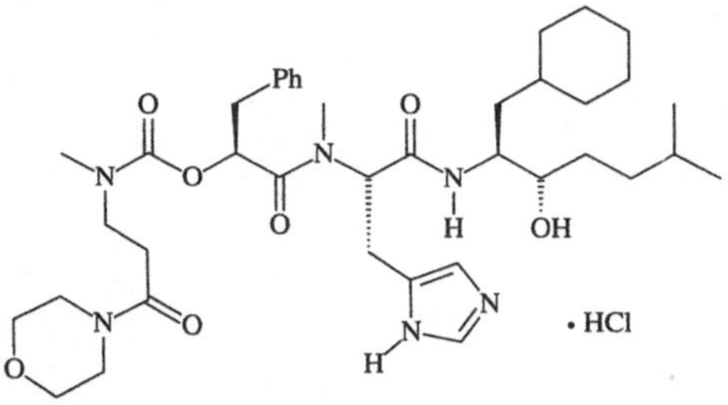		Yes

Table 2. (continued)

Compound	Structures* **RENIN**	IC$_{50}$ (nM)	Clinical study
FK-906	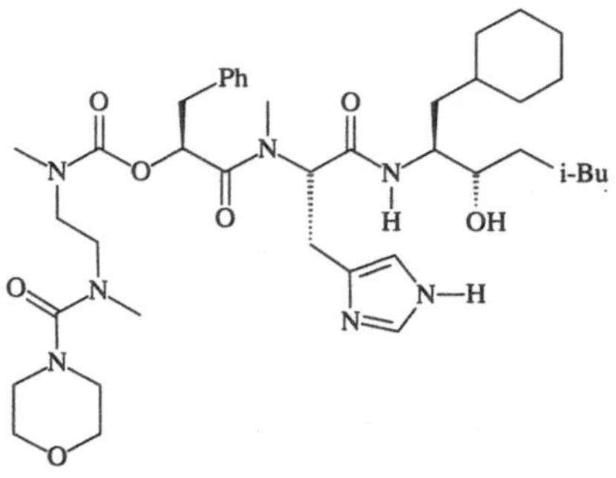		Yes (Good oral bioavail- ability) 50 mg bid
Iosartan (Dup 753; MK-954)	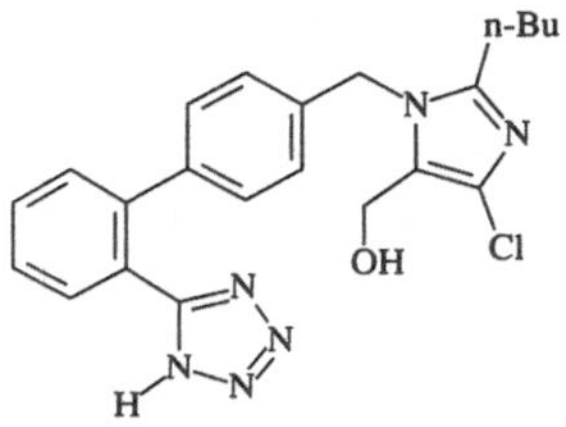		Yes (high potency and oral activity)
BW-175	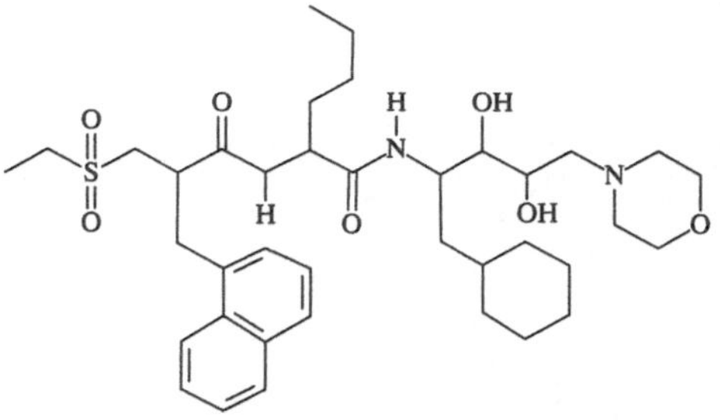	3.3	—

* S$_1$ to S$_5$ and S$_1'$ to S$_5'$ are the subsites of renin binding to the corresponding amino acids P$_1$ to P$_5$ and P$_1'$ to P$_5'$ located on the left and right of the Leu^{10}–Val^{11} cleavage site, respectively. NH$_2$-terminal amino acid sequence of human angiotensinogen and the minimal octapeptide substrate (His^6–His^{13}) cleaved by renin are indicated. Structures of various renin inhibitors with their IC$_{50}$ (nM) and current status of clinical trials are also indicated.

Table 3.
Calcium channel blockers

Generic name	Structure (year introduced)	Trade name	Indication(s)	Year marketed
Verapamil	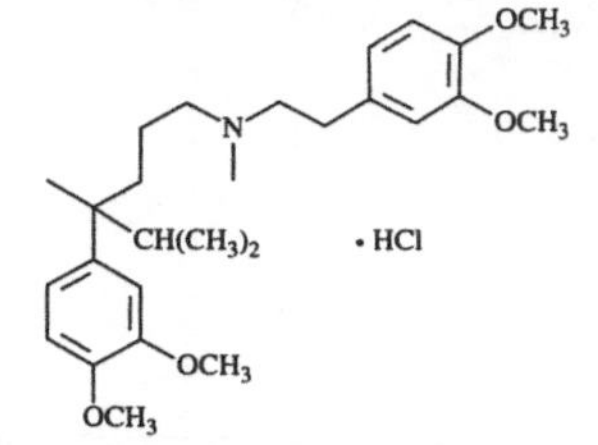 $C_{27}H_{38}N_2O_4 \cdot HCl$; MW = 491.08 (1962)	Calan (Searle) Isoptin (Knoll) Calan SR (Searle) Isoptin (Knoll) Verelan (Lederle)	1. Antiarrhythmic 2. Antihypertensive 3. Antianginal Antihypertensive	1981
Nifedipine	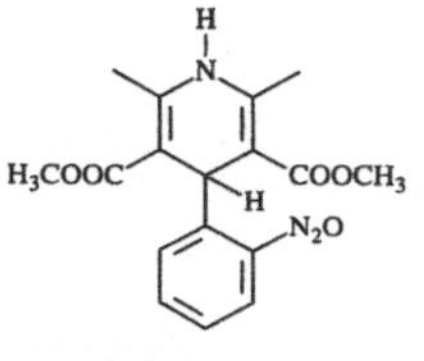 $C_{17}H_{18}N_2O_6$; MW = 364.34 (1968)	Adalat (Miles) Procardia (Pfizer) Procardia XL (Pfizer)	Antianginal 1. Antihypertensive 2. Antianginal	1982
Diltiazem HCl	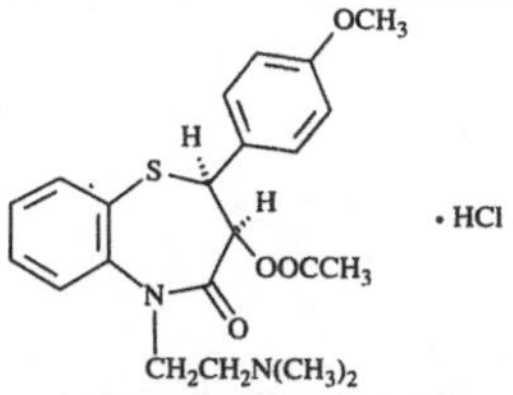 $C_{22}H_{26}N_2O_4S \cdot HCl$; MW = 450.98 (1969)	Cardizem (Marion-Merrell Dow) Cardizem CD Cardizem SR (Marion-Merrell Dow) Dilacor XL (Rhone-Poulenc Rorer)	Antianginal Antihypertensive	1982 1991
Nicardipine HCl	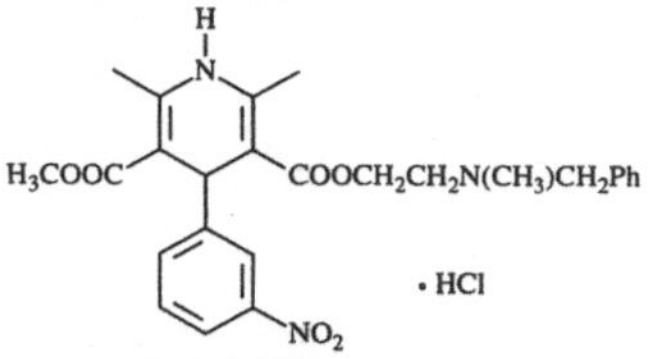 $C_{26}H_{29}N_3O_6 \cdot HCl$; MW = 515.99 (1974)	Cardene (Syntex)	1. Antianginal 2. Antihypertensive	1988
Nimodipine	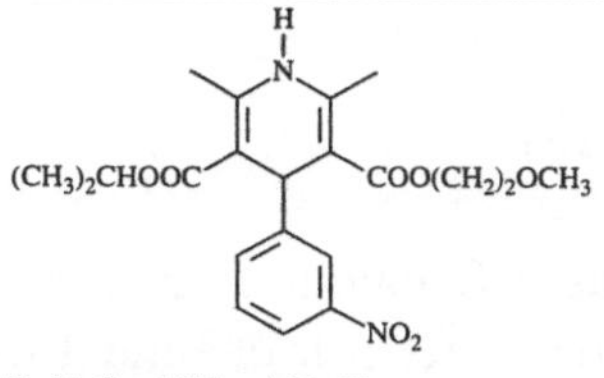 $C_{21}H_{26}N_2O_7$; MW = 418.45 (1972)	Nimotop (Miles)	Agent for neurological defects due to spasm following subarachnoid hemorrhage	1989

Table 3. (continued)

Generic name	Structure (year introduced)	Trade name	Indication(s)	Year marketed
Bepridil HCl	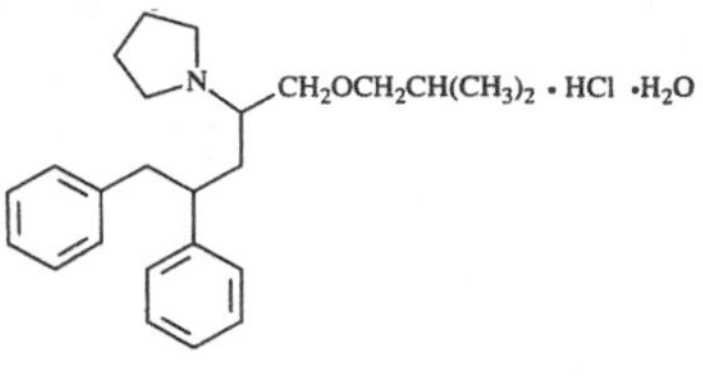 $C_{24}H_{34}N_2O \cdot HCl \cdot H_2O$; MW = 421.0 (1972 free base) (1977 HCl salt)	Vascor (McNeil)	Antianginal	1991
Isradipine	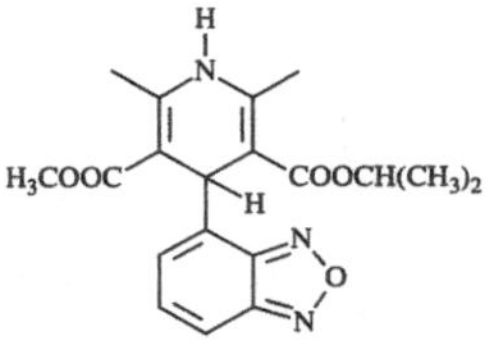 $C_{19}H_{21}N_3O_5$; MW = 371.39 (1980)	Dynacirc (Sandoz)	Antihypertensive	1991
Felodipine	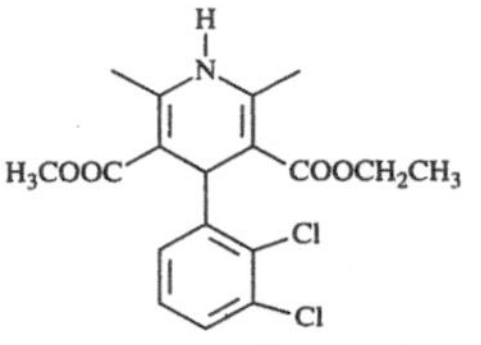 $C_{18}H_{19}Cl_2NO_4$; MW = 384.26 (1980)	Plendil (MS&D)	Antihypertensive	1991
Amlodipine besylate	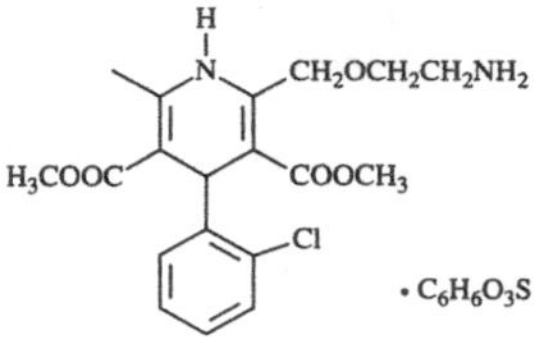 $C_{20}H_{25}ClN_2O_5 \cdot C_6H_5SO_3H$; MW = 567.1 (1983)	Norvasc (Pfizer)	1. Antihypertensive 2. Antianginal	1992

2.1   Amlodipine besylate [12–18]

Amlodipine besylate is classified as 1-S calcium channel blocker with antihypertensive and antianginal effects. Its full chemical name is 2-[(2-Aminoethoxy)methyl]-4-(2-chloropenyl)-1,4-dihydro-6-methyl-3,5-pyri-dinedicarboxylic acid 3-ethyl-5-methyl ester.

Structure-activity relationship
Amlodipine is a dihydropyridine derivative substituted at the 2-position by a basic side chain; it is comparable in potency to nifedipine and has an elimination $t_{1/2}$ of 30 hrs in dogs, and 34 hrs in humans, respectively. The (–) isomer is the more active isomer (eutomer).

Biopharmaceutics and pharmacokinetics
Oral administration of amlodipine produced peak plasma concentrations between 6 and 12 hrs. Absolute bioavailability has been estimated to be between 64 and 90%, and not altered by the presence of food. About 90% of the drug is converted to inactive metabolites *via* hepatic metabolism with 10% of the parent compound and 60% of the metabolites excreted in the urine. Steady state plasma levels of amlodipine are reached after 7 to 8 days of consecutive daily dosing.

Pharmacology and indication(s)
Amlodipine inhibits calcium ion influx across cell membranes selectively, with a greater effect on vascular smooth muscle cells than on cardiac muscle cells. It is a peripheral arterial vasodilator that acts directly on vascular smooth muscle to cause a reduction in peripheral vascular resistance and in blood pressure. The drug is indicated for the treatment of hypertension, chronic stable angina and vasospastic angina.

Dosage form(s) and dosage
Its dosage forms are in 2.5 mg, 5 mg, and 10 mg tablets. The dosages are 5 mg/day, maximum 10 mg/day, 2.5 mg/day for hepatic insufficient patient and for co-administration with other antihypertensive drugs in hypertensive patients, and 5 to 10 mg/day in anginal patients.

Adverse reactions
The adverse reactions which were reported with an incidence greater than 1% are: headache, edema, fatigue, nausea, abdominal pain, somnolence. Other adverse reactions reported are: arrhythmia, bradycardia, chest pain, hypotension, peripheral ischemia, syncope, tachycardia, palpitation, hyposthesia, parethesia, dysphagia, diarrhea, flatulence, vomiting, asthenia, back pain, hot flushes, malaise, pain, rigors, weight gain, pruritus, rash, abnormal vision, conjunctivitis, diplopia, eye pain, tinnitus, muscle cramps, dry mouth, etc.

Interactions with other drugs
Amlodipine has been safely administered with thiazide diuretics, beta-blockers, angiotensin converting enzyme inhibitors, long-acting nitrates, sublingual nitroglycerin, digoxin, warfarin, non-steroidal anti-inflammatory drugs, antibiotics, and oral hypoglycemic drugs.

2.2   Bepridil HCl [19–27]

Bepridil is classified as 1-B antianginal agent. Its full name is β-[(2-Methylpropoxy)methyl]-N-phenyl-N-(phenylmethyl)-1-pyrrolidineethan-amine.

Structure-activity relationship
Bepridil is a novel substance with antianginal and specific antiarrhythmic activities. It inhibits slow calcium as well as fast sodium channels, it interferes with calcium binding to calmodulin and blocks both voltage and receptor operated calcium channels. It is chemically not related to drugs having similar cardioactivity, e.g. diltiazem, nifedipine and verapamil. It can be considered as an ethylenediamine derivative with a 2-methyl-pro-poxymethyl group attached on one of the ethylene carbons.

Biopharmaceutics and pharmacokinetics
The drug is rapidly and completely absorbed after oral administration in healthy volunteers. It reaches peak plasma concentration in 2–3 hrs. Over a 10-day period, about 70% of a single dose of the drug is excreted in the urine and 22% in the feces as metabolites. Excretion of unmetabolized drug is negligible. The drug follows a biphasic elimination, with a distribution $t_{1/2}$ of 2 hrs, and terminal elimination $t_{1/2}$ of 42 hrs.

Pharmacology and indication(s)
Bepridil HCl is a calcium channel blocker antianginal agent with type 1 antiarrhthmic and minimal antihypertensive properties. The drug is indicated for the treatment of chronic stable angina (classic effort-associated angina) in patients resistant to or intolerant of other antianginal medications.

Dosage form(s) and dosage
Its dosage forms are 200 mg, 300 mg, and 400 mg tablets. The dosage should be individualized with a usual starting dose of 200 mg once daily.

Adverse reactions
The reported adverse reactions include asthenia, headache, flu-like syndrome, palpitations, dyspnea, G.I. distress, dry mouth, anorexia, diarrhea, constipation, drowsiness, insomnia, dizziness, tremor, nervousness, ventricular tachycardia, agranulocytosis, syncope, etc.

Interactions with other drugs
It can be used with betablocking agents and nitrates in patients without heart failure. Antiarrhythmics and tricyclic anti-depressants could exaggerate the prolong-action of the QT interval observed with bepridil HCl. Cardiac glycosides could exaggerate the depression of AV nodal conduction observed with bepridil HCl.

2.3   Felodipine [28–33]

Felodipine,   4-(2,3-dichlorophenyl)-1,4-dihydro-2,6-dimethyl-3,5-pyridinedicarboxylic acid ethyl methyl ester, is classified as 1-C calcium ion influx inhibitory antihypertensive agent.

Structure-activity relationship
It is a calcium channel blocker belonging to the dihydropyridine derivatives, and competes with nitrendipine and/or other calcium channel blockers for dihydropyridine binding sites. The drug is a racemic mixture.

Biopharmaceutics and pharmacokinetics
The drug is almost completely absorbed after oral administration, and undergoes extensive first-pass metabolism. The systemic bioavailability of the drug is approximately 20%, reaching mean peak level in 2.5 to 5 hrs. Both peak plasma concentration and AUC curve increase linearly with doses up to 20 mg. It is bound to plasma proteins greater than 99%. The renal elimination accounts for 70% of radioactivity while fecal elimination accounts for 10% after oral or IV dosing of ^{14}C-labelled felodipine.

Pharmacology and indication(s)
It blocks voltage-dependent Ca^{++} currents in vascular smooth muscle and cultured rabbit atrial cells, and also blocks potassium-induced contraction of the rat portal vein. Its effect on blood pressure is mainly a consequence of a dose-related decrease of peripheral vascular resistance in man, with a modest reflex increase in heart rate. The drug is indicated for the treatment

of hypertension, either alone or concomitantly with other antihypertensive agents.

Dosage form(s) and dosage
The dosage forms for this drug are 5 mg, 10 mg, and extended release tablets. The recommended initial dose is 5 mg once a day, and should be adjusted individually.

Adverse Reactions
The reported adverse reactions in monotherapy are peripheral edema, headache, flushing, dizziness, upper respiratory symptoms, asthenia, cough, paresthesia, dyspepsia, chest pain, nausea, muscle cramps, abdominal pain, constipation, diarrhea, pharyngitis, rhinorrhea, back pain, rash, etc.

Interactions with other drugs
Cimetidine may increase the AUC and C_{max} of felodipine. It is, therefore, recommended that low doses of felodipine be used when given concomitantly with cimetidine. Felodipine may increase the C_{max} of digoxin but not the AUC.

2.4   Isradipine [34–39]

Isradipine, 3,5-pyridinedicarboxylic acid 4-(4-benzofurazanyl)-1,4-dihydro-2,6-dimethyl methyl 1-methylethyl ester, is classified as 1-C calcium channel blocking antihypertensive agent.

Structure-activity relationship
It is a dihydropyridine derivative with a benzofurazanyl group attached at the 4-position and two carboxyl groups at the 3,5-positions, one of which is converted to an isopropyl ester, thus the name isradipine. It binds to calcium channels with high affinity as well as specificity, and inhibits calcium flux into cardiac and smooth muscle.

Biopharmaceutics and pharmacokinetics
The drug is 90–95% absorbed and is subject to extensive first-pass metabolism, yielding a bioavailability of 15–24%. It is 95% bound to plasma protein. After dosing, peak plasma concentration is reached in 1.5 hrs. The elimination of the drug is biphasic with a distribution $t_{1/2}$ of 1.5–2 hrs, and

a terminal $t_{1/2}$ of about 8 hrs. The drug is completely metabolized before it is excreted.

Pharmacology and indication(s)
The drug has diuretic activity and can dilate arterioles leading to reduced systemic resistance and lower blood pressure with a small increase in resting heart rate. It has negative inotropic effects *in vitro*. In intact anesthetized animals the vasodilating effect occurs at doses lower than those which affect contractility. It is indicated in the management of hypertension, either alone or used concurrently with thiazide diuretics.

Dosage form(s) and dosage
The dosage forms for this drug are 2.5 mg and 5 mg capsules. The recommended initial dose is 2.5 mg twice a day, the dosage should be individualized.

Adverse reactions
Headache, dizziness, edema, palpitation, fatigue, flushing chest pain, nausea, dyspnea, abdominal discomfort, tachycardia, rash, pollakiuria, weakness, vomiting, diarrhea, etc. have been reported as adverse reactions.

Interactions with other drugs
Fentanyl anesthesia and concomitant use of beta-blockers may result in severe hypotension. Co-administration of propranolol and isradipiine may increase the total bioavailability of propranolol.

2.5   Nicardipine HCl [40–48]

Nicardipine HCl is classified as 1-C antianginal and antihypertensive agent.

Structure-activity relationship
It is structurally related to an older calcium channel blocker nifedipine (Procardia®), both are 1,4-dihydro-2,6-dimethyl-4-phenyl-3,5-pyridine dicarboxylate derivatives. The differences in structure include the position of the nitro group on the phenyl ring (m- vs. o-position) and one of the carboxylates 2-[methyl(phenylmethyl)amino]ethyl ester vs. methyl ester, for the new and old compounds, respectively.

Biopharmaceutics and pharmacokinetics

The drug is completely absorbed after oral dosing of the capsules, giving maximal plasma levels within 30 min. to two hrs (mean $T_{max} = 1$ hr). Nicardipine is subject to saturable first-pass metabolism, giving a systemic bioavailability of about 35% following a 30 mg oral dose at steady state. Less than 1% of the intact drug is detected in the urine due to extensive hepatic metabolism.

Pharmacology and indication(s)

Nicardipine is a calcium entry blocker, also known as slow channel blocker or calcium ion antagonist. It inhibits the transmembrane influx of calcium ions into cardiac muscle and smooth muscle without changing serum calcium concentrations. The drug has more selectivity to vascular smooth muscle than to cardiac muscle, thus produces relaxation of coronary smooth muscle at drug levels which cause little or no negative inotropic effect of the heart. The drug is indicated for the management of chronic stable angina (effort-associated angina) and for the treatment of hypertension.

Dosage form(s) and dosage

The dosage forms for this drug are 20 mg and 30 mg capsules and Cardene® SR 30 mg, 45 mg and 60 mg. The recommended dose of the capsule is 20–40 mg three times a day and should be individualized. The dose of Cardene SR is 30–60 mg twice a day.

Adverse reactions

The following adverse reactions have been reported in some patients: pedal edema, dizziness, headache, asthenia, flushing, increased angina, palpitations, nausea, dyspepsia, dry mouth, somnolence, rash, tachycardia, myalgia, other edema, parethesia, sustained tachycardia, syncope, constipation, dyspnea, abnormal ECG, malaise, nervousness, tremor, insomnia, nocturia, vomiting, etc.

Interactions with other drugs

Combination with β-blocker is well tolerated, however, it gives no protection against the danger of abrupt β-blocker withdrawal, any such withdrawal should be by gradual reduction of the dose of β-blocker (over 8–10 days). Cimetidine may increase the plasma level of nicardipine. Serum levels of digoxin should be evaluated after concomitant therapy with nicardipine. Concomitant administration of nicardipine and cyclosporin may result in elevated plasma cyclosporin levels.

2.6   Nimodipine [49–55]

Nimodipine, 3,5-pyridinedicarboxylic acid, 1,4-dihydro-2,6-dimethyl-4-(3-nitrophenyl)-2-methoxyethyl-1-methylethyl ester, is classified as 1-A calcium influx inhibitor for the improvement of neurological deficits following subarachnoid hemorrhage.

Structure-activity relationship
It is structurally closely related to nicardipine, an older calcium channel blocker, the only difference being a MeO group taking the place of a -N(CH3)CH2Ph on one of the side chains attached to the dihydropyridine ring. Nimodipine is used for subarachnoid hemorrhage while nicardipine is used as antiangina and antihypertensive. Because of the unique application nimodipine was approved by FDA as a class 1-A drug. Being fairly lipophilic, the drug has a greater effect on cerebral arteries than on arteries elsewhere in the body due to its ability to cross the blood-brain barrier.

Biopharmaceutics and pharmacokinetics
After oral administration nimodipine is rapidly absorbed in man, reaching peak concentrations in one hr. The earlier and terminal $t_{1/2}$ values are 1–2 hrs and 8–9 hrs, respectively. The drug is bound to plasma protein over 95%, and is eliminated almost exclusively as metabolites (<1% unchanged in the urine). When the drug was given three times a day for seven days, no signs of accumulation were observed.

Pharmacology and indication(s)
Nimodipine inhibits calcium ion transfer into smooth muscle cells, thus inhibits contractions of vascular smooth muscle. It is indicated for the improvement of neurological deficits due to spasm following subarachnoid hemorrhage from ruptured congenital aneurysms in patients who are in good neurological condition post-ictus, e.g. Hunt and Hess grades I-III. It is not indicated for more severe cases.

Dosage form(s) and dosage
The dosage form is 30 mg capsule. Oral dosage is 60 mg every 4 hrs for 21 consecutive days. Therapy should commence within 96 hrs of the subarachnoid hemorrhage.

Adverse reactions
Decreased blood pressure, abnormal liver function test, edema, diarrhea, rash, headache, G.I. symptoms, nausea, dyspnea, abnormal EKG, tachycardia, bradycardia, muscle pain/cramp, acne, depression, etc. have been reported in some patients receiving nimodipine treatment.

Interactions with other drugs
Nimodipine may enhance the cardiovascular action of other calcium channel blockers, or other antihypertensive drugs.

3   β-Adrenergic blockers

Various Beta adrenergic blockers have a total of six different therapeutical applications, namely, angina, hypertension, arrhythmias, treatment after acute myocardiac infarction, glaucoma and migraine headache (see Table 4 and the individual new drugs marketed during 1986–1993). For the drugs marketed between 1980–1986, reference 56 should be consulted.
From Table 4 it is apparent that lipophilicity as measured by LogP (or LogP') plays an important role in cardioselectivity. It appears that a Log P range of 0.4–2.3 is necessary but not sufficient condition for a β-adrenergic blocker to be cardioselective, other steric and electronic factors are also involved in cardioselectivity.

3.1   Betaxolol HCl [57–63]

Betaxolol   HCl,   1-{4-[2-(cyclopropylmethoxy)ethyl-phenoxy}-3[(1-methylethyl)amino]-2-propanol-hydrochloride, is classified as antihypertensive β_1-adrenergic blocker. It is cardioselective and has antiglaucoma activity.

Structure-activity relationship
Betaxolol is β_1-selective cardioselective adrenergic blocker. It has the essential pharmacophore present in most β-adrenergic blockers, namely Ar-OCH$_2$CHOHCH$_2$NHR, where the Ar has a p-cyclopropylmethoxyethyl group and R is an isopropyl group. It is available as tablets for the treatment of hypertension, and as ophthalmic solutions or suspension for the treatment of ocular hypertension and chronic open-angle glaucoma.

Biopharmaceutics and pharmacokinetics

The drug is completely absorbed in man after oral administration, with a small first-pass effect resulting in an absolute bioavailability of $89 \pm 5\%$. In healthy volunteers, a 10-mg oral dose of the drug gives mean peak blood concentration of 21.6 ng/ml in about 3 hrs (1.5–6 hrs). Steady state plasma concentrations are attained with once-daily oral dosing in 5–7 days in subjects with normal renal function. It is about 50% plasma protein bound. The drug is eliminated primarily by hepatic metabolism and secondarily by renal excretion.

Pharmacology and indication(s)

The tablet dosage form is indicated in the management of hypertension, either alone or concomitantly with thiazide diuretics. The ophthalmic preparations are for the treatment of ocular hypertension and chronic open-angle glaucoma, either alone or with other antiglaucoma agents.

Dosage form(s) and dosage

The dosage forms are 10 mg, 20 mg tablets. The initial dose of the tablets in hypertension is 10 mg once daily. Ophthalmic solution is available in 0.5% as base, and in suspension 0.25% as base.

Adverse Reactions

The following adverse reactions have been reported: bradycardia, edema, headache, dizziness, fatigue, lethargy, insomnia, nervousness, bizarre dreams, depression, impotence, dyspnea, pharyngitis, upper respiratory symptoms, dyspepsia, nausea, diarrhea, chest pain, arthralgia, myalgia, rash, paresthesia, etc. For the ophthalmic preparations, tearing, decreased corneal sensitivity, erythema, itching sensation, corneal punctate staining, keratitis, anisocoria, photophobia, blurred vision, decreased visual acuity, crusty lashes, etc, have been reported.

Interactions with other drugs

Catecholamine-depleting drugs like reserpine may have an additive effect when given with beta-blockers. Betaxolol is contraindicated in patients with sinus bradycardia, heart block greater than first degree cardiogenic shock, overt cardiac failure, and bronchospastic diseases.

Table 4.
Beta adrenergic blockers: Compounds have the same essential pharmacophore but different auxopharmacores and physicochemical properties

Generic name	Trade name	Structural formula	U.S. supplier (Year of introduction)	Actual (or proposed) uses	MW	log P	log P pK$_a$ (log D)	β-Blockade potency ratio propranolol = 1.0	Extent of absorption[a] (% of dose)	Protein binding,[a] (%)	Cardio-select-ivity
Acebutolol	Sectral	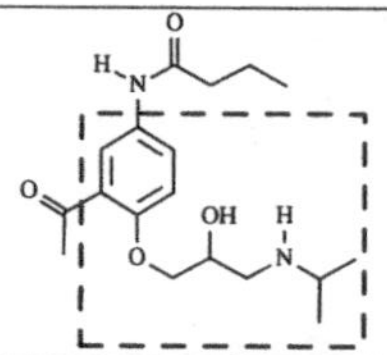	Ives (1985)	Angina, hypertension, arrhythmias	336	1.77[b]	-0.17[c] 9.20[b]	0.3	≈ 70	30-40	Yes
Atenolol	Tenormin	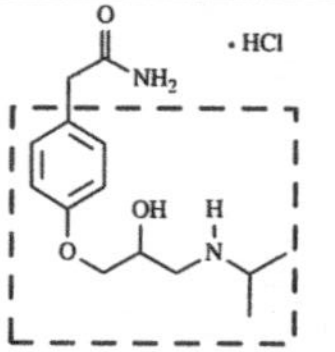	Stuart (1981)	Hypertension and (treatment after heart attack)	266 (base) 303 (salt)	0.43[e] 0.17[g]	-1.82[c] -1.62[e] -1.94[g] 9.6[g]	1.0	≈ 50	< 5	Yes
Betaxolol	Betopic / Kerlone	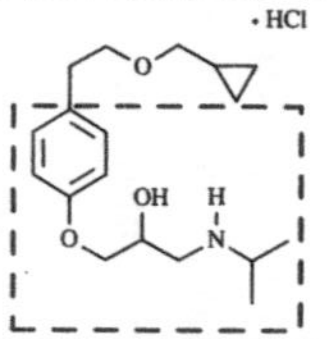	Alcon (1990) Searle (1990)	β-adrenergic blocker for glaucoma ophthalmic hypertension	307 (base) 344 (salt)	2.17[k] (calcd)	0.59[l] 9.39[n]	4.0[o]	89[l]	≈ 50[l]	Yes
Bisprodol	Zebeta	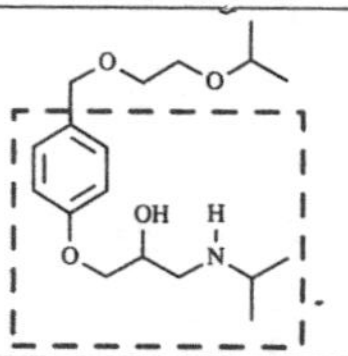	Lederle (1992)	Hypertension	325	1.69[k] (calcd)	0.04[q] (pH 7.0) 0.41[q] (pH 7.4)		< 90[q] 85[r]	30[q]	Yes

Generic name	Trade name	Structure	Company (year)	Indication	MW	logP		pKa				
Carteolol	Cartrol	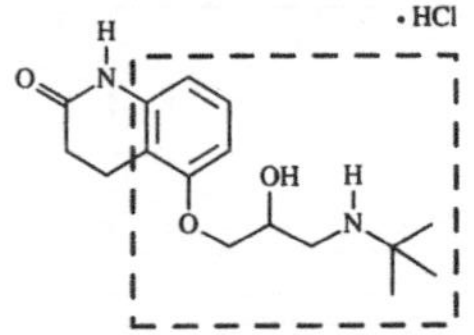 [structure] ·HCl	Abbott (Late 1988 approved)	Hypertension	292 (base) 329 (salt)	1.17[k] (calcd)	−0.46[k] (pH 7.4)			85[l]	20–30[l]	No
Esmolol	Brevibloc	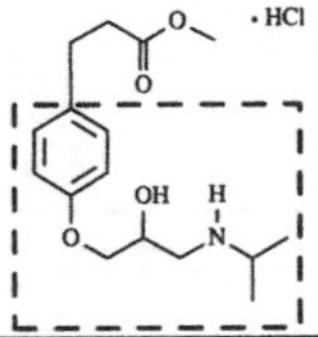 [structure] ·HCl	DuPont (1987)	Anti-arrhythmic for supra-ventricular tachycardia	295 (base) 332 (salt)	1.53[k] (calcd)					55	Yes
Labetalol	Normodyne / Trandate	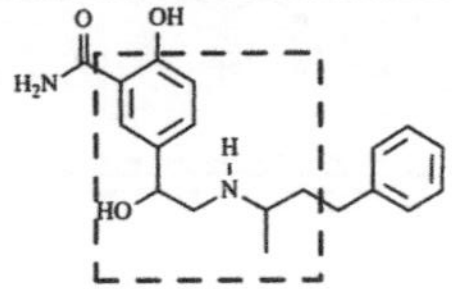 [structure]	Scherin-Plough (1984) / Allen and Hanburys (1984)	Angina Hypertension	365	3.18[e]	1.13[e] 1.06[c]	9.45[e]	0.3	> 90	≈ 50	No
Levobunolol	Betagan	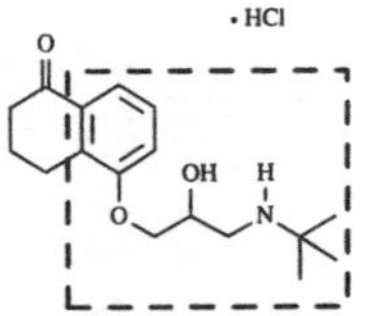 [structure] ·HCl	Allergan (1986)	Glaucoma	291 (base) 328 (salt)	2.40[k] 2.26 (calcd)		9.2[k]		≈ 75 (po)[m]		No[p]
Metipranolol	Opti-Pranolol	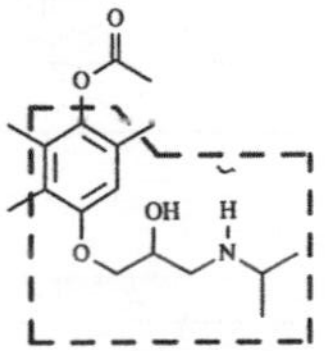 [structure]	Bausch & Lomb (Late 1989 approved)	Glaucoma	309	2.68[k] (calcd)						No[p]

64   Eric J. Lien et al.

Table 4. (continued)

Generic name	Trade name	Structural formula	U.S. supplier (Year of introduction)	Actual (or proposed) uses	MW	log P	log P (log D)	pKa	β-Blockade potency ratio[a] propranolol = 1.0	Extent of absorption[a] (% of dose)	Protein binding[a] (%)	Cardio-selectivity
Metroprolol	Lopressor	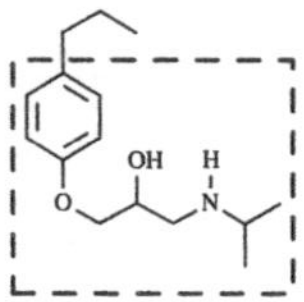	Ciba-Geigy (1978)	Hypertension and (treatment after heart attack)	267	2.04[e] 2.34[g]	-0.01[c] -0.25[e] 0.04[g]	9.60[g] 9.68[e]	1.0	> 90 50[l]	12	Yes
Nadolol	Corgard	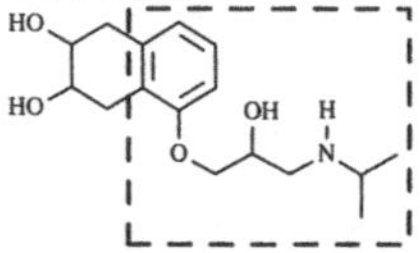	Squibb (1979)	Angina, Hypertension	309	1.09[f] 0.93[b]	-1.18[c]	9.67[h] 9.39[b]	1.0	≈ 30	≈ 30	No
Oxprenolol	Trasicor	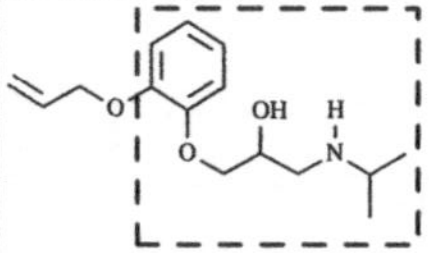	Ciba-Geigy (1983)	Angina, Hypertension	265	2.37[b]	-0.37[d] 0.36[c]	9.32[b]	0.1–1.0	≈ 90	80	No
Penbutolol	Levatol	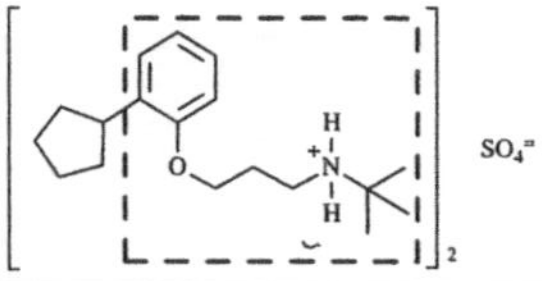	Reed & Carnirick (1988)	Hypertension	291 (base) 681 (salt)	4.15[k] 4.04[k] (calcd)			4.0	~ 100[l]	50–70[l] 80–98	No
Pindolol	Visken	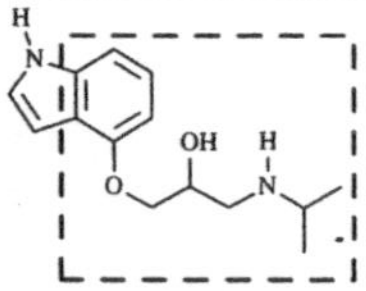	Sandoz (1982–83)	Angina, Hypertension, (treatment after heart attack)	248	1.61[f]	-0.09[c]	8.81	6.0	> 90	57	No

Propranolol	Inderal		Ayerst (1967) (1973) (1976) (1979) (1982)	Arrhythmias, Angina, Hypertension, Migraine and (treatment after heart attack) Treatment after acute MI	259	3.29[d] 3.14[g]	0.73[d] 1.30[c] 1.41[g]	9.60[g] 9.45[e,n]	1.0	>90	93	No
Sotalol	Betapace		Berlex (1992) —	(Arrhythmias, treatment after heart attack	272	0.08[f] 0.26[d]	-1.96[d] -1.40[c]	9.05[j]	0.3	≈ 70	0	No
Timolol	Timoptic Blocadren		Merck (1978) Merck (1981)	Glaucoma Treatment after heart attack, hypertension, and (angina)	316	1.91[b]	-0.06[c]	9.21[b]	6.0	>90	10	No

[a] From W. H. Frishman. In: Clinical Pharmacology of the β Adrenoreceptor Blocking of Drugs, p. 13, W. H. Frishman (ed.), Appleton-Century Crofts, 1984.
[b] From R. D. Schoenwald, H. H. Huang and J. L. Lach: J. Pharm. Sci. 72, 1273, 1983.
[c] From P. B. Woods and M. L. Robinson: J. Pharm. Sci. 33, 172, 1981. n-octanol-phosphate buffer pH 7.4, not ion-corrected.
[d] From D. Hellenbrecht, B. Lemmern, G. Wiethold and H. Grobecker: Naunyn-Schmiedebergs Arch. Pharmac. 277, 211, 1973. n-octanol-phosphate buffer pH 7.4, not ion-corrected.
[e] From P.H. Wang and E. J. Lien: J. Pharm. Sci. 69, 662, 1980. n-octanol-phosphate buffer pH 7.4, not ion-corrected.
[f] Calculated from log P = log P' − log (1−α), where α = ¹/(1 + antilog [pH − pKa]).
[g] From H. Lullmann and M. Wehling: Biochem. Pharmac. 28, 3409, 1979.
[h] From M. Windholz (ed.): The Merck Index, Merck Sharp & Dohme Resemich Laboratories, Rahway, New Jersey, 1983.
[i] From G.S. Avery (ed.): Drug Treatment, p. 890. Publishing Sciences Group, Inc., Littletown, MA, 1976.
[j] From C. Hansch and A. Leo: The Log P Database, from the Polona College Medicinal Chemistry Project. Technical Database Services, Inc., New York, 1983. n-octanol-phosphate buffer pH 7.4, not ion-corrected.
[k] From P. N. Craig: Drug Compendium. In: C. Hansch, P.G. Sammes and J.B. Taylor (edits.): Comprehensive Medicinal Chemistry, Vol. 6, Pergamon Press, New York, pp. 237–965, 1990.
[l] From AMA Division of Drugs and Toxicology, Chapter 22, Beta-adrenergic blocking drugs, AMA, Drug Evaluations Annal 1993. American Medical Association, Chicago, IL., pp. 517–528, 1993.
[m] From E. U. Kölle, H. Hengy and P. Thomann: Naunyn-Schmiedeberg's Arch. Pharmacol. 322 (suppl.), Abstract 34, 1983.
[n] From B.J. Davis and P. Turner: Brit. J. Clin. Pharmacol. 8, 405P, 1979.
[o] From J.F. Giudicelli, M. Chauvin, C. Thvillez et al.: Brit. J. Clin. Pharmacol. 10, 41, 1980.
[p] From M.A. Duffy: Physician's Desk Reference for Ophthalmology, 21 edition. Medical Economics Data, Montvale, NJ, 1993.
[q] From B.N.C. Prichard: Europ. Heart J. 8 (Suppl. M) 121–129, 1987.
[r] From G. Leopold, J. Pabst, W. Ungethüm and K.U. Bühring, Clin. Pharmacol. Ther. 31, 243, 1982.

3.2   Carteolol HCl [64–70]

Carteolol HCl, 2(1H)-quinolinone, 5-{3-[1,1-dimethylethyl)-amino]-2-hy-droxy-propoxy}-3,3-dihydro, monohydrochloride, is classified as 1-C an-tihypertensive β-adrenergic blocker.

Structure-activity relationship
It is a synthetic, nonselective β-adrenergic blocker with intrinsic agonist activity. It has the typical pharmacophore of a β-blocker, i.e. Ar-OCH2CH(OH)CH2NHC(CH3)3. The aromatic ring is a bicyclic quinolinone ring. Both the structure and pharmacological activity of carte-olol are similar to those of pindolol, having intrinsic sympathomimetic activity as well as β-blocking activity.

Biopharmaceutics and pharmacokinetics
Carteolol is well absorbed after oral administration, it reaches peak level in 1–3 hrs. The bioavailability of carteolol tablets is about 85% compared to i.v. dosing. The plasma $t_{1/2}$ of the drug is approximately 6 hrs. In patients with normal renal function, steady-state serum levels are reached within 1–2 days. The drug is 23–30% protein bound in humans. Its metabolites include 8-hydroxycarteolol and the glucuronides of both the parent drug and 8-hydroxy derivative. The 8-hydroxy derivative is active in man, with a $t_{1/2}$ of 8–12 hrs. It represents about 5% of the given dose excreted in the urine.

Pharmacology and indication(s)
Being a partial agonist, it does not reduce resting β-agonist activity as much as other β-blockers lacking the intrinsic activity. The drug competes with β-adrenergic receptor agonists for both $β_1$-receptors in cardiac muscle and $β_2$-receptors in the bronchial and vasculature, blocking the chronotropic, inotropic, and vasodilator response to β-adrenergic stimulation. The drug interferes with endogenous adrenergic bronchodilator activity and diminishes the response to exogenous bronchodilators, this may be critical in patients subject to bronchospasm (e.g. asthma patients). The drug is indicated in the management of hypertension. It may be used alone or in combination with thiazide diuretics.

Dosage form(s) and dosage
The dosage forms for this drug are 2.5 mg and 5 mg tablets. The initial dose is 2.5 mg as a single dose, either alone or with a diuretic.

Adverse reactions
The following adverse reactions have been reported: asthenia, abdominal pain, back pain, chest pain, diarrhea, nausea, abnormal laboratory test, peripheral edema, arthralgia, muscle cramps, lower extremity pain, insomnia, paresthesia, nasal congestion, pharyngitis, skin rash, etc. The drug is contraindicated in patients with bronchial asthma, severe bradycardia, greater than first degree heart block, cardiogenic shock, and congestive heart failure.

Interactions with other drugs
Catecholamine-depleting drugs like reserpine may have additive effect when given with β-blockers. β-blockers may exaggerate the hypotensive effect of general anesthetics. When the heart function is normal oral calcium antagonists may be used in combination with β-blockers, but should be avoided in patients with impaired cardiac function. Concomitant use of insulin or oral antidiabetic agents with β-blockers may be associated with hypoglycemia or possibly hyperglycemia. The dosages should be adjusted accordingly.

3.3   Esmolol HCl [71–75]

Esmolol HCl, (±)-Methyl p-[2-hydroxy-3-(isopropylamino)-propoxy]hydrocinnamate hydrochloride, is classified as 1-B antiarrhythmic β-adrenergic blocker.

Structure-activity relationship
It is a β_1 cardioselective adrenergic blocker with a very short duration of action (elimination $t_{1/2}$ about 9 min). Due to the presence of a chiral center it exists as an enantiomeric pair, the racemic mixture is used in the commercial product. The trade name of Brevibloc suggests the short duration of action. The drug possesses the general pharmacophore found in most β-blockers, namely, Ar-OCH$_2$CH(OH)CH$_2$NHR, where R being a branched alkyl group. The presence of the easily hydrolyzable ester function at the p-position of the Ar ring contributes to its very short duration of

action. The ester linkage in esmolol is rapidly hydrolyzed by red blood cell cytosol esterases.

Biopharmaceutics and pharmacokinetics
The total body clearance of this drug is about 20 l/kg/hr, higher than that of the cardiac output. The metabolism is therefore not limited by the rate of blood flow. It has a rapid distribution $t_{1/2}$ of about 2 min and an elimination $t_{1/2}$ of about 9 min. Steady-state blood levels of esmolol increase linearly over the dose range (50–300 mcg/kg/min) and elimination kinetics are dose-dependent. Steady-state levels are maintained during the i.v. infusion but decrease quickly after termination of infusion. The drug has been shown to be 55% bound to plasma protein, while the acid metabolite is bound only to the extent of 10%.

Pharmacology and indication(s)
Esmolol inhibits the β_1 receptors located mainly in cardiac muscle. At higher doses the drug also inhibits β_2 receptors in the bronchial and vascular tissues. It is indicated for the rapid control of ventricular rate in patients with atrial fibrillation or atrial flutter in preoperative, postoperative, or other emergency cases where short duration of drug action is desirable. It is also indicated in noncompensatory sinus tachycardia. The drug is not intended for use in chronic settings.

Dosage form(s) and dosage
The dosage forms are 10 mg/ml and 250 mg/ml injections. The average infusion rate is 100 mcg/kg/min, and the dosage should be individualized.

Adverse reactions
The following adverse reactions have been reported: symptomatic hypotension (diaphoresis, dizziness) (12%), asymptomatic hypotension (25%), peripheral ischemia (1%), pallor, flushing, bradycardia, chest pain, syncope, pulmonary block, serious coronary artery disease, severe bradycardia, sinus pause, asystole, somnolence (3%), confusion, headache, agitation (2%), fatigue (1%), paresthesia, asthenia, depression, abnormal thinking, anxiety, anorexia, lightheadedness, one brief grand mal seizure (30 sec.), bronchospasm, wheezing, dyspnea, nasal congestion, rhonchi, rales, nausea (7%), vomiting (1%), dyspepsia, constipation, dry mouth, abdominal discomfort, taste perversion, inflammation and induration of infusion site (8%), edema, erythema, skin discoloration, burning at infusion site, urinary

retention, speech disorder, abnormal vision, midscapular pain, rigors and fever.

Interactions with other drugs
Reserpine may have an additive effect with a β-blocker. Esmolol may increase the digoxin blood levels by 10–25% when administered concomitantly. The duration of neuromuscular blockade by succinylcholine may be prolonged from 5 min to 8 min.

3.4   Metipranolol HCl [76–84]

Metipranolol, 4-{2-Hydroxy-3-[(1-methylethyl)-amino]-propoxy}-2,3,6-trimethylphenol 1-acetate, is classified as 1-C antiglaucoma agent.

Structure-activity relationship
It is the 4th β-adrenergic blocker to be used topically in the treatment of ocular disorders like ocular hypertension and chronic open-angle glaucoma. It appears to be as effective as the other three agents, i.e. betaxolol, levobunolol and timolol. Structurally, metipranolol has the typical essential pharmacophore present in most β-adrenergic blockers, namely Ar-$OCH_2CH(OH)CH_2NHCHR$, where Ar is substituted with three CH_3 and one CH_3COO group and R is i-propyl group.

Biopharmaceutics and pharmacokinetics
The onset of action of metipranolol occurs within 30 min after administration and the maximum effect occurs in about two hrs. It should be applied in the affected eye(s) twice a day.

Pharmacology and indication(s)
Metipranolol acts primarily by reducing aqueous humor production resulting in reduced intraocular pressure. The drug is indicated for the treatment of ocular hypertension and chronic open-angle glaucoma.

Dosage form(s) and dosage
The dosage form is 0.3% ophthalmic solution. The recommended dosage is one drop of the solution in the affected eye(s) twice a day.

Adverse reactions
The following adverse reactions have been reported in some patients: local

discomfort, conjunctivitis, eyelid dermatitis, blepharitis, blurred vision, photophobia, edema, dyspnea, bronchitis, coughing, headache, dizziness, anxiety, somnolence, nervousness, nausea, arthritis, myalgia, allergic reactions, rash, hypoglycemia in diabetic patients, and masking signs of hyperthyroidism resulting in thyroid storm upon abrupt withdrawal.

Interactions with other drugs
The drug is contraindicated in patients with bronchial asthma or severe chronic obstructive pulmonary disease (COPD). The drug is also contraindicated in patients with symptomatic sinus bradycardia, greater than a first-degree atrioventricular block, cardiogenic shock, or overt cardiac failure because of the potential for cardiovascular complications. Metipranolol is a nonselective β-blocker.

3.5   Penbutolol sulfate [85–92]

Penbutolol sulfate, (S)-1-tert-butylamino-3-(o-cyclopentyl-phenoxy)-2-propanol sulfate, is an antihypertensive, nonselective β-adrenergic blocker with the common essential pharmacophore found in many β-blockers $Ar\text{-}OCH_2CH(OH)CH_2NHC(CH_3)_3$. The (S)-levorotatory isomer is the one used clinically, thus the trade name levatol. The generic name carries the ending common to most β-blockers, namely -olol, representing the 2-propranol moiety. The β-blocking potency of penbutolol is about 4 times that of propanolol.

Biopharmaceutics and pharmacokinetics
Penbutolol is rapidly and completely absorbed after oral administration. Peak plasma level are reached in 2–3 hrs, and are proportional to single and multiple doses of 10–40 mg once a day. The average plasma elimination $t_{1/2}$ is about 5 hrs. The drug is about 80–98% bound to plasma protein. It is metabolized via oxidation and conjugation in humans, the metabolites are excreted in the urine.

Pharmacology and indication(s)
Penbutolol is a β_1, β_2-nonselective adrenergic blocker, it antagonizes the heart rate effects of exercise and infused isoproterenol. It is indicated in the treatment of mild to moderate arterial hypertension, and can be used alone or in combination with thiazide diuretics.

Dosage form(s) and dosage
The dosage form is 20 mg tablet. The usual recommended dose is 20 mg once a day.

Adverse reactions
The following adverse reactions have been reported in some patients: asthenia, chest pain, pain in limbs, diarrhea, nausea, dyspepsia, dizziness, fatigue, headache, insomnia, cough, dyspnea, upper respiratory symptoms, sweating, impotence, etc.

Interactions with other drugs
Combination of penbutolol and alcohol may increase the number of errors in the eye-hand psychomotor function test. Penbutolol may increase the volume of distribution of lidocaine. Calcium antagonist may have synergistic hypotensive effects, bradycardia and arrhythmias in patients receiving β-blockers. The drug should not be used in patients receiving catecholamine-depleting drugs.

4   α-Adrenergic blockers

The older β-haloalkylamine type of irreversible α-adrenergic blockers have too many side effects, and have been replaced by milder quinazoline derivatives like doxazosin and terazosin (see Table 5).

4.1   Doxazosin mesylate [93–100]

Doxazosin mesylate, 1-(4-amino-6,7-dimethoxy-2-quinazolinyl)-4-[(2,3-dihydro-1,4-benzodioxin-2-yl)carbonyl]-piperazine monomethanesulfonate, is classified as 1-C antihypertensive agent.

Structure-activity relationship
It is a new once-daily cardioselective α_1-adrenergic blocker belonging to the quinazoline derivatives, and is, therefore, contraindicated in patients with a known hypersensitivity to quinazolines.

Biopharmaceutics and pharmacokinetics
In six healthy normotensive subjects, i.v. administration of doxazosin (12 μg/kg) resulted in a significant fall in erect blood pressure, with a corre-

Table 5.
α-Adrenergic blockers

Generic name (trade name)	Structure	Indication(s)	Year marketed
Doxazosin mesylate [Cardura (Roerig)]	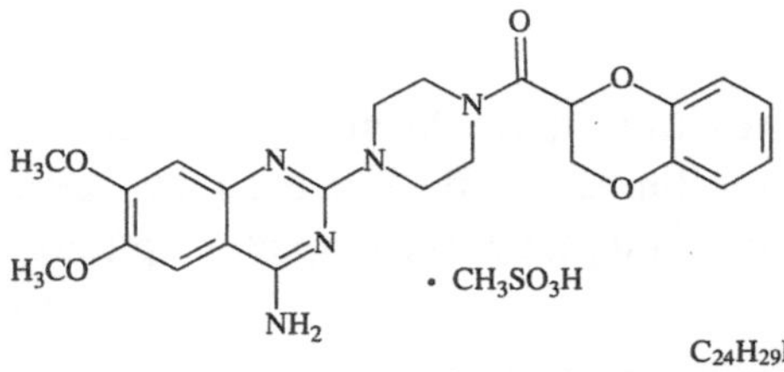 $C_{24}H_{29}N_5O_8S$; MW = 547.59	Antihypertensive	1991
Terazosin HCl [Hytrin (Abbott)]	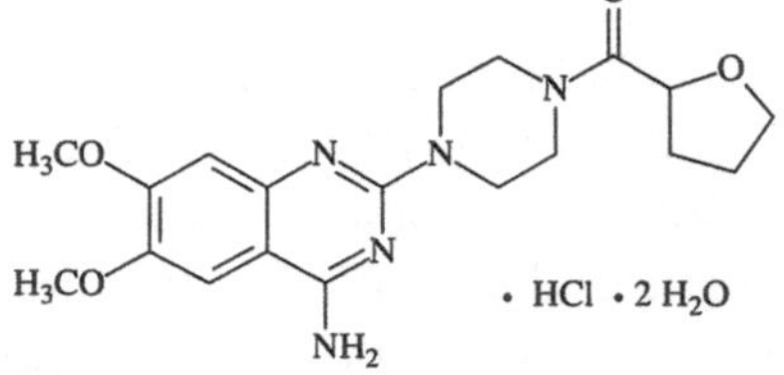 $C_{19}H_{25}N_5O_4 \cdot HCl \cdot 2H_2O$; MW = 459.93	Antihypertensive For treating symptomatic benign prostatic hyperplasia (BPH)	1987

sponding increase in heart rate, with no significant changes in supine blood pressure or heart rate. The changes in blood pressure and heart rate were maximal at 6 hrs after i.v. dosing. The mean elimination $t_{1/2}$ of doxazosin was 11 hrs as compared with a $t_{1/2}$ of 2.5 hrs for prazosin.

Pharmacology and indication(s)
This drug is a cardioselective α_1-adrenergic blocker, indicated for the treatment of hypertension. It may be used alone or in combination with diuretics or β-adrenergic blocking agents.

Dosage form(s) and dosage
The dosage forms for this drug are 1 mg, 2 mg, 4 mg, and 8 mg tablets. The initial dose is 1 mg once daily, and should be adjusted slowly, with increase in dose every two weeks if needed, up to 16 mg/day.

Adverse reactions
The most common side effects reported are dizziness, somnolence, and fatigue. Increase in dose beyond 4 mg increases the likelihood of excessive postural effects e.g. syncope, dizziness, vertigo, and hypotension.

Interactions with other drugs
Limited studies have been done with doxazosin mesylate in combination with ACE inhibitors or calcium channel blockers. The drug has been reported to reduce total serum cholesterol by 2–3% and LDL by 4% while increasing HDL to total cholesterol ratio by 4% in normal cholesterolemic patients. The clinical significance is not certain.

4.2   Terazosin [101–107]

Terazosin, piperazine, 1-(4-amino-6,7-dimethoxy-2-quinazolinyl)-4-[(tetrahydro-2-furanyl)carbonyl]-, monohydrochloride, dihydrate, is an antihypertensive α-adrenoceptor blocker.

Structure-activity relationship
It is a quinazoline derivative with an acylated piperazine attached to the 2-position. It is an α_1 selective adrenoceptor blocker. It causes blood pressure lowering by decreasing total peripheral vascular resistance, primarily due to α_1-adrenoceptor blockade. It is closely related to prazosin, the only difference being a tetrahydrofuran in place of a furan ring.

Biopharmacetics and pharmacokinetics
Terazosin tablet is essentially completely absorbed in man, with little or no effect by the presence of food. First-pass hepatic effect is minimal with nearly all of the circulating dose in the form of the parent drug. The plasma levels reach the peak in about one hour followed by an elimination $t_{1/2}$ of about 12 hrs. Protein binding in plasma is extensive. Approximately 10% of the oral dose can be found in the urine as the unchanged drug and 20% in the feces.

Pharmacology and indication(s)
Terazosin decreases blood pressure gradually within 15 min after oral dosing. The magnitude of blood pressure lowering was similar to that of prazosin and less than that of hydrochlorothiazide. The heart rate was unchanged 24 hrs after dosing of terazosin. The drug is indicated for the treatment of hypertension. It can be used alone or in combination with other antihypertensive drugs like diuretics or β-adrenergic blockers. FDA has recently approved terazosin HCl for the treatment of symptomatic benign prostatic hyperplasia (BPH).

Dosage form(s) and dosage
The dosage forms are 1 mg, 2 mg, 5 mg, and 10 mg tablets. The initial dose at bed time is 1 mg, subsequent dose range from 1 mg to 5 mg, up to 20 mg/day if needed.

Adverse reactions
The following adverse reactions have been observed in some patients: asthenia, back pain, headache, palpitation, postural hypotension, tachycardia, nausea, edema, peripheral edema, weight gain, pain in extremities, depression, dizziness, decreased libido, nervousness, paresthesia, somnolence, dyspnea, nasal congestion, sinusitis, blurred vision, and impotence.

Interactions with other drugs
When terazosin is given concomitantly with other antihypertensive drugs like calcium antagonists, caution should be observed to prevent excessive hypotension. When adding a diuretic or other antihypertensive, dosage reduction and careful titration may be necessary.

5   ACE inhibitors

ACE inhibitors have only three therapeutical applications, i.e. as antihypertensive, for the treatment of congestive heart failure and for the treatment after a heart attack (see Table 6 and the individual drugs listed). ACE is a peptidyl dipeptidase catalyzing the conversion of angiotensin I to the vasoconstrictor, angiotensin II which also stimulates aldosterone secretion by the adrenal cortex (see Fig. 2).

5.1   Benazepril HCl [108–116]

Benazepril HCl, 3-{[1-(ethoxy-carbonyl)-3-phenyl-(1S)-propyl]amino}-2,3,4,5-tetrahydro-2-oxo-1H-1-(3S)-benzazepine-1-acetic acid monohydrochloride, is classified as 1-C antihypertensive ACE inhibitor.

Structure-activity relationship
It is a prodrug of benazeprilat, and a long-acting angiotension-converting enzyme (ACE) inhibitor useful for the treatment of essential hypertension. Benazeprilat is a non-sulfhydryl ACE inhibitor.

Table 6.
ACE inhibitors

Generic name [trade name]	Structure (year introduced)	Indication(s)	Year marketed
Captopril [Capoten (Squibb)]	HS $C_9H_{15}NO_3S$; MW = 217.28 $pK_1 = 3.7$, $pK_2 = 9.8$ (1977)	1. Antihypertensive 2. Congestive heart failure 3. Treatment after a heart attack	1981 (approved in 1993)
Enalapril maleate [Vasotec (MS & D)]	$C_{20}H_{28}N_2O_5 \cdot C_4H_4O_4$; MW = 492.53 $pK_{a1} = 3.0$, $pK_{a2} = 5.4$ (1980)	1. Antihypertensive 2. Congestive heart failure	1986
Lisinopril [Prinivil (MS & D)] [Zetril (Stuart)]	$C_{21}H_{31}N_3O_5S \cdot 2H_2O$; MW = 441.52 $pK_{a1} = 2.5$, $pK_{a2} = 4.0$, $pK_{a3} = 6.7$, $pK_{a4} = 10.1$ (1980)	Antihypertensive	1988
Fosinoril sodium [Monopril (Mead Johnson)]	$C_{30}H_{45}NNaO_7P$; MW = 585.65 (1982)	Antihypertensive	1991
Ramipril [Altace (Hoechst-Roussel)]	$C_{32}H_{32}N_2O_5$; MW = 416.52 (1983)	Antihypertensive	[j] 1991
Benazepril HCl [Lotensin (Ciba)]	$C_{24}H_{28}N_2O_5 \cdot HCl$; MW = 460.96 (1990)	Antihypertensive	1991

Table 6. (continued)

Generic name [trade name]	Structure (year introduced)	Indication(s)	Year marketed
Quinapril hydrochloride [Accupril (Parke-Davis)]	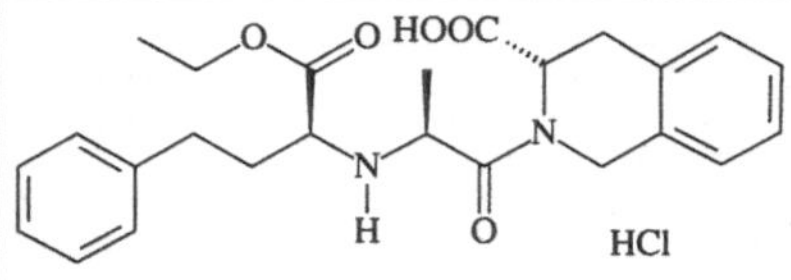 $C_{25}H_{30}N_2O_5 \cdot HCl$; MW = 474.98 (1982)	1. Antihypertensive 2. Congestive heart failure	1992 (approved in 1993)

Biopharmaceutics and pharmacokinetics

After oral administration, peak plasma levels of benazepril are reached within 0.5–1.0 hr. Approximately 37% of the dose is absorbed. It is converted to benazeprilat by hepatic cleavage of the ester group. Peak plasma levels of benazeprilat are reached 1–2 hrs after dosing in fasting subjects and 2–4 hrs in nonfasting state. The serum protein binding is about 96.3% for the active metabolite. The effective $t_{1/2}$ of accumulation of benazeprilat following multiple dosing of prodrug is 10–11 hrs, thus providing steady-state concentrations of the active metabolite after 2 or 3 doses of the prodrug given once daily.

Pharmacology and indication(s)

Inhibition of ACE by the active metabolite results in a decreased plasma angiotensin II, leading to decreased vasopressor activity and to decreased aldosterone secretion. Benazepril is indicated for the treatment of hypertension, either alone or in combination with thiazide diuretics.

Dosage form(s) and dosage

The dosage forms are 5 mg, 10 mg, 20 mg and 40 mg base' tablets. Initial dose is 10 mg once a day. The usual maintenance dosage is 20–40 mg/day as a single dose or in two equally divided doses.

Adverse reactions

The following adverse reactions have been reported: headache, dizziness, fatigue, cough, nausea, symptomatic hypotension, postural hypotension, syncope, increased serum creatinine, increased blood urea nitrogen, angioedema, constipation, gastritis, vomiting, melena, dermatitis, pruritis, rash, flushing, anxiety, decreased libido, hypertonia, insomnia, impotence, arthralgia, arthritis, asthenia, asthma, dyspnea, sweating, etc.

Interactions with other drugs
Increased serum lithium levels and symptoms of lithium toxicity have been reported in patients under ACE inhibitor treatment. Benazepril can attenuate potassium loss caused by thiazide diuretics, potassium-sparing diuretics or potassium supplement can increase the risk of hyperkalemia.

5.2   Fosinopril sodium [117–122]

Fosinopril sodium, (2α,4β)-4-cyclohexyl-1-{[[2-methyl-1-(1-oxoprop-oxy)propoxy](4-phenylbutyl)phosphinyl]acetyl}}-L-proline, is classified as 1-C antihypertensive agent.

Structure-activity relationship
It is the sodium salt of fosinopril, which is the ester prodrug of ACE inhibitor, fosinoprilat. The drug contains a phosphate group capable of specific binding to the active site of ACE.

Biopharmaceitics and pharmacokinetics
The absorption of fosinopril is 36% after oral dose. It is highly protein-bound ($\geq 95\%$), has a relatively small volume of distribution. Times to peak levels are independent of dose and are achieved in about 3 hrs. After oral administration of radiolabeled fosinopril, 75% of radioactivity in plasma was present as active fosinoprilat, 20–30% as a glucuronide conjugate of fosinoprilat, and 1–5% as a p-hydroxy metabolite of fosinoprilat. Approximately half of the absorbed dose is excreted in the urine, and the remainder in the feces. The terminal elimination $t_{1/2}$ of an i.v. dose of fosinopril is 12 hrs in healthy subjects, 11.5 hrs in hypertensive patients.

Pharmacology and indication(s)
Monopril is hydrolyzed by esterases to the pharmacologically active fosino-prilat, a specific competitive inhibitor of ACE. Inhibition of ACE results in decreased plasma angiotension II, which leads to decreased vasopressor activity and to decreased aldosterone secretion. The latter decrease may result in a small increase of serum potassium. Fosinoril sodium is indicated for the treatment of hypertension.

Dosage form(s) and dosage
The dosage forms are 10 mg and 20 mg tablets. Initial dose is 10 mg once a day and the maintenance dose is 20–40 mg/day up to 80 mg/day if needed.

Adverse reactions
The following adverse reactions have been reported: angioedema, symptomatic hypotension, hyperkalemia, neutropenia, agranulocytosis, eosinophilic pneumonitis, pancytopenia, anemia, thrombocytopenia, acute renal failure, hepatic failure, jaundice, symptomatic hyponatremia, urticaria, rash, photosensitivity, pruritis, abdominal pain, flatulence, constipation, heartburn, dry mouth, drowsiness, memory disturbance, gout, decreased libido, tinnitus, taste disturbance, eye irritation, chest pain, excessive sweating, palpitations, cerebrovascular accident, and renal insufficiency.

Interactions with other drugs
Patients on diuretics may experience an excessive reduction of blood pressure after initiation of therapy with Fosinopril. The drug can attenuate potassium loss caused by thiazide diuretics. Potassium-sparing diuretics (spironolactone, amiloride, triamterene etc.) or potassium supplements can increase the risk of hyperkalemia. Increased serum lithium levels and symptoms of lithium toxicity have been reported in patients receiving ACE inhibitors during therapy with lithium.
Coadministration of an antacid (aluminum hydroxide, magnesium hydroxide, and simethicone) with fosinopril reduced serum levels and urinary excretion of fosinopril as compared with fosinopril administrated alone suggesting that antacid may impair absorption of fosinopril.

5.3   Lisinopril [123–127]

Lisinopril, 1-[N^2-[(S)-1-carboxy-3-phenylpropyl]-L-lysyl]-L-proline dihydrate, is classified as 1-C antihypertensive agent.

Structure-activity relationship
It is the lysine analog of enalapril. It is a long-acting, non-sulfhydryl ACE inhibitor. Lisinopril does not have to be metabolically activated. Both lisinopril and enalapril lack the SH group that is present in captopril. The presence of the SH group in captopril has been thought to be associated with the rash, proteinuria and neutropenia seen with captopril administration. The antihypertensive activity of lisinopril in man is more prominent when given with thiazide diuretics. ACE inhibitors act by chelating zinc in the enzyme, thus preventing the formation of vasoconstricting angiotensin II, block the secretion of volume-expanding aldosterone, and prevent the breakdown of vasodilating bradykinin.

Biopharmaceutics and pharmacokinetics
Lisinopril shows variable absorption (6–60%) at all dosages tested (5–80 mg), absorption does not appear to be affected by food. Peak serum levels occur approximately 7 hrs after administration. The $t_{1/2}$ is about 30 hrs, with multiple dosing the effective $t_{1/2}$ of accumulation is about 12 hrs. Saturable binding is responsible for dose-independent declining serum concentrations with a prolonged terminal phase. The drug is excreted unchanged entirely in the urine. Renal impairment decreases elimination, the decrease is clinically important when the glomerular filtration rate falls below 30 ml/min.

Pharmacology and indication(s)
The ACE inhibitor acts on the renin-angiotensin-aldosterone system to reduce both systolic and diastolic blood pressure in patients with uncomplicated mild to moderate essential hypertension. Lisinopril has been shown in clinical studies to be effective as a single agent in up to 50% of patients with hypertension. Concomitant administration of a thiazide diuretic with lisinopril increases success rate up to 90%. Lisinopril is indicated for the treatment of hypertension, either alone as initial therapy or together with other antihypertensive agents. Like other ACE inhibitors, it can be used in the treatment of hypertension with concomitant conditions, e.g. diabetes mellitus, gout, asthma, heart block, peripheral vascular disease, and congestive heart failure.

Dosage form(s) and dosage
The dosage forms are 5 mg, 10 mg and 20 mg tablets. Initial dose is 10 mg once a day, and the usual dose ranges from 20 to 40 mg administered in a single daily dose.

Adverse reactions
Lisinopril has fewer adverse effects, e.g. malaise and drowsiness, than other antihypertensive agents. The following adverse reactions have also been reported: dizziness, headache, fatigue, diarrhea, upper respiratory symptoms and cough.

Interactions with other drugs
Excessive hypotension may occur in patients on diuretics after initiation of lisinopril, which may be minimized by discontinuing the diuretic or initiating therapy with 5 mg of lisinopril.

5.4   Quinapril HCl [128–133]

Quinapril HCl, [3S-[2[R*(R*)], 3R*]]-2-[2-[[1-(ethoxy-carbonyl)-3-phenylpropyl]amino]-1-oxopropyl]-1,2,3,4-tetrahydro-3-isoquinolinecarboxylic acid, monohydrochloride, is classified as 1-C antihypertensive agent.

Structure-activity relationship
Quinapril hydrochloride is the HCl salt of the ethyl ester of quinaprilat, which is a non-SH containing ACE inhibitor. It is deesterified to the active metabolite quinaprilat *in vivo*.

Biopharmaceutics and pharmacokinetics
The drug exerts antihypertensive actions even in patients with low renin hypertension; its major mechanism of action is thought to be through the renin-angiotensin-aldosterone system. Peak plasma concentrations of quinapril are obtained within one hour following oral administration. At least 60% of the administered drug is absorbed. It is deesterified to its major active metabolite, quinprilat (38% of oral dose), and to other minor inactive metabolites. The drug is mainly eliminated by renal route (96% of i.v. dose), and has an elimination $t_{1/2}$ of 2 hrs, and terminal $t_{1/2}$ of 25 hrs.

Pharmacology and indication(s)
Single doses of 20 mg of quinapril HCl provide over 80% inhibition of plasma ACE for 24 hrs. It is indicated for the treatment of hypertension, either alone or in combination with thiazide diuretics, and for treating congestive heart failure (approved by FDA in late 1993).

Dosage form(s) and dosage
The dosage forms are 5 mg, 10 mg and 40 mg tablets. The recommended initial dosage of quinapril HCl in patients not on diuretics is 10 mg once daily. Dosage should be adjusted according to the blood pressure.

Adverse reactions
The following adverse reactions have been reported: back pain, malaise, palpitation, vasodilation, tachycardia, heart failure, hyperkalemia, myocardial infarction, cerebrovascular accident, hypertensive crisis, angina pectoris, orthostatic hypotension, cardiac rhythm disturbances, dry mouth or throat, constipation, G.I. hemorrhage, pancreatitis, abnormal liver func-

tion, somnolence, vertigo, syncope, nervousness, depression, sweating, pruritus, exofoliative dermatitis, photosensitivity, acute renal failure, amblyopia, pharyngitis, sinusitis, bronchitis, agranulocytosis, thrombocytopenia, angioedema, etc.

Interactions with other drugs
Concomitant diuretic treatment should be carefully monitored to avoid excessive blood pressure reduction. Simultaneous administration of tetracycline with quinapril HCl may reduce the absorption of tetracycline by 28–37%, probably due to high magnesium content of the quinapril tablets. The drug may enhance lithium toxicity.

5.5 Ramipril [134–139]

Ramipril, [2S-[1[R*(R*)],2α,3αS,6αS]]-1-[2-[[1-(ethoxycarbonyl)-3-phenylpropyl]amino]-1-oxopropyl]octahydrocyclopenta-[b]pyrrole-2-carboxylic acid, is classified as 1-C antihypertensive agent.

Structure-activity relationship
It is a new prodrug of a non-sulfhydryl ACE inhibitor. It is hydrolyzed *in vivo* to give the active diacid metabolite ramiprilat, which has about 6 times the ACE inhibitory activity of ramipril.

Biopharmaceutics and pharmacokinetics
Peak plasma levels are reached within one hour following oral dosing of ramipril. The extent of absorption is 50–60%. The ester group is hydrolyzed primarily in the liver to its active metabolite ramiprilat, which reaches peak level in 2–4 hrs after dosing. The serum protein binding of ramipril is approximately 73% and that of ramiprilat about 65%. About 60% of the drug and its metabolites are excreted in the urine and 40% in the feces.

Pharmacology and indication(s)
Ramipril and ramiprilat inhibit ACE *in vivo*. The drug also has an effect on patients with low-renin hypertension. It is indicated for the treatment of hypertension, either alone or in combination with thiazide diuretics.

Adverse reactions
The following adverse reactions have been reported in controlled studies: headache, dizziness, asthenia (fatigue), nausea. Others include hypoten-

sion, angina pectoris, arrhythmias, chest pain, palpitation, myocardial infarction, increase in blood urea nitrogen and serum creatinine, angioneurotic edema, cough, abdominal pain, anorexia, constipation, diarrhea, dry mouth, dyspepsia, gastroenteritis, increased salivation, taste disturbance, dermatitis, pruritis/rash, anxiety, amnesia, convulsions, depression, hearing loss, insomnia, nervousness, neuralgia, etc.

Interactions with other drugs

Changes in renal function may be anticipated in susceptible individuals. In patients with renal impairment or collagen-vascular disease, a drug such as captopril (ACE inhibitor) may cause agranulocytosis.

References

1   F. Gross: Am. J. Cardiol., *34*, 471–475 (1974).
2   G. Gross. In: Handbuch der experimentellen Pharmakologie XXXIX, Chapter I. Antihypertensive Drugs. F. Gross (ed.). Springer Verlag, Berlin, pp. 1–11 (1977).
3   W.J. Greenlee and P.K.S. Siegl. In: Annual Reports in Medicinal Chemistry, Chapter 7, J.A. Bristol (ed.): Angiotensin/renin modulators. Academic Press, Inc. New York *26*, 63–72 (1991).
4   W.J. Greenlee and P.K.S. Siegl. In: Annual Reports in Medicinal Chemistry, Chapter 7, J.A. Bristol (ed.): Angiotensin/renin modulators. Academic Press, Inc. New York *27*, 59–68 (1992).
5   W.J. Greenlee: Med. Res. Rev. *10,* 173–236 (1990).
6   H.D. Kleinert, W.R. Baker and H.H. Stein: Adv. Pharmacol. *22*, 207–250 (1991).
7   R.A. Buchholz, B.A. Lefker and M.A. Ravi Kiron. In: Annual Reports in Medicinal Chemistry. Chapter 8. Hypertension Therapy, what next? J.A. Bristol (ed.). Academic Press, Inc., New York *28*, 69–78 (1993).
8   D.J. Triggle. In: Calcium in Drug Action. Chapter 6. The chemistry of calcium channel agonists and antagonists. P.F. Baker (ed.). Springer Verlag, Berlin, pp. 115–199 (1988).
9   L.H. Opie. In: International Encyclopedia of Pharmacology and Therapeutics. Chapter 5. Calcium ions drug action and the heart – with special reference to calcium channel blockers (calcium antagonist dugs). M.A. Denborough (ed.). Pergamon Press, New York, pp. 103–125 (1987).
10   E.J. Lien, H. Gao, and F. Wang: Med. Chem. Res. *1*, 173–184 (1991).
11   E.J. Lien: Prog. Drug Res. *40*, 163–189 (1993).
12   J.E. Arrowsmith, S.F. Campbell, P.E. Cross et al.: J. Med. Chem. *29*, 1696–1702 (1986).
13   R.A. Burges, D.G. Gardiner, M. Gwilt, et al.: J. Cardiovascul. Pharmacol. *9*, 110–119 (1988).
14   A.P. Beresford, D. McGibney, M.J. Humphrey, et al.: Xenobiotica *18*, 245–254 (1988).
15   G.P. Reams, A. Lau, A. Hamory and J.H. Bauer: Am. J. Kidney Dis. *10*, 446–451 (1987).
16   J. Webster, O.J. Robb, T.A. Jeffers et al.: Br. J. Clin. Pharmacol. *24*, 713–719 (1987).

17   J.K. Faulkner, D. McGibney, L.F. Chasseaud et al.: Br. J. Clin. Pharmacol. 22, 21–25 (1986).
18   D.B. Zurich, Physician's Desk Reference, 47 ed Medical Economics Co. Inc., Montvale, N.J., pp.1836–1838 (1993).
19   S. Vogel, R. Crampton and N. Sperelakis: J. Pharmacol. Exp. Ther. 210, 378–385 (1979).
20   C. Labrid, A. Grosset, G. Dureng et al.: J. Pharmacol. Exp. Ther. 211, 546–554 (1979).
21   G.R. Hasegewa: Clin. Pham. 7, 97–108 (1988).
22   F.P. Zeller and S.A. Spinler: Drug Intell. Clinic. Pharm. 21, 487–492 (1987).
23   P.W. Pflugfelder, D.P. Humen, P.A. O'Brien et al.: Am. J. Cardiol. 59, 1283–1288 (1987).
24   J.O. Parker and B. Farrell: Am. J. Cardiol. 58, 449–452 (1986).
25   R. DiBianco, J. Alpert, R.J. Katz et al.: Am. J. Cardiol. 53, 35–41 (1984).
26   G. Forche, H. Kopera and H.J. Marsoner: Int. J. Clin. Pharmacol. Ther. Toxicol. 21, 234–240 (1983).
27   M.A. Duffy, Physicians' Desk Reference, 46 ed. Medical Economics Data, Montvale, pp.1383–1385 (1992).
28   B. Edgar, K.J. Hoffman, P. Lundborg et al.: Drugs 29 (suppl. 2), 9–15 (1985).
29   O. Ronn, B. Bengtsson, B. Edgar and S. Raner: Drugs 29 (suppl. 2), 16–25 (1985).
30   B. Ljung: Drugs 29 (suppl. 2), 46–58 (1985).
31   B. Edgar, C.G. Regardh, P. Lundborg et al.: Biopharm. Drug Dispos. 8. 235–248 (1987).
32   H.E. Sluiter (on behalf of the Dutch Multicentre Study Group): Drugs 34 (suppl. 3), 97–106 (1987).
33   M.A. Duffy, Physicians' Desk Reference. 46 ed. Medical Economics Inc. Montvale, pp.1526–1528 (1992).
34   F.L. Tse and J.M. Jaffe: Eur. J. Clin. Pharmacol. 32, 361–365 (1987).
35   K. Simonsen and C.D. Sundstedt: Am. J. Med. 86, 91–93 (1989).
36   C.D. Sundstedt, P.C. Rueegg, A. Keller and R. Waite: Am. J. Med. 86, 98–102 (1988).
37   H.F. Schran, J.M. Jaffe and L.M. Gonasun: Am. J. Med. 84 (suppl 3B), 80–89 (1988).
38   L.R. Krusell, L.T. Jespersen, A. Schmit et al.: Hypertension 10, 577–581 (1987).
39   Anony: New DynaCirc® (isradipine), Pharmacy Fact Sheet, Sandoz Pharm. Co. East Hanover, NJ (1991).
40   T. Takenaka and J. Handa: Int. J. Clin. Pharmacol. Biopharm. 17, 1–11 (1979).
41   T. Seki and T. Takenaka: Int. J. Pharmacol. 15, 267–274 (1977).
42   T. Takenaka, S. Usuda, T. Nomura, H. Maeno and T. Sado: Arzneim.-forsch. 26, 2172–2178 (1976).
43   S. Higuchi and Y. Chiobara: Xenobiotica 10, 447–454 (1980).
44   S. Higuchi, H. Sasaki and T. Seki: Xenobiotica 10, 897–903 (1980).
45   Anonymous: Cardene® (nicardipine hydrochloride) capsules, Package insert, Syntex Lab., Inc. Palo Alto (1988).
46   K. Satoh, T. Yanagisawa and N. Taira: Clin. Exp. Pharmacol. 7, 249–262 (1980).
47   K.A. Conrad, T.C. Fagan, P. Mayshar, T.P. Davis and D.G. Johnson: Clin. Pharmacol. Ther. 42, 113–118 (1987).
48   E.M. Sorkin and S.P. Clissold: Drugs 33, 296–345 (1987).
49   S. Kazda, B. Garthoff, H.P. Krause and K. Schlossmann: Arzneim.-Forsch. 32, 331–338 (1982).

50   R. Towart, E. Wehinger, H. Meyer and S. Kazda: Arzneim.-Forsch. *32*, 338–346 (1982).
51   S. Kazda: Neurochirug. *28* (suppl. 1), 70–73 (1985).
52   K.-D. Rämsch, G. Ahr, D. Tettenborn and L.M. Auer: Neurochirug. *28* (suppl. 1), 74–83 (1985).
53   G.S. Allen, H.S. Ahn, T.J. Preziosi et al.: N. Engl. J. Med. *308*, 619–624 (1983).
54   Anonymous: Nimotop® (nimodipine/Miles) capsules, Package insert, Miles Inc., West Haven (1989).
55   Anonymous: Am. Pharm. NS *29*, 58 (1989).
56   E.J. Lien: US New Drug Digest 1980–1986, Aurora Publishers, Inc., Nashville (1987).
57   R. Barnhart: Physicians' Desk Reference, 45 ed. Medical Economics Co. Inc., Oradell, N.J., pp.2074–2076; 572–574 (1991).
58   H. Bourgeois: Ophtalmologie *4*, 323–325 (1990).
59   M.T. Dorigo, O. Cerin, G. Fracasso and R. Altafini: Int. J. Clin. Pharmacol. Res. *10*, 163–166 (1990).
60   R.N. Winreb, D.R. Caldwell, S.M. Goode et al.: Am. J. Ophthalmol. *110*, 189–192 (1990).
61   S.G. Chrysant, C. Chrysant, I.S. Bal et al.: Hemodynamic Aspects Chest *96*, 499–504 (1989).
62   M.E. Davidov, N. Glazer, G. Wollam et al.: Am. J. Hypertens. *1*, 206S–210S (1988).
63   W.J. Mroczek, J.F. Burris, L.B. Hogan et al.: Am. J. Cardiol. *61*, 807–811 (1988).
64   S. Morita, Y. Irie, S. Sakuragi, H. Kohri and H. Nishino: Folia Pharmacol. Japan *73*, 229–237 (1977).
65   S. Morita, M. Iinuma, M. Kido, s. Sakuragi, H. Kohri and N. Nishino: Arzneim.-Forsch. *27*, 2380–2383 (1977).
66   W.H. Fennell, J.A. Farmer, J.B. Young et al.: Clin. Res. *28* (5), 817 (1981).
67   P.J. Schmitz, G.A. Walker, W.M. Barker and R.W. Stoll: Clin. Res. *29* (2), 23A (1981).
68   A. Tarkiainen, K. Saraste, T. Seppala: Eur. J. Clin. Pharmacol. *19*, 239–244 (1981).
69   L. Alcocer, J. Aspe, E. Arce and J. Vieyra: Curr. Ther. Res. *31*, 67–73 (1982).
70   E.R. Barnhart, Physicians' Desk Reference 44 ed. Medical Economics, Co. Inc., Oradell, N.J., pp.510–512 (1990).
71   R. J. Gorczynski, J.E. Shaffer and R.J. Lee: J. Cardiovasc. Pharmacol. *5*, 668–677 (1983).
72   A. Yacobi, R. Kartzinee, C.M. Lai and C.Y. Sum: J. Pharm. Sci. *72*, 710–711 (1983).
73   R.C. Byrd, R.J. Sung, J. Mark et al.: Clin. Res. *31*, 172A (1983).
74   D. Dickerson, M. Paulos, J. Klein and A. Yacobi: Clin. Res. *31*, 179A (1983).
75   E.R. Barnhart, Physicians's Desk Reference, 42 ed., Medical Economics Co. Inc., Oradell, N.J., pp.914–916 (1988).
76   O. Mayer, V. Čepelák, J. Vitouš and J. Potmešíl: Int. J. Clin. Pharmacol. Ther. Toxic. *18*, 113–120 (1980).
77   B. de Galleani: Ophthalmologie *3*, 220–222 (1989).
78   C.L. Le Jeunne, F.C. Hugues and J.L. Dufier: J. Clin. Pharmacol. *29*, 97–101 (1989).
79   P.E. Battershill and E.M. Sorkin: Drugs *36*, 601–615 (1988).
80   G.K. Krieglstein, G.D. Novak, E. Voepel et al.: Br. J. Ophthalmol. *71*, 250–253 (1987).
81   O. Mueller and H.R. Knobel: Klin. Monatsbl. Augenheilkd. *188*, 62–63 (1986).
82   K.B. Mills and G. Wright: Br. J. Ophthalmol. *70*, 39–42 (1986).
83   D.A. Hussar: Am. Pharm. NS *31*, 54–84 (1991).

84   E.R. Barnhart: Physicians's Desk Reference for Ophthalmology, 19 ed., Medical Economics Co. Inc., Oradell, N.J., pp.258–260 (1991).
85   V.G. Härtfelder, H. Lessenich and K. Schmitt: Arzneim.-Forsch. 22, 930–932 (1972).
86   V.J. Kaiser, G. Härtfelder, E. Lindner and B. Schölkens: Arzneim.-Forsch. 30, 420–427 (1980).
87   H.W. Jun, S.L. Hayes, J.J. Vallner, I.L. Honigberg, A.E. Rojos and J.T. Stewart: J. Clin. Pharmacol. 19, 415–423 (1979).
88   S.D. Sharma, A.D. Mehra and B.J. Vakil: Curr. Ther. Res. 27, 576–583 (1980).
89   P.L. Sharma and R.P. Sapru: Int. J. Clin. Pharmacol. 16, 83–85 (1978).
90   E.R. Von Leitner and G. Biamino: Eur. J. Cardiol. 12, 121–128 (1980).
91   W.S. Hillis, A.C. Tweddel, R.G. Murray and T.D.V. Lawrie: Arzneim.-Forsch. 30, 1595–1599 (1980).
92   Anonymous: Tablets Levatol, penbutolol sulfate, Package insert, Reed & Carnrick, Piscataway, N.J. (1988).
93   H.L. Elliott, P.A. Meredith, D.J. Sumner et al.: Br. J. Clin. Pharmacol. 13, 699–703 (1982).
94   H. Shionoiri, G. Yasuda, H. Yoshimura et al.: J. Cardiovasc. Pharmacol. 10, 90–95 (1987).
95   P. Hjortdahl, H. von Krogh, L. Daae et al.: Acta. Med. Scand. 221, 427–434 (1987).
96   P.W. de Leeuw, P.N. van Es, R. de Bos et al.: Hypertension 9 (III), 210–212 (1987).
97   K. Hayduk and H.T. Schneider: Am. J. Cardiol. 59, 95G–98G (1987).
98   D.T. Nash, G. Schonfeld, R.L. Reeves et al.: Am. J. Cardiol. 59, 87G–90G (1987).
99   H.L. Elliott, P.A. Meredith and J.L. Reid: Am. J. Cardiol. 59, 78G–81G (1987).
100   Anonymous: Am. Pharm. NS 31, 12 (1991).
101   J.J. Kyncl, R.E. Hollinger, K.O. Oheim and M. Winn: Pharmacologist 22, 272 (1980).
102   H.F. Oates: N. Zeal. Med. J. 94, 67 (1981).
103   S. Mizogami and M. Hanazuka: Jap. J. Pharmacol. (suppl.), 174P (1982).
104   F.L. Fort, S. Tekeli, K. Majors et al.: Drug Chem. Toxicol. 7, 435–449 (1984).
105   J.H. Mersey and U. Elkayam: Clin. Res. 32, 688A (1984).
106   A.J. Dietz, Jr., E. Magarian, D. Freeman and J. Carlson: J. Clin. Pharmacol. 24, 416 (1984).
107   Anonymous: Hytrin® (terazosin hydrochloride tablets) package insert, Abbott Health Care Products, Inc., North Chicago, Ill. (1987).
108   A. Salvetti: Drugs 6, 800–828 (1990).
109   J. G. Kelly and K. O'Malley: Clin. Pharmacokinetics 19, 177–196 (1990).
110   M.H. Winberger, H.R. Black, K.C. Lasseter, et al.: Clin. Pharmacol. Ther. 47, 608–617 (1990).
111   G. Kaiser, R. Ackermann, S. Brechbuehler and W. Dieterle: Biopharm. Drug Dispos. 10, 365–367 (1989).
112   J. Insel, S.M. Mirvis, M.J. Boland et al.: Clin. Pharmacol. Ther. 45, 312–320 (1989).
113   E. Valvo, P. Casagrande, V. Bedona et al.: J. Hypertens. 8, 991–995 (1990).
114   M. Bellet, J.J. Whalen, F. Bodin et al.: J. Hypertens. 4 (suppl. 8), S43–48 (1990).
115   M.H. Winberger, H.R. Black, K.C. Lasseter et al.: Clin. Pharmacol. Ther. 47, 608–617 (1990).
116   D.B. Eurich: Physicians' Desk Reference, 47 ed., Medical Economics Co. Inc., Montvale, pp. 902–904 (1993).
117   G. Waldemar, H. Ibsen, S. Strandaard et al.: Am. J. Hypertens. 3, 464–470 (1990).

118 S.M. Singhvi, K.L. Duchin, R.A. Morrison et al.: Br. J. Clin. Pharmacol. *25*, 9–15 (1988).

119 K.L. Duchin, A.P. Waclawski, J.I. Tu et al.: J. Clin. Pharmacol. *31*, 58–64 (1991).

120 R.J. Anderson, T.M. Nolen, P. Wolfson et al.: Hypertens. *17*, 636–642 (1991).

121 P.A. Sullivan, M. Dineen, J. Cervenka and D.T. O'Connor: Am. J. Hypertens. *1*, 280S–283S (1988).

122 M.A. Duffy, Physicians' Desk Reference, 46 ed., Medical Economics data, Montvale, pp.1406–1409 (1992).

123 D.B. Brunner, G. Desponds, J. Biollaz et al.: Br. J. Clin. Pharmacol. *11*, 461–467 (1981).

124 E.H. Ulm, M. Hichens and H.J. Gomez: Br. J. Clin. Pharmacol. *14*, 357–362 (1982).

125 M.S. Kochar, G. Bolek, J.H. Kalbfleisch and P. Olzinski: J. Clin. Pharmacol. *27*, 373–377 (1987).

126 K. Bolzano, J. Arriaga, R. Bernal et al.: J. Cardiovas. Pharmacol. *9* (suppl. 3), S43–47 (1987).

127 C. Mörlin, H. Baglivo, J.K. Boeijinga et al.: J. Cardiovas. Pharmacol. *9* (suppl. 3), S48–52 (1987).

128 G.J. Frank, K.E. Knapp and R.W. McLain: Angiology *40*, 405–415 (1989).

129 D. Maclean: Angiology *40*, 370–381 (1989).

130 A.J. Sedman and E. Posvar: Angiology *40*, 360–369 (1986).

131 S.C. Olson, A.M. Horvath, B.M. Micaniewicz et al.: Angiology *40*, 351–359 (1989).

132 J.J. Ferry, A.M. Horvath, M. Easton-Talyor et al.: J. Chromatog. *421*, 187–191 (1987).

133 P. Holt, J. Najm and E. Sowton: Eur. J. Clin. Pharmacol. *31*, 9–14 (1986).

134 R.A. Becker and B. Schoelkens: Am. J. Cardiol. *59*, 3D–11D (1987).

135 K. Felder and P.U. Witte: Arzneim.-Forsch. *34*, 1452–1454 (1984).

136 H.G. Eckert, M.J. Badian and D. Gantz: Arzneim.-Forsch. *34*, 1435–1447 (1984).

137 P.W. de Leeuw and W.H. Birkenhaeger: Am. J. Cardiol. *59*, 79D–82D (1987).

138 M.A. Duff, Physicians' Desk Reference, 46 ed., Medical Economics Data, Montvale, pp.1086–1089 (1992).

139 M. Aurell, K. Delin, H. Herlitz et al.: An. J. Cardiol. *59*, 65D–69D (1987).

Progress in Drug Research, Vol. 43 (E. Jucker, Ed.)
© 1994 Birkhäuser Verlag, Basel (Switzerland)

The natural polyamines and the immune system

by N. Seiler[1] and C. L. Atanassov[2]

[1]Groupe de Recherche en Thérapeutique Anticancéreuse URA CNRS 1529 DRED1266, Faculté de Médecine, Université de Rennes, 2, Avenue du Professeur Léon Bernard, F-35043 Rennes Cédex (France); and
[2]Laboratory of Immunochemistry, I.B.M.C. of the C.N.R.S., 15 rue René Descartes, 67084 Strasbourg Cédex (France)

[1]I dedicate this work to Abel Lajtha, Center of Neurochemistry, Division of the Nathan S. Kline Institute for Psychiatric Research, Orangeburg, N.Y. in remembrance of our 25-year-long friendship and in appreciation of his incessant support.

1   Introduction

The natural polyamines putrescine, spermidine and spermine (Fig. 1) are constituents of all eukaryotic cells. Their biochemistry [1–7] and different aspects of their functional roles [8–16] have been reviewed in recent years. However, in spite of a considerable number of pertinent publications, immunological aspects of the polyamines seem not to have been reviewed, with the exception of a short essay on the potential modulatory functions of the polyamines on Ca^{2+}-dependent immune processes [17]. It is hoped that a critical synopsis of the published observations will contribute to the clarification of an important but somewhat controversial area of research. Since the ultimate target is the development of drugs directed against human immune-related diseases, we confine our considerations to experiments with mammals.

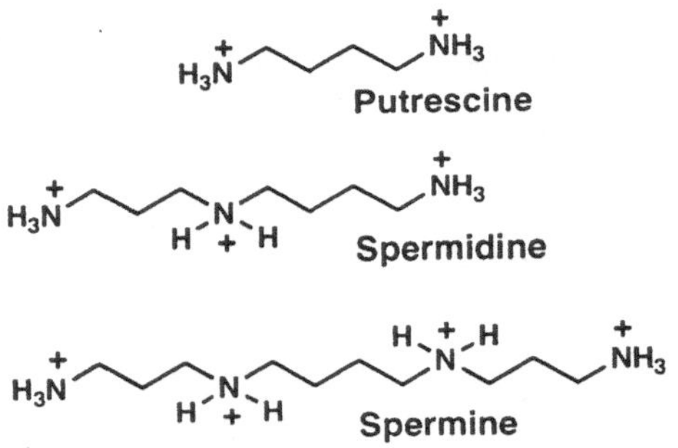

Fig. 1
Structural formulae of the natural polyamines

It is beyond the scope of the present review to give accounts on basic aspects of the immune system, or on polyamine metabolism. The reader is referred to the above-mentioned reviews and the following texts, respectively: Alberts et al. [18], Roitt et al. [19], Paul [20], Klein [21]. However, in order to illustrate at least the most important metabolic reactions of the poly-

> Fig. 2
Reactions involved in intracellular polyamine metabolism and polyamine exchange between intra- and extracellular compartments.
Enzymes: (1) Ornithine decarboxylase (ODC); (2) S-adenosylmethionine decarboxylase (AdoMet DC); (3) Spermidine synthase; (4) Spermine synthase; (5) AcetylCoA: polyamine N^1-acetyltransferase (cytosolic); (6) AcetylCoA: spermidine N^8-acetyltransferase (nuclear); (7) N^8-acetylspermidine deacetylase; (8) Polyamine oxidase (PAO); (9) Arginase; (10) Ornithine aminotransferase; (11) 5'Methylthioadenosine phosphorylase. Reproduced from Seiler [12].

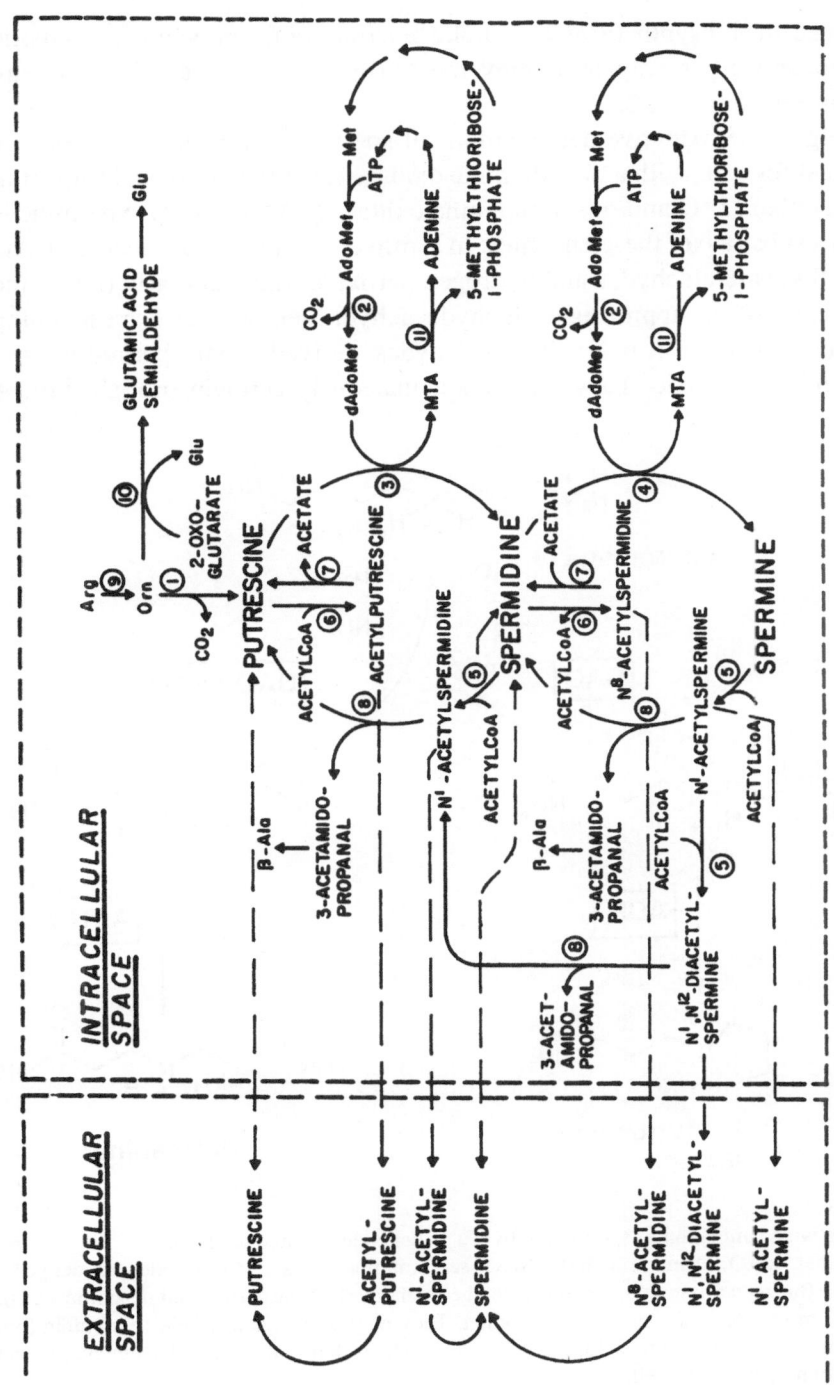

amines, the biosynthetic and catabolic reactions of the polyamine metabolic cycle, as well as polyamine movements (release and uptake by cells) are summarized in Fig. 2.

In Fig. 3 the oxidative deaminations of spermidine are shown. These are typical for cells with a high diamine oxidase (DAO) activity and for serum with either DAO and/or serum amine oxidase (SAO) activity. Spermine is also a substrate of these enzymes. In serum or plasma the products of DAO and SAO are aldehydes and hydrogen peroxide. Intracellularly (i.e. in the presence of an appropriate aldehyde dehydrogenase) the corresponding amino acids are formed. The aldehydes derived from spermidine and spermine are toxic. They release spontaneously acrolein (not shown). A

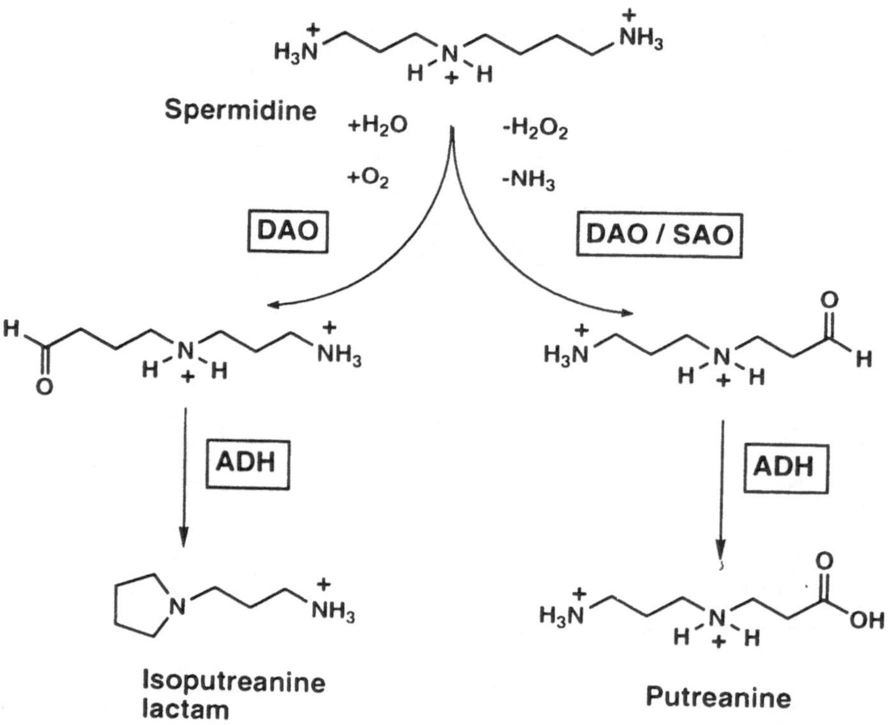

Fig. 3
Oxidative deamination of spermidine by Cu^{2+}- dependent amine oxidases.
Enzymes: DAO: Diamine oxidase; SAO: serum amine oxidase; ADH: aldehyde dehydrogenase (or and oxidase suited to transform the aldehydes into the corresponding amino acids). In serum the aldehydes are an end-product. They may spontaneously release acrolein (not shown). In cells the amino acids are the major products, but reduction of the aldehydes to an alcohol may occur as well.

frequent misunderstanding is based on the belief that SAO and polyamine oxidase (PAO) are not different enzymes. The latter, a flavin enzyme, is responsible for the oxidative splitting of the acetylderivatives of spermidine and spermine in tissues (Fig. 2). A detailed account on the enzymes and reactions involved in polyamine catabolism was published by Seiler [22].

Depletion of putrescine and spermidine prevents eukaryotic cells from dividing. Selective inactivators of enzymes involved in the biosynthesis of the polyamines were, therefore, expected to be useful in the therapy of diseases characterized by pathologic cell division [8, 10, 23, 24]. The clinical results did not fulfil all expectations [12, 25]. However, several inactivators of polyamine metabolic enzymes, which were developed in the course of the years as potential drugs, turned out to be excellent tools. Among these α-difluoromethylornithine (DFMO) [26] (Fig. 4) had by far the greatest importance. DFMO reacts with ornithine decarboxylase (ODC) as a pseudosubstrate, i.e. it forms a Schiff-base with pyridoxalphosphate within the active site of the enzyme, and is decarboxylated. By elimination of F$^-$ a chemically reactive species is formed from the decarboxylated DFMO which reacts with a (nucleophilic) cysteine residue of the enzyme and irreversibly inactivates it (Fig. 5) [27]. Inactivation of ODC by DFMO is a time-dependent process ($\tau_{1/2} = 3$ min).

One should bear in mind that the decrease of intracellular polyamine stores after inactivation of ODC occurs due to cell division, release, and catabolism, and takes several hours. Putrescine is depleted first, followed by spermidine. Spermine concentrations are usually not diminished. (For the time-relationship of polyamine depletion in a proliferating cell line, see e.g. [28]).

Among the pharmacological properties of the polyamines [12], antihistamine effects were observed early on [29–31], although they were also found to be histamine releasers [32]. In view of the importance of cell proliferation in cell-mediated immune response, and the established role of the polyamines in growth processes, the main emphasis of research during the last fifteen years was on lymphocyte proliferation, especially since DFMO became available as a tool suitable to selectively deplete putrescine and spermidine in cultured cells [33] and tissues *in vivo* [34].

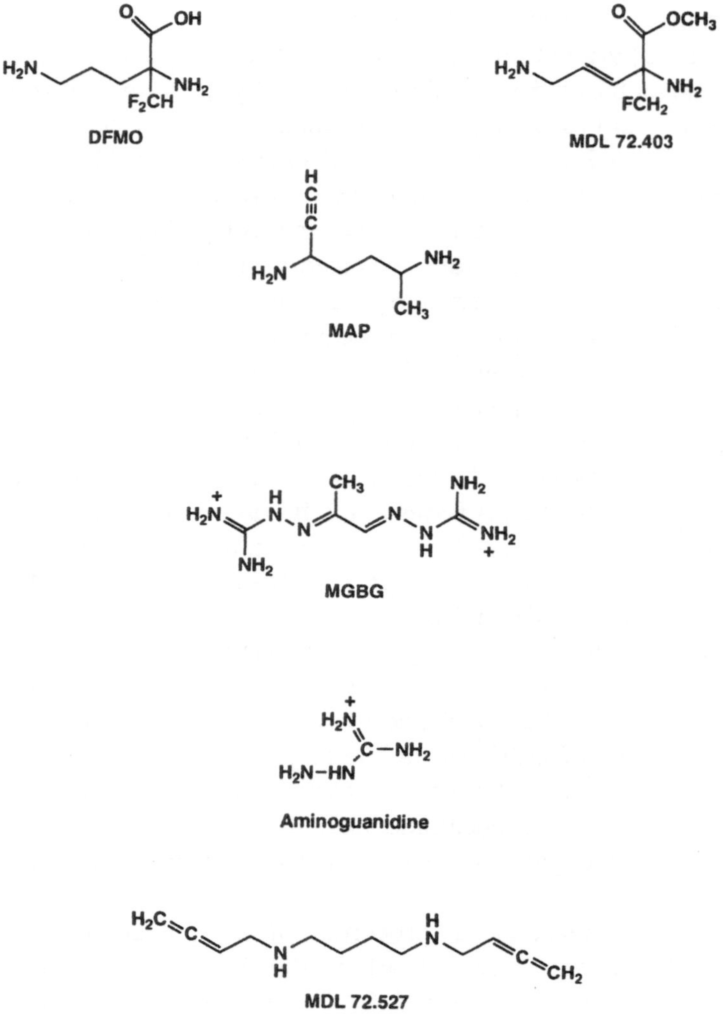

DFMO

MDL 72.403

MAP

MGBG

Aminoguanidine

MDL 72.527

Fig. 4

Inhibitors of polyamine metabolism.

DFMO (α-(difluoromethyl)ornithine) and MAP (6-heptyne-2,5-diamine) are inactivators of ornithine decarboxylase (ODC).

MDL 72,403 is a prodrug (methyl ester) of the ornithine decarboxylase inactivator α-(fluoromethyl)dehydro-ornithine [26].

MGBG (methylglyoxal-bis(guanylhydrazone)) is a competitive inhibitor of S-adenosylmethionine decarboxylase (AdoMet DC) [252]. Aminoguanidine is an inhibitor of Cu^{2+}-dependent amine oxidases, with selectivity for diamine oxidase (DAO) [142], but it is also an inhibitor of serum amine oxidase (SAO) [22, 253].

MDL 72,527 (N^1, N^4-Bis(2,3-butadienyl)1,4-butanediamine) is a selective inhibitor of polyamine oxidase (PAO) [253, 254].

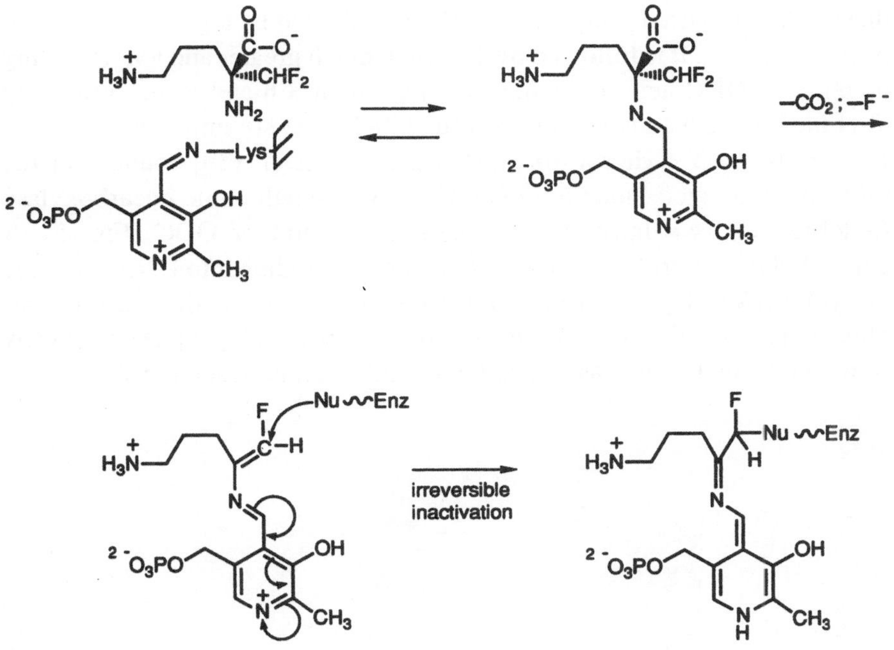

Fig. 5
Reactions involved in the inactivation of ornithine decarboxylase (ODC) by α-difluoro-methylornithine.
Mechanism proposed by Poulin et al. [27]. Reproduced from Seiler [12].

2 Proliferation and maturation of immunocompetent cells

2.1 Polyamines and lymphocyte proliferation

Upon stimulation with mitogenic ligands, unfractionated lymphocytes (both B and T cells) resume DNA synthesis and proliferate. Concomitantly polyamine metabolism changes dramatically, and many enzymes and their corresponding mRNAs (e.g. thymidine kinase [35], pyruvate kinase isozymes [36], casein kinase II [37]) and enzymes of carbohydrate metabolism [38] are enhanced, indicating functional maturation.

Resting lymphocytes have a very low ODC activity [39, 40]. Stimulation, for instance with the T-cell mitogenic lectin concanavalin A, causes an activation of ODC within minutes. This first burst of ODC, with a maximum around 20 min is insensitive to cycloheximide, showing that protein synthesis is not required. In this case ODC is activated by a post-translational process [40, 42]. It is followed by a second, much greater and longer lasting increase of ODC activity, which starts at about 3 h and wanes gradually after having reached a maximum around 48 h after stimulus (Fig. 6).

In contrast with earlier work [43], Bachrach et al. [39] found that the mitogen-stimulated induction of S-adenosyl-L-methionine decarboxylase (AdoMetDC) is a later event than the induction of ODC (Fig. 5). It paralleled the incorporation of radiolabelled thymidine into DNA. The role of cyclic AMP-dependent protein kinase for ODC induction during lymphocyte proliferation was pointed out by Klimpel et al. [44]. (For a review of the molecular events associated with cell activation, see [45].)

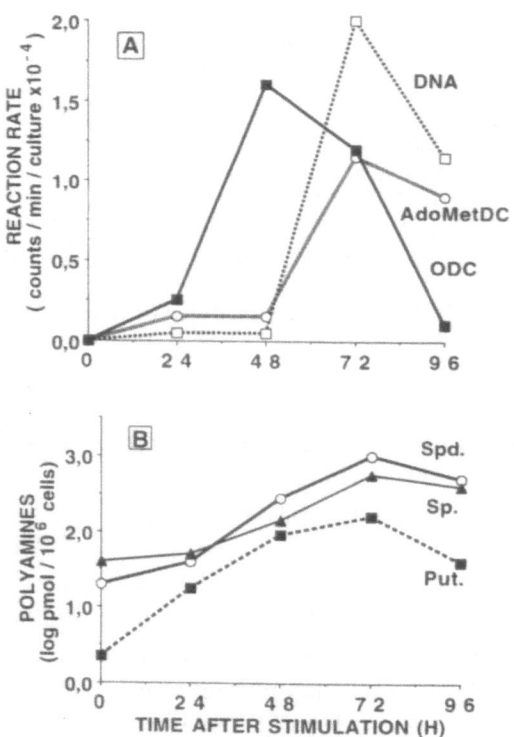

Fig. 6
Ornithine decarboxylase (ODC) and S-adenosylmethionine decarboxylase (AdoMetDC) activities, DNA synthesis rate (A), and polyamine concentrations (B) in peripheral blood lymphocytes, after stimulation with 1 μg/ml phytohemagglutinin.
Data from Bachrach et al. [39].

While polyamine concentrations are not changed significantly during the early ODC, activation [40], putrescine, spermidine and spermine concentrations increase with the second increase of ODC, and remain high even at times when ODC activity has returned near to basal levels. At this time (96 h after stimulation), AdoMetDC activity and DNA synthesis rate are also still high (Fig. 5). It was, therefore, suggested that elevated concentrations of spermidine or spermine are required for optimal DNA synthesis in lymphocytes after activation by concanavalin A [46]. Other characteristics of polyamine metabolism in mitogenic lymphocytes (in comparison with resting cells) are the excessive release of N^1-acetylspermidine, and the enhanced oxidative splitting of N^1-acetylspermidine by PAO to putrescine [39]. The enhancement of N^1-acetylation is indicative for a participation of the interconversion pathway in the regulation of intracellular polyamine concentrations [2].

As most other cells, lymphocytes are capable of taking up polyamines from the environment by an active, carrier-mediated process [7]. It was shown recently that B lymphocytes initiate transport as they enter the G1 stage of the cell cycle [47]. Active uptake and release are part of a refined system of intracellular polyamine regulation and makes cells partially independent of *de novo* polyamine synthesis.

Further evidence for a role of the polyamines in lymphocyte proliferation comes from the effects of biosynthesis inhibitors. It was reported [48, 49] that DFMO reduced the rate of DNA replication in activated peripheral blood lymphocytes, by preventing the cells to traverse from G1 into S-phase. Another example is the suppression of DNA synthesis in colonic lamina lymphocytes by DFMO [50, 51]. Under comparable conditions the reduction in the number of Golgi apparatus and its swelling, as well as a reduction in the activity of galactosyltransferase activity was observed in bovine lymphocytes and mouse small intestine epithelium [52], indicating the impairment of post-translational protein modifications due to the polyamine deficit.

MGBG (methylglyoxal-bis(guanylhydrazone)) is a well-known inhibitor of AdoMetDC (Fig. 4). It inhibits protein, RNA and DNA synthesis in lectin-stimulated lymphocytes [53]. Abdel-Monem et al. [54] found similar effects using inhibitors of AdoMetDC which are structural analogs of AdoMet. Although these compounds are not entirely selective for AdoMetDC, there is little doubt that they prevent lymphocyte proliferation by preventing spermidine and spermine formation.

Although DNA synthesis is inhibited due to polyamine depletion, it is probably not an immediate consequence of polyamine deficiency. Both in rat hepatoma tumor cells [28], and in human lymphocytes [50], the first observable consequence of spermidine depletion by DFMO was the impairment of polyribosome formation and of protein synthesis. The decrease in thymidine incorporation into DNA was detectable at later times and paralleled the decrease in the thymidine kinase activity in the polyamine-depleted cells [50].

A role of extracellular polyamines in the regulation of lymphocyte activation was recently demonstrated [55]. The increase of extracellular polyamines impaired the mitogen-stimulated transmembrane Ca^{2+} mobilization in murine T cells. This observation suggests an immunosuppressive role of the polyamines via a Ca^{2+}-signal-transduction pathway, thereby affecting T cell proliferation and differentiation. In contrast with most other observations concerning *in vitro* polyamine effects, putrescine was most potent in blocking the transmembrane Ca^{2+}-influx. The polyamine-related impact was restricted to the $CD4^+$ T (helper) subpopulation. $CD8^+$ cells did not respond; thus this polyamine effect seems to be membrane-specific.

2.2   B lymphocytes and immunoglobulin formation

It is well established that B cell stimulation of immunoglobulin (Ig) synthesis is both T cell and macrophage dependent [56], and mimicks the *in vivo* immune response. Following contact between T helper cells and B lymphocytes cyclic AMP (second messenger), and ODC are induced as early markers of B cell activation. In this process ODC mRNA is enhanced in the absence of protein synthesis, suggesting that ODC belongs to the early gene family [57].

Ig formation by normal human B lymphocytes, activated by pokeweed mitogen, appears to be a suitable model for the *in vivo* immune response. It was, therefore, used to study the effects of ODC inactivators on IgM and IgG production. Both, DFMO [58] and a more potent inactivator of ODC (2R, 5R)-6-heptyne-2,5 diamine (MAP) (Fig. 4) [59] were effective in blocking polyamine accumulation, DNA synthesis and IgM and IgG production. MAP prevented Ig production completely at 100 µM, an effect not achieved to the same extent by DFMO even at 5 mM. That the effect of the ODC inhibitors was indeed the result of the prevention of polyamine formation, was demonstrated by addition of the ODC inhibitors together with 10 µM putrescine or spermidine (in the presence of 50 µM aminoguanidine (Fig. 4)) to the culture medium. Under these conditions the impairment of IgM formation by the ODC inhibitors was completely prevented.

Methotrexate and the tumor-promoting agent 12-O-tetradecanoylphorbol-13-acetate (TPA) inhibit B cell proliferation and differentiation. The effects of methotrexate are known to be mediated primarily through inhibition of dihydrofolate reductase, which results in the inhibition of purine and pyrimidine base synthesis. More recently, evidence was presented that other folate-dependent reactions may be affected as well. One such pathway is the regeneration of methionine from homocysteine, with subsequent formation of AdoMet. In pokeweed mitogen-stimulated mononuclear cells from healthy donors incubation with methotrexate resulted in a decreased rate of proliferation and a decreased rate of IgG, IgM and IgM-rheumatoid factor synthesis. Addition of methionine, S-adenosylmethionine or spermidine to the culture medium prevented the methotrexate-mediated inhibition, suggesting that an important effect of methotrexate is due to the inhibition of a methionine salvage pathway, which affects polyamine formation [60].

In unfractionated spleen cells (containing macrophages, and T and B lymphocytes) polyamine depletion by 0.1 mM DFMO prevented the TPA-induced inhibition of proliferation of antibody-forming cells in a 5-day *in vitro* immunization procedure, as measured by hemolytic plaque assay. However, DFMO did not prevent the TPA-mediated inhibition of antibody production in these cells. In the absence of TPA, DFMO reduced antibody formation. This latter effect of DFMO could be prevented by addition of 0.1 mM putrescine to the culture medium on day 4 of immunization. Putrescine, however, did not abrogate the DFMO-suppression of TPA-mediated inhibition of proliferation of antibody-forming cells [61]. It appears that the effect of TPA on the number of plasma cells can be mediated indirectly through effects on T lymphocytes and/or macrophages. These effects are antagonized by DFMO. However, a direct effect of TPA on B lymphocytes is also possible, as was shown with enriched cultures. This direct effect of TPA on B cells was not prevented by putrescine and spermidine depletion [61].

Exposure to DFMO did not affect the expression of Epstein-Barr virus encoded nuclear antigens, when human B lymphocytes were infected. However, other steps in the virus-induced transformation were inhibited, such as DNA and immunoglobulin synthesis [62], in agreement with the above-mentioned effects of polyamine depletion on pokeweed mitogen-induced differentiation.

2.3   Cytolytic T cell and natural killer cell activation

Owing to the central role of T cells in cell-mediated immune reactions, factors involved in the maturation and activation of T cells attract great interest. The molecular events in T cell activation are rather numerous and complex [63]. A multiple role of the natural polyamines in these processes becomes more and more apparent.

2.3.1   Polyamines and programmed cell death

Cells undergoing programmed cell death (apoptosis) must first differentiate and then they undergo DNA fragmentation. This suggests that polyamines may participate in this process in several ways. Brüne et al. [64] demonstrated that spermine (but not putrescine and spermidine) prevented Ca^{2+}-induced endonuclease activation, and DNA fragmentation in thymocytes from immature rats, and thus prevented apoptosis. It was assumed that the stabilization of chromatin [16] is the mechanism underlying the protective effect of spermine.

Among the many genes, whose expression has been shown to coincide with cell death, belongs transglutaminase [65]. This enzyme is induced during apoptosis [66]. The polyamines are natural substrates of transglutaminases, capable of forming covalent links and cross links with certain proteins (see section 5.2, Polyamine binding to macromolecules). Hence, there is a potential role of the polyamines in programmed cell death, that requires scrutiny.

Putrescine, spermidine and spermine are a source of hydrogen peroxide, which is formed as a product of their oxidative deaminations (Fig. 3) [22]. Owing to its ability to form oxygen radicals, hydroperoxide is currently considered to cause apoptotic cell death [67]. Experimental support to this notion comes, among others, from the presence of polyamine oxidases in the mammalian epidermis, where they are supposed to control the production of tissue mass.

In order to assess the presumed relationship between resting cells, proliferating cells, and cell death, the changes of ODC mRNA and of sulfated glycoprotein 2 (a marker of programmed cell death) were compared in human peripheral blood lymphocytes [68]. After stimulation with phytohemagglutinin, in parallel to the increase of ODC mRNA, the repression of sulfated glycoprotein 2 was observed. This indicates an inverse transcriptional regulation of these two proteins during the transition from quiescence to mitosis.

The striking difference between the signal-transduction pathways of immature and mature T cells is an important feature in the suppression of autoimmune processes during T cell maturation. The T cell receptor of many thymocytes can reorganize antigens present within the host organism. These cells have the potential to initiate a dangerous autoimmune response. Therefore, they are removed by apoptosis during negative selection in the thymus. Apoptosis is normally initiated when the T cell receptor is engaged by antigen presented in association with a major histocompatibility complex (MHC). *In vitro,* cell death may be induced by CD3 stimulation (a T cell receptor associated molecule), by glucocorticoids, or by ionizing irradiation. In mature peripheral T cells, the same stimuli do not initiate apoptotic death, but rather mitosis and anergy, depending on the presence of other stimuli [65]. It will be interesting to study details of how the polyamines are involved in T cell selection by apoptosis, and the development of the mature signal-transduction pathways.

2.3.2   *Immunostimulating and immunosuppressing effects of the polyamines*

Several years ago Häcker-Shahin and Dröge [69] reported that injections of putrescine strongly augment *in vivo* priming for secondary *in vitro* responses to syngeneic T cell lymphoma (ESb-D) cells and minor histocompatible allogeneic spleen cells. A similar effect was achieved with ornithine, the precursor of putrescine. The state of immune memory after *in vivo* priming reflects the reactivity of helper T cells and cytolytic T lymphocytes. Mechanisms for the enhancement of the immune response by putrescine (and ornithine) are at present speculative. A likely explanation is the promotion of specific clones since putrescine in the presence of DAO is known to inhibit mitogen-induced cell proliferation [70]. In analogy to this observation, the presence or absence of a suitable oxidase in certain cells could be a mechanism for selecting and promoting specific clones. Another possibility for specific clone promotion is the enhanced spermidine formation by certain cells.

A more likely possibility is the transglutaminase-catalyzed formation of putrescine conjugates. Activated lymphocytes have elevated transglutaminase activity [71]. Putrescine, a natural substrate of transglutaminases [72], is suited to modify physical and biological properties of proteins. (For more details, see section 5.2 on polyamine binding to macromolecules). The proteins modified by conjugation with a polyamine may function as modulators of a variety of regulatory pathways.

The effects of selective inactivators of ODC suggested the requirement of the polyamines in T cell activation:

The concanavalin A-mediated polyclonal induction of cytolytic T lymphocytes was inhibited by inactivation of ODC, using DFMO or MAP, and could be reversed by addition of putrescine to the culture medium [73, 74]. The generation of interleukin-2 (IL-2) by T helper cells was markedly reduced by MAP [74], but DFMO had no effect on IL-2 production under the experimental conditions [75]. Exogenous IL-1, IL-2, IL-4 and γ-interferon (IFN-γ) failed to abrogate the effect of DFMO on cytolytic T lymphocyte activation, but putrescine (1 mM), and more efficiently spermidine (0.01 mM) did prevent the effects of DFMO. It was concluded from these observations that the reduction of polyamine biosynthesis has a greater effect on the differentiation of cytolytic T lymphocytes than on proliferation of these cells.

The effect of DFMO on cytolytic T cell activation can be enhanced by the immunosuppressive agent cyclosporin A, both *in vitro* and *in vivo* [76]. DFMO (0.2 mg.ml^{-1}) or cyclosporin A (10 ng.ml^{-1}) in the culture medium inhibits mitogen and alloantigen-induced cytolytic T lymphocyte generation by 50–60%. Combined treatment with the two drugs reduced induction by 80–90%. *In vivo,* DFMO had no effect on alloantigen-induced cytolytic T lymphocyte generation. However, in combination it potentiated the immunosuppressive effect of cyclosporin A, and IL-2 levels were reduced. Since the combined administration had no greater effect on cellular putrescine and spermidine concentrations than DFMO alone, it is evident that the two drugs inhibit different processes required for activation of cytolytic T lymphocytes.

The retarded rejection of a skin allograft in mice by treatment with DFMO [77] has been considered as an argument for the interference of the polyamines with T cell functions. However, polyamine depletion by the same agent prolonged and modified both, the specific cytotoxic T lymphocyte, and antibody responses to grafted allogeneic mastocytoma P815 cells [78]. A rather interesting observation was made by Thomas et al., [79] using an animal model of lupus: T-cells of MRL-lpr/lpr mice show aberrant surface markers. At 14 weeks of age, a stage of clinical disease expression, $40 \pm 13\%$ of the thymocytes lacked both, CD4 and CD8 and only $25 \pm 14\%$ had both these cell surface markers. Treatment with DFMO decreased the cell population which lacked CD4 and CD8 to $19 \pm 4\%$ and increased the cells with the correct surface markers to $47 \pm 10\%$. Since in T cells of MRL-lpr/lpr mice a two-fold increase of the putrescine and spermidine

concentrations was determined, which was abolished by DFMO, a pathogenetic role of the polyamines in T cell maturation seems evident.

In view of the apparent role of the natural polyamines in cytolytic T
lymphocyte maturation, the inhibition of the differentiation of this cell type
by ornithine [80, 81] appears paradoxical, especially since one of these
groups also reported that immune reactivity was enhanced by ornithine [69].
The following *in vitro* experiments were reported: ornithine prevented the
development of cytolytic T lymphocytes in unfractionated lymphocyte
cultures, but it had no effect on proliferative T cell responses, or on the
production of IL-2 and IFN-γ. If unfractionated lymphocyte cultures were
depleted of accessory cells, so that cytolytic lymphocyte activation was
dependent upon addition of lymphokines, activation still was susceptible to
inhibition by ornithine.

Evidence for an immunosuppressive effect of ornithine *in vivo* was obtained
as follows:

Cyclophosphamide-treated C3H mice were injected with ornithine immediately before immunization with trinitrophenylated syngeneic cells. Subsequently, the cytolytic effect of the inguinal and axillary lymph node cells
of these animals was reduced, in parallel with the dose of ornithine injected
to the mice.

In unfractionated lymphocytes obtained from ornithine-treated mice, cytolytic T lymphocyte precursors were undergoing clonal expansion, but their
maturation was arrested in a precytolytic stage. Thus, ornithine, as well as
depletion of cellular polyamines, seem to prevent maturation of the precursor cells.

Since the immunosuppressive effect of ornithine was selective, and had no
toxic component, it was speculated that elevated ornithine levels may represent a physiological signal that triggers processes which affect cytolytic T
lymphocyte maturation. However, in view of the high (9 mM) concentration
of ornithine needed to produce the immunosuppressive effect *in vitro*, [80]
and the low concentrations of ornithine present in tissues (20–700 µM; [82]),
a physiological function of ornithine in cellular immune regulation is not
very likely. The long-term elevation of tissue ornithine concentrations by
selective inactivation of ornithine aminotransferase [82] seems a suitable
experimental approach to study the role of ornithine in T-cell function.

2.3.3   *Natural killer cells and tumor growth*
In Lewis lung carcinoma bearing mice tumor growth (and formation of lung
metastases) can be extensively inhibited, if all major polyamine sources are

blocked [83]. This was done by combining a polyamine-deficient diet and decontamination of the gastrointestinal tract with the administration of DFMO and an inactivator of polyamine oxidase (PAO) (MDL 72,527) (Fig. 4). The latter prevents the formation of putrescine from spermidine, and of spermidine from spermine (Fig. 2).

In contrast with L1210 leukemia cells [84], the putrescine and spermidine-depleted cells of the solid tumor did not prolong their cell cycle time, although tumor growth was inhibited by about 80%. Therefore, it was concluded that under the treatment conditions cell death was enhanced due to stimulation of the immune system [85]. Evidence for this notion was recently obtained by Chamaillard et al. [86]. In mice with Lewis lung carcinoma grafts a dramatic decrease in the cytotoxic activity of their natural killer cells was observed. Treatment with the above-mentioned regimen, i.e. extensive depletion of putrescine and spermidine in all tissues, restored natural killer cell activity. DFMO alone, which is not capable of depleting *in vivo* tissue spermidine concentrations as profoundly as the systematic blockade of all polyamine sources, did not affect natural killer cell activity after their activation by IFN-γ [87].

The mechanisms involved in the restoration of natural killer cell activity in tumor-bearing animals by global depletion of endogenous polyamines awaits clarification. The possibility that the enhanced blood polyamines in tumor-bearing animals and humans [88] may act as natural immunosuppressive agents is considered as a suitable working hypothesis.

2.4   Polyamines and monocytes/macrophages

Under certain conditions the monocytes undergo differentiation to macrophages which become capable of phagocytosis. The term monocytes/macrophages will be used in the following, because cells with different degrees of differentiation have been used in most investigations.

The role of polyamines in monocytes/macrophages was studied in relation with activation, differentiation, mechanisms of phagocytosis and antitumor activity.

Resident peritoneal macrophages and peritoneal macrophages activated by a lymphoreticular agent (*Corynebacterium parvum*) express unique ectoenzyme phenotypes, while bone marrow-derived macrophages and thioglycolate-elicited peritoneal macrophages exhibit a similar ectoenzyme phenotype. All these macrophage populations differ in polyamine accumulation patterns [89]. One of the conclusions from these observations is that ectoenzyme phenotypes do not serve as completely selective markers of cell differentiation. However, the combined use of both ectoenzymes and intracellular polyamine patterns as cellular characteristics may allow one to distinguish between macrophage populations.

When monocytes are kept in culture until they acquire characteristics of mature macrophages, they diminish spontaneous respiratory burst activity. (For a review of the respiratory burst of macrophages and its physiological role, see [90]). If these cells are activated (e.g. by bacterial lipopolysaccharides (LPS) or by IFN-γ, they induce ODC mRNA [91]. Stimulation with tumor necrosis factor (TNF) also induces ODC and causes the enhancement of the respiratory burst, i.e. the cells release superoxide at an enhanced rate (from which hydrogen peroxide is formed by reaction with water). Polyamine biosynthesis inhibitors (DFMO and MGBG (Fig. 4)) prevent the stimulated release of superoxide [92], together with other responses of activation [93–97]. However, not only superoxide formation, but also the polyamine-dependent production of lymphocytotoxic amounts of ammonia by human peripheral blood monocytes has been reported [98], indicating immunosuppressive potentials of ammonia.

The fact that spermine and spermidine stimulate the phagosome-lysosome fusion and the polymerization of G-actin in murine macrophages [99] argues in favor of a role of the polyamines in phagocytosis.

The involvement of polyamines in functional aspects of monocytes/macrophages has been studied mainly with respect to malignant processes and their treatment with inhibitors of polyamine biosynthesis. Macrophage-mediated tumoricidal activity directed against B 16 melanoma cells is transiently augmented after 6, but not after 18 days of treatment with DFMO [100]. Treatment with *Corynebacterium parvum* enhanced the DFMO effect *in vivo* [101], and reduced the polyamine levels in macrophages, but had no effect on the tumoricidal macrophage activation that is promoted by other agents, i.e. by IFN-α/β [100].

The comparison of the effects of three ODC inhibitors, DFMO, MAP and α-(fluoromethyl)dehydro-ornithine methylester (MDL 72,403; Fig. 4) demonstrated a difference with regard to IFN-stimulated tumoricidal activity: the structural analog of ornithine (MDL 72,403) but not the structural analog of putrescine (MAP) enhanced the effect of IFN-γ, although all compounds depleted putrescine and spermidine in macrophages [102]. It turned out that LPS-stimulated macrophages isolated from mice treated with MDL 72,403 produced more TNF and IL-1 than macrophages from MAP-treated mice.

It is known that MAP and another ODC inactivator with putrescine like structure ((E)-α-(fluoromethyl)-dehydroputrescine (MDL 72,197)), in contrast with DFMO blocked the formation of "neurite-like processes" in primary cultures of neurons [103], although polyamine depletion by all three compounds was comparable. This indicates that ODC inhibitors which are structural analogs of putrescine may exert effects on cell differentiation, which are not shared by the ornithine-type structures. Whether this effect is mediated via the putrescine binding sites on the plasma membrane surface [104], is an open question. The above-mentioned increased secretion of TFN is, however, most probably a major cause for the enhanced tumoricidal activity of LPS- and IFN-stimulated, polyamine-depleted macrophages.

Owing to a high arginase activity in intratumoral macrophages of mastocytoma-P815 bearing mice, a high rate of ornithine production was observed in these cells. Tumor rejection in P815-preimmunized mice was accompanied by a decreased arginase activity [105]. It was, therefore, suggested that the capability of the immune system to stimulate or inhibit tumor growth is attributable (at least in part) to the capability of the macrophages to produce polyamines.

Polyamines are also involved in the 1-α,25-dihydroxyvitamin-D3-driven fusion of mouse alveolar macrophages into multinucleated giant cells [106]. Multinucleated giant cells occur in inflamed tissues and are thought to represent a specialized form of macrophages activated by lymphokines and 1-α,25-dihydroxyvitamin-D3 in conditions of chronic inflammation [107]. Fusion of mouse alveolar macrophages is significantly inhibited when cells are incubated with 1-α,25-dihydroxyvitamin-D3 and 5 μM MGBG, suggesting that 1-α,25-dihydroxyvitamin-D3-induced synthesis of polyamines precedes fusion. The inhibition by MGBG of 1-α,25-dihydroxyvitamin-D3-induced fusion is restored by adding 1 μM spermidine or spermine, and 100 μM putrescine [106].

Three proteins (with mol. masses of 98 kD, 78 kD and 50 kD), which need the presence of spermidine for synthesis, have been shown to take part in the fusion of mouse alveolar macrophages induced by 1-α,25-dihydroxyvitamin-D3 and Interleukin-4 [108]. Spermidine synthesis in this study was inhibited by MGBG. Polyamine depletion was accompanied by a concomitant decrease in the synthesis of some proteins, and by inhibition of fusion. Supplementation with spermidine restored protein synthesis and macrophage fusion as well [108]. Pulmonary alveolar macrophages have a greater rate of putrescine and spermidine uptake than the total lung cell population.

Uptake in these cells is apparently mediated by multiple polyamine transporter systems [109].

3   Cytokines and complement

3.1   Interrelations between polyamine metabolism and the cytokines

In previous sections effects of polyamine deprivation on cytokine formation, as well as effects of cytokines on polyamine synthesis have repeatedly been mentioned. Key observations concerning polyamine cytokine interrelations are summarized below.

The induction of ODC by cytokines seems a rather general phenomenon: along with IL-1α, IL-1β, TNF-α, TNF-β, granulocyte/macrophage colony-stimulating factor and granulocyte-colony stimulating factor, induce ODC in hematopoetic cells of bone marrow, spleen and liver [110]. Unfortunately, as in many related cases, ODC determinations are not sufficient to establish an important function of the polyamines.

Interleukin-1 is a pleiotropic cytokine produced primarily by activated monocytes/macrophages, but also by a number of other cell types, including natural killer cells, B lymphoblasts and B and T cell lines. It exists in two forms, IL-1α and IL-1β, which display similar activities: they induce fever, sleep, hepatic acute-phase protein expression, and T and B cell activation and proliferation. IL-1 mediates host responses to injury, infection and antigenic challenge in combination with other cytokines whose bioactivities overlap with those of IL-1, i.e. TNF-α and IL-6 [20, 111, 112]. ODC activity is suppressed by IL-1 in non-immune cells which do not proliferate in response to IL-1 (e.g. human melanoma and malignant human mammary gland cell lines), but ODC activity is stimulated in cells originating from the immune system whose proliferation is enhanced by IL-1, such as a mouse helper T cell line, and natural killer-like cell lines. Putrescine reverses most antiproliferative effects of IL-1 in melanoma cells, but not in mammary tumor cells. In contrast, putrescine and IL-1, exhibit a co-mitogenic activity on mouse helper T cells. Analogous experiments with TNF-α and the same cell lines gave similar results, and putrescine again overcame partially the inhibitory effect of TNF-α. The regulation of ODC activity is most probably a key component in the antiproliferative and proliferative actions of IL-1 and TNF in certain tumor cell types [113].

Combined treatment of the histiocytic lymphoma cell line U937 with TPA and 1-α,25-dihydroxyvitamin-D3 for 72 h, followed by incubation with LPS for 24 h, induced ODC, as well as the release of IL-1β by 65%. Similar results have been obtained with DFMO during the differentiation of the U937 cells up to the monocyte or macrophage stage [114].

Interleukin-2 (IL-2, formerly "T-cell growth factor") is produced by T lymphocytes. Its major biological effects are the stimulation of T cell proliferation and differentiation, the enhancement of cytolytic activity of natural killer cells and the promotion of proliferation and immunoglobulin secretion of activated B cells [20, 115]. Several lines of evidence suggest that DFMO interferes with IL-2-mediated effects [116–121].

CTLL-20 cells (a murine cytotoxic T cell line) are absolutely dependent on IL-2. Stimulation with IL-2 will produce an eight-fold increase of ODC activity. Inactivation of ODC not only caused the depletion of putrescine and spermidine, and a reduction of IL-2 dependent proliferation, but also a decrease of the ability of these cells to take up IL-2. All these effects can be abrogated by addition of micromolar concentrations of putrescine to the culture medium, demonstrating the specificity of the polyamine requirement. Quite analogous observations were reported for FDC-P1 cells, an IL-3 dependent murine cell line [116]. (IL-3 is a factor produced by T cells, mast cells, neurons and keratinocytes. It promotes the proliferation of pluripotential progenitor cells, monocytes/macrophages and some non-immune blood cells [20].)

Concanavalin A-induced IL-2 production of T cells is enhanced by treatment with DFMO, both *in vitro* and *in vivo* (in C57 BL/6 mice) [118]. The concanavalin A-mediated expression of IL-2 receptors in human peripheral blood mononuclear leukocytes is, however, unaffected under conditions of polyamine depletion, which causes a reduction by 80–100% of the responsiveness of the cells to IL-2 stimulation [117]. The notion that polyamine biosynthesis is a prerequisite for IL-2 dependent proliferation, but not for the expression of the high affinity receptors of this cytokine, was confirmed by Yukioka et al. [119] using concanavalin A-stimulated mouse splenic mononuclear cells. Furthermore, it was demonstrated that the DFMO-driven inhibition of proliferation of human lymphocytes (stimulated by concanavalin A, phytohemagglutinin, phorbol-myristate acetate, or ionomycin-60) can be reversed by spermidine, without decreasing IL-2 production [121].

Exposure of EL-4 lymphoma cells with TPA induces the production of IL-2, which can be further augmented ("superinduced") by exposing the cells to DFMO. However, glycolytic activity, general protein synthesis and mitosis are inhibited by DFMO [120] in agreement with the mentioned primary effects of spermidine depletion.

Although most findings are somewhat preliminary and not entirely convincing, there is little doubt that the relationship between polyamines and the cytokines is not only confined to immune competent cells, but is also important for non-immune cells [122–124]. It seems also evident that cytokine production and release and cellular polyamine metabolism (and release) are mutually interdependent in events of immune stimulation, in which several cell types are associated to achieve immune reactions.

3.2   Polyamines and complement

The complement system [125, 126] is the principal means by which antibodies defend vertebrates against most bacterial infections. Besides its role in antibody-mediated cell lysis, complement attracts phagocytic cells to sites of infections and enhances the ability of these cells to destroy microorganisms. In view of its paramount importance it is astounding that only one study has been dedicated to potential interactions of polyamines with the complement system. Lysine and some homologous diamines (1,2-ethanediamine, 1,3-propanediamine, 1,4-butanediamine (putrescine), and 1,5-pentanediamine (cadaverine)) inhibit spontaneous and antibody-dependent complement C1 activation, and are able to dissociate C1 into its two entities, Clq and the calcium-dependent Clr2-Cls2 complex. The polyamines spermine and spermidine dissociate C1 with a higher efficiency than lysine and putrescine [127]. The *in vitro* diamine- and polyamine-induced dissociation of the first component of human complement C1 lends support to the assumption that complement-mediated immune reactions *in vivo* can also be affected by extracellularly circulating polyamines.

4   Oxidative deamination of the polyamines and immunomodulating effects

A controversy existed for many years concerning the role of polyamines in lymphocyte proliferation. It was repeatedly suggested that lymphocyte proliferation in cell cultures is inhibited by polyamines. However, the authors of these reports had overlooked the oxidative deamination of the polyamines by SAO (Fig. 3), an enzyme especially rich in ruminant serum. (Ruminant serum is often used to supplement cell culture media.) Since the products of this reaction, hydrogen peroxide, ammonia, and the aldehydes are cytotoxic, most pertinent observations can be explained by the cell-independent formation of these products in the culture medium. In the absence of SAO polyamines do normally not affect lymphocyte proliferation [70]. However, as is shown in Fig. 3, spermidine (and spermine) are substrates of DAO as well. This mainly cytosolic and releasable enzyme is also capable of oxidatively deaminating polyamines to the same aldehydes, that are formed by SAO [22]. Therefore, it needs to be excluded from the culture medium as well. As was pointed out by Smith et al. [128], some cells are a source for polyamine-oxidizing enzymes, which may be excreted or exert their functions intracellularly. For example, the immunologic barrier which protects the fetus against maternal immune rejection is presumably a result of the oxidative deamination of the polyamines by placental DAO [129]. Likewise, the immunosuppressive effect of seminal plasma relies on the oxidative deamination of spermine by an amine oxidase [130]. Furthermore, the stimulated secretion by mast cells of serotonin and histamine was blocked by the products of SAO-catalyzed oxidation of the polyamines [131]. Another example of considerable importance for a potential role of polyamine oxidation is the regulation of IL-2 production.

Based on the observation that IL-2 production was increased in murine and human lymphocytes after depletion of the intracellular putrescine and spermidine by exposure to DFMO [117, 118], it was assumed that not only prostaglandin E but also polyamines may be involved in the downregulation of IL-2 production. The following hypothesis was suggested [132]: Polyamines are secreted by activated T cells [133]. Macrophages secrete a polyamine oxidase [128, 134]. The products of the oxidative deamination of spermidine and spermine (H_2O_2, NH_3, aldehydes) constitute an inhibitory signal to activated T cells, and regulate in this way cell 'proliferation [134], and IL-2 production [132]. A scheme of the major aspects of this hypothesis is shown in Fig. 7. In pursuit of this idea the following observations were reported [135]:

a) Hydrogen peroxide produced by phytohemagglutinin-activated peripheral blood mononuclear cells inhibited IL-2 production. (Oxygen radicals formed from hydrogen peroxide are presumably the reactive species in this process.) It appeared that the observed effect could not be entirely explained by hydrogen peroxide formation from spermidine and SAO added to the culture medium.

b) N^1,N^4-Bis(2,3-butadienyl)-1,4-butanediamine (MDL 72,527) (Fig. 4), quinacrine, and benadryl increased significantly IL-2 production in the

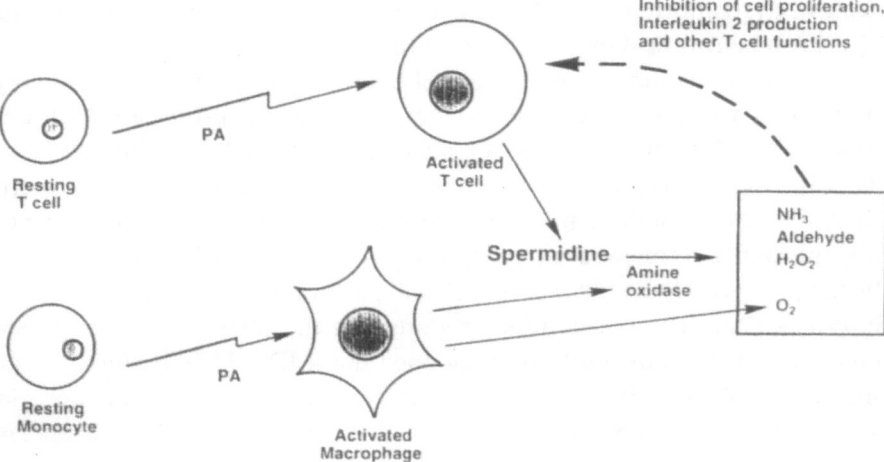

Fig. 7
Potential mechanisms involved in the regulation of T cell activity and Interleukin-2 production by macrophages.
Spermidine (and spermine) released from activated T cells serve as substrate for an amine oxidase released by macrophages. The products of this reaction, together with superoxide (from which hydrogen peroxide is formed) are assumed to constitute an inhibitory signal which regulates cell proliferation. (Hypothesis of Talal and Flescher, [132]). PA indicates the role of polyamines in the process of resting T cell and monocyte activation.

presence of monocytes even in the absence of fetal calf serum (i.e. in the absence of SAO). This indicates that the monocytes were the source of an amine oxidase. Withdrawal of the monocytes abolished the effect of MDL 72,527.
Rheumatoid arthritis is associated with decreased IL-2 production [136]. The concentration of polyamines in peripheral blood monocytes from patients with rheumatoid arthritis and in synovial fluid mononuclear cells was 2-20-fold higher than in normal cells [137]. Elevated putrescine concentrations in synovial fluid and tissues [138], and a polyamine-oxidizing enzyme in rheumatoid arthritis synovial fluid [139] were also reported. The above-described hypothesis on the downregulation of IL-2 production by polyamines became, therefore, quite attractive, especially since changes in IL-2 production in rheumatoid arthritis peripheral blood monocytes could be produced by polyamine depletion and by amine oxidase inhibitors [137], as was described above for normal human peripheral blood monocytes. Moreover, the defect in phytohemagglutinin-stimulated IL-2 production

seen in systemic lupus erythematosus [140] and in rheumatoid arthritis [137] can be reversed by resting the cells in culture for 2–3 days.

In a previous section the production of cytotoxic amounts of ammonia by monocytes was mentioned. Surprisingly, the excessive formation of ammonia was inhibitable by the PAO inactivator MDL 72,527 [98].

This and the above-mentioned reports obviously contain important experimental facts. But at the same time certain details need clarification. First of all, the oxidase released by macrophages [134] must be characterized, because spermidine and spermine are substrates of several oxidative enzymes [22]. The observations reported in the above experiments are confusing: It has already been mentioned that MDL 72,527 (Fig. 4) is an inactivator of tissue PAO, the flavin enzyme of the polyamine interconversion cycle (Fig. 2), not an inactivator of SAO and related Cu^{2+}-dependent amine oxidases. Spermine, and acetylderivatives of spermidine and spermine are substrates of PAO; spermidine is not a substrate. Hydrogen peroxide and aldehydes (3-acetamidopropanal and 3-aminopropanal) are products of PAO, but ammonia is not formed. The fact that quinacrine was also effective in the experiments of Flescher et al. [98], argues in favor of a flavin enzyme. However, benadryl is an inactivator of SAO [141].

Aminoguanidine (Fig. 4) is a very potent inactivator of DAO [142], but less active against SAO [143]. Furthermore, N^1, N^{12}-diacetylspermine is a substrate of PAO, but not of SAO and DAO [144]. Thus, the tools exist which allow us to clarify the confusion and misunderstandings in the cited papers, which in part are due to the lack of a standardized nomenclature of the polyamine-related oxidases.

5   Polyamine antigenicity and immunogenicity

5.1   Natural and injection-elicited antibodies

Due to their low molecular weight the polyamines have long been considered as haptens which become immunogenic when administered in a complex with a carrier molecule. Using this approach polyclonal and monoclonal antibodies against polyamines have repeatedly been prepared by injection of covalent polyamine-protein conjugates [145–151]. They have mainly been used to determine the polyamines in serum [149, 150, 152]. All available information [149, 151, 152, 153] indicates that both polyclonal and monoclonal spermine antibodies cross-react to some extent with spermidine, but practically not with putrescine. This indicates that the antibody paratope is directed towards the aminopropyl residue present on both spermine and spermidine (Fig. 1).

Recently, it was observed that repeated injections of spermine in rabbits are sufficient to induce the formation of spermine and spermidine antibodies [153]. This indicates that the injection of polyamines covalently bound to protein is not a prerequisite for inducing polyamine antibodies. Spermine is not expected to interact with immunocompetent cells as such, but as complex with some protein or a nucleic acid fragment which was formed *in vivo*. As presented in section 5.2, binding could occur by electrostatic or Van der Waals interactions, or by a transglutaminase-catalyzed reaction. Along with the possibility of selection of new immunocompetent clones, the injections of spermine could trigger the proliferation and differentiation of pre-existing clones. The latter assumption implies the presence of (natural) spermine antibodies in normal serum.

Indeed, in the course of the isolation of polyamine antibodies several groups found that normal human and rabbit serum contains spermine antibody [154–156]. The natural IgG-like spermine binding component of Furuichi et al. [155] had the same physicochemical properties as the spermine antibody obtained from rabbits immunized with spermine-thyroglobulin conjugate. However, it did not precipitate a spermine-bovine serum albumin complex, nor did it bind to a spermine-sepharose column. In contrast, the natural Ig-like spermine-binding materials of Bartos et al. [156] did bind to spermine-sepharose and were released from the gel by decreasing the pH of the eluent. In this way several populations of antibodies to spermine were distinguished. One may speculate that a function of the natural spermine antibody is to remove the toxic spermine [12] from the circulation [155]. However, it has been demonstrated that polyamine antibodies obtained by immunization exert cytotoxic effects on cells in culture. Morphological changes, and increase of the number of lysosomes, a decreased proliferation rate, and cytolysis were observed [157]. In view of these properties of polyamine antibodies there is an obvious interest in the exploration of potential physiological and pathophysiological roles of the population of endogenous spermine antibodies.

5.2   Polyamine binding to macromolecules and cationization

It is highly unlikely that the free polyamines are antigenic. We have to assume that conjugates are formed with macromolecules from spermidine and spermine released from cells, as well as from the exogenous spermine in the experiments of Atanassov et al. [153].

Owing to their positive charges at physiological pH electrostatic interactions of the polyamines with anionic sites of macromolecules are the basis for most of their functions. Polyamine-DNA interactions have attracted most interest in the past [158]. Recently, more refined structural considerations became possible by new methodology [159].

Several groups have reported that polyamines can affect DNA function by causing transition from one form of DNA into another. Spermine and spermidine are known to induce the transition of certain polynucleotides at near physiologic conditions from the B- to the left-handed Z-conformation [160]. This fact induced Thomas and Messner [161] to speculate that the beneficial effect of DFMO on lupus in MRL-lpr/lpr mice may rely on the prevention of DNA from assuming an immunogenic Z-DNA conformation. It was shown more recently [162] that polyamines stabilize the Z-conformation of poly(dA-dC)poly(dG-dT), and of related alternating pyrimidine sequences. Immunization with poly(dA-dC)poly(dG-dT) complexed with spermidine or spermine produced antibodies reacting with Z-DNA (in addition to antibodies binding poly(dA-dC)poly(dG-dT) and ssDNA). Since antibodies having a high affinity toward Z-DNA are present in the sera of patients with systemic lupus erythematosus and lupus-prone strains of mice [163], the above-mentioned assumptions receive experimental support.

Another aspect of DNA-polyamine interactions is the facilitation of DNA-IgG complex formation: In the presence of quantities of polyamines sufficient to increase the melting temperature of DNA, and to produce a partial resistance to DNase, the amount of IgG needed to form DNase-resistant DNA-IgG complexes was 100 times less than that required in the absence of polyamines [164].

Stabilization of certain conformations of macromolecules by the polyamines is a general principle that may also play an important role in immune diseases. Electrostatic interactions of the polyamines with proteins are known. In general, binding to proteins is less tight than to polynucleotides. (Owing to the enormous variations in the distribution of negative charges along polypeptide chains, it is not possible to make general predictions concerning electrostatic interactions between polyamines and proteins.) Therefore, changes in the immunogenicity of proteins by electrostatically bound polyamines are less likely than in the case of polynucleotides. However, polyamines can bind covalently to proteins. As a result the ratio of positive/negative charges is increased, and considerable changes in conformation and in other physical properties of the proteins can be predicted.

Cationization has been shown to alter among others the immunogenic properties of proteins [165–168]. For example, the enhanced immunogenicity of cationized bovine serum albumin is due to an increase of its affinity for negatively charged membrane components of the antigen-presenting cells. This may result in a more intensive antigen uptake [169]. Effects of cationization of proteins by the natural polyamines on structural and immunogenic properties is today a virtually unexplored topic of presumably great importance.

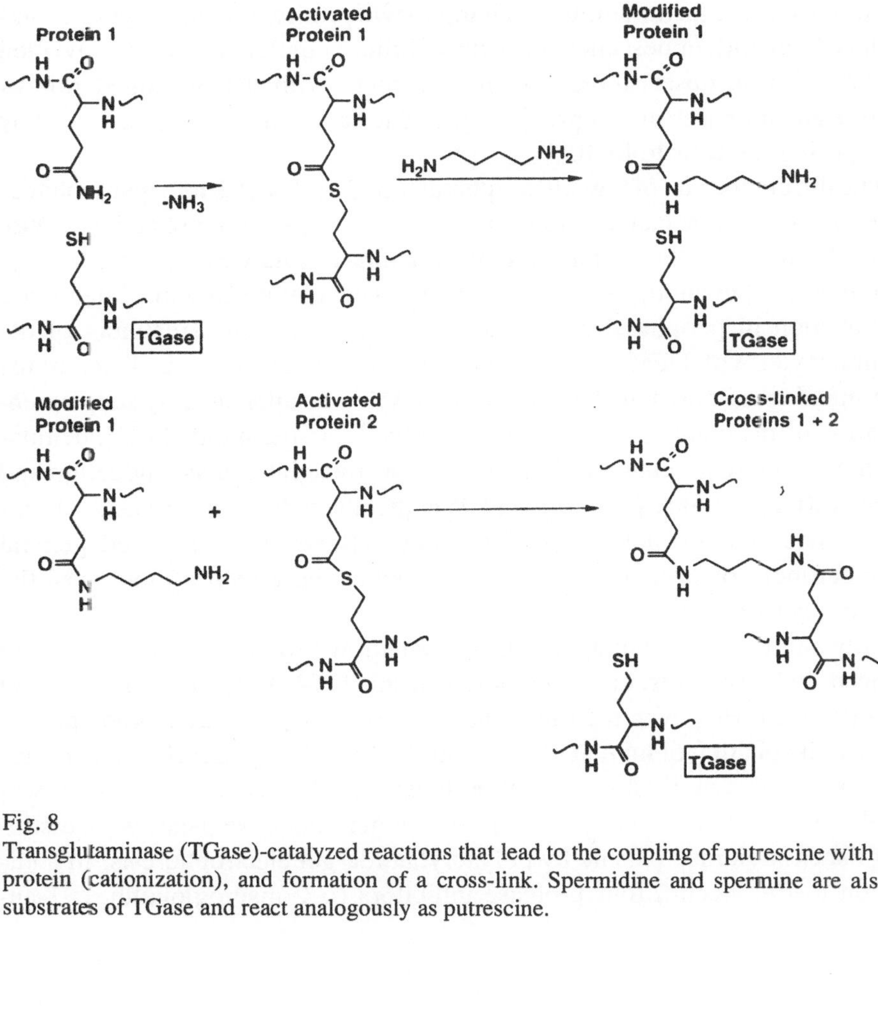

Fig. 8
Transglutaminase (TGase)-catalyzed reactions that lead to the coupling of putrescine with a protein (cationization), and formation of a cross-link. Spermidine and spermine are also substrates of TGase and react analogously as putrescine.

Among the reactions which generate covalent bonds between polyamines and proteins the transglutaminase-catalyzed amide bond formation is most important [170, 171]. The polyamines are physiological substrates of trans-glutaminases [71]. Fig. 8 illustrates how proteins are modified by exchanging the amido-group of a glutamyl residue against putrescine (or spermidine and spermine), and how cross-links can be formed between proteins, owing to the two primary amino groups of the natural polyamines.

As compared with resting cells, in mitogen-induced lymphocytes the Ca^{2+}-dependent transglutaminase-catalyzed binding of putrescine to proteins is strongly enhanced [71]. Evidence for cross-link formation in these cells was not found, but occurs in extracellular compartments (e.g. seminal plasma) [72].

If transglutaminase was competitively inhibited by dansyl cadaverine, allogeneic and lectin-stimulated lymphocyte proliferation and zymosan-induced chemiluminescence of neutrophilic granulocytes was prevented [172]. These observations are in agreement with the presumed role of transglutaminases in cell proliferation. The same effects were achieved by exposing the cells to MGBG.

The differentiation of human peripheral blood monocytes into macrophages has also been associated with an increase of transglutaminase activity. With this finding, and the enhanced transglutaminase-catalyzed binding of poly-amines [71] in mind, the effect of polyamine depletion on transglutaminase induction in peripheral blood monocytes was studied. Treatment of the monocytes with DFMO significantly reduced retinoic acid-mediated trans-glutaminase induction. The effect of DFMO was abolished by supplementation of the culture medium with putrescine or spermidine [173], demonstrating the requirement of polyamines for transglutaminase induction and cell differentiation by retinoic acid. Whether the reduction of transglutaminase induction by polyamine deficiency reflects the mentioned general impairment of protein synthesis, or whether the effect is more specific, needs clarification.

Polyamine-protein conjugates have been known for more than ten years to occur in body fluids, including blood plasma [174–177] and in mammalian cells [178]. However, the functions of these conjugates are unknown.

After incubation of human plasma with ^{14}C-labelled putrescine, incorporation of radioactivity into several proteins was observed, one of which was fibronectin [179]. Subsequently 15 different radioactive bands were distinguished in human plasma by polyacrylamide-gel electrophoresis. In addition to fibronectin, four protease inhibitors (α-2-macroglobulin, α-1-antitrypsin, α-1-antichymotrypsin and antithrombin III) were identified among these bands as substrates of transglutaminases [180].

The concentrations of non-covalently bound polyamines in serum under physiologic conditions are low [152].

Putrescine	0.13 ± 0.15 µM
Spermidine	0.30 ± 0.50 µM
Spermine	0.04 ± 0.06 µM

However, in the above-described labelling experiments of Roch et al. [179], the ^{14}C-putrescine concentration ranged from 90–600 µM. Therefore, one has to conclude from these facts that at physiological serum polyamine concentrations the transglutaminase-catalyzed coupling of the polyamines to proteins will be slow.

Although total spermidine and spermine concentrations are much higher in mammalian cells than in plasma, it can be assumed that the greatest part is electrostatically bound to anionic sites; the pool of free (i.e. neither covalently, nor electrostatically bound) polyamines is presumably comparable to plasma concentrations. However, the intracellular pools of the free polyamines can be modulated more rapidly than in plasma by changing the activity of rate-limiting enzymes (ODC; AdoMetDC; acetylCoA:spermine/spermidine N^1-acetyltransferase), and of transport activities (Fig. 2); i.e. cells have the means to adjust concentrations of substrates of the transglutaminases to physiological requirements.

Although the significance of the *in vitro* labelling experiments is not conclusive with regard to physiologic or pathologic consequences of cationization of plasma proteins by the natural polyamines, they demonstrate at least the presence of a multitude of substrates that may undergo this reaction. Undoubtedly, transglutaminase-catalyzed reactions offer a considerable potential for profound structural and functional post-translational modifications of numerous proteins.

6   Polyamines in immune-related pathology

6.1   Polyamines in body fluids as markers of pathologic events

Since the pioneering work of D.H. Russell [181] numerous attempts have been made to utilize polyamines as markers of malignancy [182] and of other diseases [183, 184].

Humans excrete polyamines mainly as monoacetyl derivatives. Since poly-amine patterns in urine and body fluids are not specific for certain diseases, and are dependent of nutritional and metabolic parameters, and of drug treatment, the diagnostic value of polyamine determinations is restricted. Nevertheless, in some diseases consistent aberrations from normal values exist, and may help in identifying pathogenetic aspects. Thus, the fact that elevated concentrations of serum polyamines were found in children with systemic lupus erythematosus [185] and in the synovial fluid [138] and urine [186] of patients with rheumatoid arthritis, was taken as a hint for a pathogenetic role of the polyamines in these autoimmune diseases.

Longitudinal studies of the polyamines in individual patients following surgery, or other therapies, were even more successful; e.g. brain tumor regrowth was indicated by enhanced cerebrospinal fluid polyamine levels considerably earlier than by standard clinical diagnostic methods [187].

Allograft rejection is associated with enhanced rates of T lymphocyte proliferation, and changes in cell loss. These could be detected by altera-tions of polyamine concentrations in body fluids. Both in non-immuno-suppressed dogs, as well as in cyclosporin- and steroid-treated dogs with cervical heterotopic heart transplantations, an increase of putrescine levels and of total urinary polyamines preceded histologically diagnozed allograft rejection [188, 189].

In line with these experimental studies, total polyamines were found ele-vated in the urine of patients with heart transplants one to three days before rejection could be proven by biopsy [190]. One may conclude that daily monitoring of urinary polyamine levels is a useful, non-invasive method to control the cellular metabolic activity of the immune system, and allograft rejection.

6.2   Polyamines, autoimmunity, and graft-versus-host disease

Polyamines have been detected at abnormally high levels in biological fluids of patients with autoimmune disorders. Using an antibody against spermine, Puri et al. [185] quantified by RIA serum-free polyamines in children with systemic lupus erythematosus. They found approximately a two-fold elevation in the polyamine levels of lupus patients when compared to those of normal children. In another study, Yukioka et al. [138] demon-strated that putrescine levels in synovial tissues and synovial fluids of patients with rheumatoid arthritis were significantly higher than in those with non-autoimmune osteoarthritis. It has also been reported that the concentration of polyamines in the peripheral blood mononuclear cells and the synovial fluid mononuclear cells of rheumatoid arthritis patients is 2–20 fold higher than in normal cells [135]. Elevated spermidine and spermine levels have also been found in the blood of psoriasis patients [191].

As has been described in section 5.2, polyamines are positively charged and are capable of interacting with negatively charged sites of macromolecules such as proteins and nucleic acids [158, 192]. Cationic complexes are retained more firmly within articular structures than the uncomplexed proteins, as has been shown for polylysine-cationized enzymes [193]. Another target for cationic complexes with potential involvement of the polyamines is the glomerular basement membrane of kidney. Various cationic ligands bind preferentially to this membrane [194–197], and cationic antibodies are involved directly in the pathogenesis of lupus nephritis [198–202]. Polyamines are known to interact with intrinsic anions on the renal surface and modify membrane characteristics [203]. Therefore, it is conceivable that circulating polyamine-polypeptide conjugates [175–177, 184, 192, 204] participate in immune complex deposition, and contribute to renal damage. In this context one should remember that the biologically oriented research of the polyamines started with the attempt to understand their renal toxicity [205, 206].

Repeated administration of spermine induces antibodies to histones [153]. They are likely to contribute to the pathogenesis of lupus-like nephritis, because it has been demonstrated that cationic histones show a tendency to form depositions on the glomerular membrane [207]. This suggestion is further supported by the polyamine involvement in the generation of DNA antibodies by inducing the formation of immunogenic Z-DNA [208, 209]. DNA antibodies cross-react with heparan sulfate which is a major gly-cosaminoglycan component of the glomerular basement membrane [210]. In addition, antibodies in New Zealand white rabbits immunized with cationized IgG cross-react with histones [211].

The majority of lupus antibodies react strongly with Z-DNA [163, 212]. The presence of spermine or spermidine enhances the binding of lupus sera toward certain polynucleotides [213]. DNA antibodies are present in the sera of MRL-lpr/lpr mice, an animal model of lupus. Lymphoid organs (thymus, spleen, lymph nodes) of MRL-lpr/lpr mice contain 3- to 5-fold higher polyamine concentrations than BALB/c mice [214]. In these mice the percentage of T cells lacking CD4 and CD8 is higher than in normal controls, and there is a premature export of these cells in the lymph nodes [79]. The (CD4⁻, CD8⁻)-cells appear refractory to T cell stimuli (e.g.

concanavalin A); however, they are capable of producing cationic DNA antibodies, which are pathogenic autoantibodies [215].

The elevated polyamine levels in cells and body fluids of patients with autoimmune diseases, and the effects of ODC inactivation on lymphocyte proliferation and Ig formation [58, 59] prompted studies on the potential immunosuppressive effects of ODC inactivators in MRL-lpr/lpr mice. Oral administration of DFMO (1%) or of MAP (0.2%) in tap water as sole drinking fluid delayed the development of lymphadenopathy, reduced the development of splenomegaly and increased significantly the mean survival time of the mice. DFMO delayed the appearance of DNA antibodies [161], and treatment with MAP reduced plasma IgG concentrations by 50%, but in contrast, those of IgM were elevated [216]. DFMO also reduced histo-logic criteria of glomerulonephritis (interstitial and perivascular inflammation, vasculitis), but had no effect on pulmonary histologic findings [217]. MAP can prevent the development of arthritis in DBA/1 mice immunized with native type II collagen (an antigen with repetitive cationic epitopes). This effect is possibly due to the inhibition of the immune response to this antigen resulting in subsequent generation of autoantibodies to articular structures [218].

Since both DFMO and MAP are rather selective inactivators of ODC, it is apparent that the observed beneficial effects of these compounds in an autoimmune disease are based on the impaired formation of putrescine. Inhibition of lymphocyte proliferation is considered a likely mechanism, in analogy to the effects of ODC inactivation in cell cultures. Nevertheless, polyamine depletion *in vivo is* a complex phenomenon. In order to clarify underlying mechanisms detailed studies on a variety of cells involved in the immune response are required.

ODC activity was found to be constitutively elevated in the kidney of the lupus-prone mice [162], but ODC mRNA was lower than in normal strains [219]. By treatment with DFMO, ODC mRNA increased 12-fold in the kidneys of MRL-lpr/lpr mice, when ODC activity was reduced to normal activity. It was assumed that a post-translational modification which stabilizes ODC against degradation may be responsible for the elevated enzyme activity. The beneficial effect of DFMO suggests a pathogenetic role for elevated polyamine concentration in murine lupus.

The graft-versus-host disease is characterized by the proliferation of grafted immunocompetent cells. These cells attack most tissues which leads to the recruitment of a large number of host cells to inflammatory sites. The disease takes two forms, a chronic and an acute lethal form. The latter is induced for example, if cells of C57BL/6 mice are transferred into (C57BL6 × BBA/2)F1 mice. It is characterized by anemia, a diminished number of splenocytes, hypogammaglobulinemia, and the loss of T helper cell function. Depletion of putrescine and spermidine by DFMO (1,5% in the drinking water) ameliorated the clinical expression of the disease [220] similarly to the effects of polyamine depletion on some animal models of autoimmunity.

Along with their apparent capability of enhancing the immunogenicity of different molecules, the polyamines could contribute through a more direct way to antibody diversity by acting as non-specific "growth factors" that are triggering polyclonal activation of antibody-producing cells. This assumption finds support in the observed increase in antibody-forming spleen cells in mice injected with sheep red blood cells or in mice with tumors, which had been pretreated *in vivo* with polyamines [221]. It is not unlikely that polyamines activate a subset of antibody-producing cells, namely cells belonging to the $CD5^+$ B cell lineage, which are considered to produce autoantibodies and play a central role in autoimmune pathogenesis [222].

6.3   Polyamines and inflammation

The processes involved in inflammation cannot be discussed without mentioning the participation of immunocompetent cells and their products. Based on the numerous interactions of the polyamines with components of the immune system, a certain role of the polyamines in inflammatory processes had to be expected. However, the experimental results available today are scarce, mainly descriptive, and with regard to mechanisms involved, speculative. Nevertheless, it appears of interest to briefly summarize published observations, because they may induce more in-depth research.

In endotoxin-induced uveitis of rabbits the concentrations of putrescine and N^1-acetylspermidine increase significantly in the aqueous humor, indicating the enhanced degradation of spermidine (and spermine) along the interconversion pathway (Fig. 2). Since the changes of the polyamine pattern correlated with a well-known parameter of inflammation, namely with the infiltration of leukocytes, putrescine and N^1-acetylspermidine may be used as markers of inflammation [223, 224].

In analogy to these observations elevated-putrescine concentrations were found in human gingival crevicular fluid from periodontitis patients [225]. Since the putrescine concentrations were higher than in serum, its local formation due to the inflammation should be assumed. Not unlikely, the enhanced formation of putrescine in inflammatory processes is part of the cellular defense mechanisms. This assumption is supported by the following observations, although, unfortunately some of the most suggestive findings concerning the potential role of the polyamines in inflammatory processes have been published only in the form of abstracts. Bartholeyns et al. [226, 227] found that inhibition by dexamethasone of carrageenan-induced paw edema in rats requires active polyamine biosynthesis, in order to maintain protein synthesis. DFMO prevented the therapeutic effect of dexamethasone, but had no effect on indomethacin. This underlines the difference of the mechanisms which underly these prominent anti-inflammatory drugs. Interestingly, prevention of putrescine catabolism by DAO, i.e. administration of aminoguanidine sulfate 1 h prior DFMO, prevented the blocking effect of DFMO on dexamethasone. Apparently, the rate of endogenous putrescine accumulation due to DAO blockade was sufficiently high to outbalance the putrescine-depleting effect of DFMO.

According to Oyanagui [228] serotonin paw edema of mice, and carrageenan paw edema in rats can be ameliorated by oral or subcutaneous administration of the polyamines prior to the local injection of serotonin and carrageenan. The fact that local polyamine injections were not antagonizing edema formation, indicates the necessity to enhance circulating polyamines, in order to achieve the anti-inflammatory effect.

For a 30% inhibition of serotonin paw edema formation 8 mg/kg spermine, 28 mg/kg of spermidine or 55 mg/kg of putrescine had to be injected 2 h before serotonin. Antagonism of carrageenan paw edema required higher doses.

As a potential mechanism the following sequence of events was suggested [228]: Glucocorticoid induces ODC, which enhances polyamine metabolism. The polyamines are presumed to support the glucocorticoid-induced synthesis of vascular permeability inhibitory protein (vasoregulin). This idea is supported by the fact that protein synthesis inhibition by cycloheximide reversed the polyamine effect on vascular permeability.

Spermidine and spermine at 1–2 μM concentrations suppress human platelet aggregation [229, 230]. It is, therefore, not excluded that this effect also contributes to the anti-inflammatory effect of the polyamines.

The activities of ODC and AdoMetDC, and the concentrations of the polyamines increase in a characteristic, time-dependent manner in the liver of rats during the acute-phase response to inflammation, which may be elicited by turpentine injection [231, 232]. This is further support to the above-mentioned suggestion that the changes of polyamine metabolism are part of the acute-phase response. Certain drug-inducible alterations in polyamine metabolism could ameliorate inflammation processes. In agreement with this notion subcutaneous administrations of putrescine or spermidine antagonized ODC induction, decreased the synthesis of serum α-2-macroglobulin (an acute-phase protein), and diminished the inflammatory response [232].

Owing to the limitation of putrescine, DAO appears to have an antiproliferative effect on gut mucosa, which becomes especially well visible in intestinal adaptation [233]. In the mucosa of patients with active ulcerative colitis DAO activity was reduced by nearly 90%, and at the same time mucosal cells were hyperproliferative. An antiproliferative rebound effect was found in patients, which were under remission. The rebound was obviously caused by the 5–10-fold increase of DAO activity over the normal values in rectosigmoidal mucosa [234]. Patients with Crohns disease, a disease with segmental inflammation and chronic destruction of ileum and colon, also have significantly (50%) lowered DAO activity [235, 236]. In contrast, in a case of congenital inflammatory bowel disease and intestinal epithelial immaturity with fatal, intractable diarrhea, a mucosal polyamine deficiency was noticed [237]. It remains to be clarified whether the alterations in DAO activity and the consequent changes in polyamine metabolism are primary or secondary phenomena, and to what extent the inflammatory processes are polyamine-related.

The rapid proliferation and differentiation of mucosal cells of the gastrointestinal tract generates a high demand for polyamines. The gastrointestinal tract and intestinal inflammatory processes are, therefore, a case of especial interest to polyamine-directed research of pathophysiological mechanisms.

7   Polyamine derivatives, homologs and analogs

Although this review is devoted to immunological aspects of the natural polyamines, it seems nevertheless justified to consider some structural analogs and derivatives as well, especially since these may indicate new lines for the development of drugs.

For example, not only inhibitors of polyamine biosynthetic enzymes, but also the bis-acetyl derivative of putrescine and of its homolog, 1,6-hexanediamine, cause inhibition of c-myc oncogene expression in IgM-activated human B-lymphocytes [238], as well as the proliferation and Ig secretion of LPS-stimulated spleen B cells [239]. The bis-acetyl derivatives of putrescine and 1,6-hexanediamine are known to induce differentiation, and prevent growth in many types of cells by unknown mechanisms [240].

Spermidine and spermine regulate the biosynthetic decarboxylases ODC and AdoMetDC by several mechanisms [1, 3, 5, 8]. It was expected that derivatives which are capable of mimicking these and related effects of the natural polyamines, but do not support growth, may turn out to be useful in cancer therapy. N^1,N^{12}-Bis(ethyl)spermine is the most important example of this type of polyamine derivative with antiproliferative properties [241]. The compound was shown subsequently to exhibit a number of spermine-like functions [242], among which the support of globin and ODC synthesis in a cell-free system, the recovery of growth of polyamine-deficient bovine suprapharyngeal lymphocytes, and the amelioration of stress-induced gastric ulceration are most important within our context. N^1,N^{12}-Bis(ethyl)spermine is not undergoing oxidative deamination by SAO and DAO. This is presumably the reason for the fact that it is less toxic than spermine. This type of derivative has, therefore, a chance to become therapeutically useful.

Norspermidine (N-(3-aminopropyl)-1,3-propanediamine), a natural homolog of spermidine, was found to inhibit LPS-induced Ig production by splenic B lymphocytes [243]. It was excluded in these experiments that the oxidative deamination of norspermidine played a role. The most likely explanation for these results is the above-mentioned down-regulation of ODC and AdoMetDC by polyamines and structural analogs.

Singh et al. [244] studied the capability of lower (1,2-ethanediamine, 1,3-propanediamine) and higher homologs (1,5-pentanediamine (cadaverine), 1,6-hexanediamine) of putrescine (1,4-butanediamine) to prevent DFMO-mediated immune responses, including lymphocyte proliferation in response to T-cell mitogen (concanavalin A), B-cell mitogen (LPS) and alloantigen stimulation. Only putrescine and the homologs with a shorter carbon chain were effective in preventing the inhibitory effect of DFMO on normal immune response. In contrast, only putrescine and its higher homologs prevented DFMO-mediated inhibition of tumor cell growth. These observations are analogous to the above-mentioned differential effects of N^1,N^{12}-bis(ethyl)spermine on the growth of tumor cells [241, 245], and on polyamine-depleted lymphocytes [242]. Thus, it appears that the possibility exists to sustain normal immune response, and nevertheless inhibit tumor growth, if DFMO (or other inactivators of the biosynthetic enzymes) are combined with a suitable polyamine analog.

N^1,N^7-Bis[3-(ethylamino)-propyl]-1,7-heptanediamine, a higher homolog of N^1,N^{12}-bis(ethyl)spermine shows tumoricidal activity at concentrations which do not significantly deplete intracellular polyamine concentrations [246]. The most striking effect of this compound is, however, its ability to induce resistance to injected L1210 leukemia cells in mice which had been cured by this drug of L1210 leukemia [247]. From the available experimental data it appears that T cell-mediated immunity plays a pivotal role in the mechanism by which this synthetic polyamine analog prevents neoplastic growth. This is supported by the fact that in T cell-deficient nude mice the compound was not curative.

8   Conclusions

As was shown in this review, an impressive body of evidence suggests that the natural polyamines are in many ways involved in the complex phenomena related to host defense mechanisms. This is not surprising, since the polyamines participate in macromolecular syntheses, in the structural organization of numerous cell components, and they modulate and regulate the activity of enzymes. These processes are also the general basis for the functioning of the immune system. The difficulty to pinpoint polyamine functions is not due to their relative unimportance within the cellular machinery, but due to their numerous contributions to functions at many levels of cell biology.

Most of our knowledge on polyamine functions in immunocompetent cells were generated by addition of exogenous polyamines to cultured cells, and more frequently by depleting endogenous polyamine stores, using an inhibitor of ODC or AdoMetDC, mostly DFMO, and MGBG. While MGBG has severe side effects, DFMO turned out to be an excellent tool *in vitro,* owing to its selectivity and absence of toxicity. The use of pure cell populations, the careful control of the polyamine contents in cells, and culture medium, as well as the controlled depletion of putrescine and spermidine will further improve the relevance of the results obtained with DFMO. A limitation of this drug: intracellular spermine concentrations are usually not decreased by ODC inhibition, but may be increased, i.e. the observations reflect only functional changes of the cells at reduced putrescine and spermidine, but at normal or enhanced spermine concentrations.

Polyamine depletion by ODC inhibition is limited in addition *in vivo,* because spermidine depletion in most cells, even at large doses of DFMO, is modest. This is due to the difficulty to maintain constant levels of DFMO in the circulation, the high turnover rate of ODC, its induction in situations of spermidine depletion, and due to the enhanced uptake of environmental polyamines by the polyamine-depleted cells. In spite of these difficulties, inactivation of ODC was able to generate significant clinical improvements in models of autoimmune diseases [161, 209, 216–218], indicating the possibility that autoimmune diseases may become a promising target for improved *in vivo* methods of polyamine depletion.

In recent years potent and selective inactivators of AdoMetDC have become available, which are useful for the *in vivo* blockade of spermidine and spermine synthesis [248, 249]. Since these compounds preferentially deplete spermine, but cause an increase of intracellular putrescine concentrations due to induction of ODC, the functional alterations of immunocompetent cells in comparison with tumor cells could be studied under new conditions of polyamine depletion. New and unexpected insights into polyamine-related cellular functions can be expected from this work. Combined administration of ODC and AdoMetDC inhibitors, or of inhibitors of other biosynthetic enzymes of polyamine metabolism [8], as well as the N-alkylated polyamines and their homologs, mentioned in a previous section [244–246] should offer interesting tools suited for the more precise exploration of polyamine functions in immune system-related processes, but may also open new ways for therapy.

As a general theme, a deleterious effect of extracellular polyamines, especially of spermine, which is more toxic than putrescine and spermidine [12], emerges from a variety of observations in autoimmune diseases and neoplasms. Toxic effects may be produced by spermine itself, or by the toxic reaction products after oxidative deaminations of putrescine, spermidine and spermine.

Owing to its strong binding to anionic sites, spermine is under physiological conditions less likely to be released by cells than putrescine or spermidine. Its proportion in blood [88] and urine [250] is correspondingly low. However, excessive amounts of spermine are released by dying cells of tumors. If this spermine is not metabolized to non-toxic products at a sufficiently high rate, it may gradually initiate pathophysiological mechanisms.

ODC inhibitors showed a significant but limited therapeutic efficacy in models of autoimmune diseases. One reason is perhaps the relative accumulation of spermine in cells responding to ODC inhibition, which in turn is a reason for the enhanced release of this toxic amine. An animal model seems to support this notion. Long-term administrations of DFMO or of the PAO inhibitor MDL 72,527 alone are apparently not toxic. However, administration of these two drugs to normal, and even more to tumor-bearing mice, causes the dramatic accumulation of spermine in red blood cells and plasma, and lethal toxicity develops [251]. That the accumulation of spermine plays a role in this model is evident from the fact that the interruption of the treatment with the PAO inhibitor for one or two days per week diminishes spermine accumulation and prevents the development of lethal toxicity.

The new AdoMetDC inhibitors, or their combinations with ODC inhibitors, are presumably better suited as drugs for the depletion of extracellular polyamines in autoimmune diseases than ODC inhibitors. Since inactivation of AdoMetDC depletes intracellular spermine stores, but enhances putrescine concentrations [248, 249], the amount of spermine released into the circulation by unhealthy cells is expected to be decreased, while the less toxic putrescine and spermidine will be released instead.

In spite of undoubted importance, some areas of potential interest have only been touched, and others were entirely neglected by current research. For example, there is an obvious lack of insight into polyamine function in inflammation. The presumed role of the polyamines in gut mucosal immune reactions with IgA secretion has not been studied at all, although it is known that DFMO suppresses DNA synthesis in colonic lamina lymphocytes [51]. Additional evidence is necessary to confirm the contribution of the natural polyamines as factors, which modulate, and especially which increase the immunogenicity of proteins and peptides. We consider cationization of proteins by the natural polyamines as an area of future research of pivotal importance.

The vast majority of the reports on polyamine function in immune reactions are merely descriptive and concerned with isolated aspects. What is needed. is a systematic analysis of the interplay of the polyamines at various cellular and subcellular levels with the major elements of the immune system. This should permit to elucidate the functions of polyamine metabolism in immune homeostasis of the living organisms. New and unexpected treatment strategies for malignant and immune-related pathological processes are likely to emerge from such studies.

9 Acknowledgements

We are grateful to Dr. Marc H.V. Van Regenmortel (UPR 9021, Immunochimie des Peptides et des Virus, IBMC du CNRS, Strasbourg, France) and to Dr. Gérard Rebel (Centre de Neurochimie, CNRS, Strasbourg, France) for constructive criticism of the manuscript.

10   Non-standard abbreviations

AdoMetDC	S-Adenosyl-L-methionine decarboxylase
DAO	Diamine oxidase
DFMO	α-Difluoromethylornithine (ODC inhibitor)
IFN	Interferon
Ig	Immmunoglobulin
IL	Interleukin
LPS	Bacterial lipopolysaccharide
MAP	(2R,5R)-6-heptyne-2,5-diamine (ODC inhibitor)
MGBG	Methylglyoxal-bis(guanylhydrazone) (AdoMetDC inhibitor)
ODC	Ornithine decarboxylase
PAO	Polyamine oxidase
SAO	Serum amine oxidase
TNF	Tumor necrosis factor
TPA	12-O-tetradecanoylphorbol-13 acetate (tumor promotor)

References

1   Pegg, A.E.: Recent advances in the biochemistry of polyamines in eukaryotes. Biochem. J. *234*, 249–262 (1986).

2   Seiler, N.: Functions of polyamine acetylation. Can. J. Physiol. Pharmacol. *65*, 2024–2035 (1987).

3   Seiler, N. and Heby O.: Regulation of cellular polyamines in mammals. Acta Biochim. Biophys. Hung. *23*, 1–36 (1988).

4   Bachrach, U. and Heimer, Y.M. (eds.): The Physiology of Polyamines. Two volumes. CRC Press, Boca Raton (1989).

5   Heby, O. and Persson, L.: Molecular genetics of polyamine synthesis in eukaryotic cells. TIBS *15*, 153–158 (1990).

6   Seiler, N.: Polyamine metabolism. Digestion *46* (Suppl. 2), 319–330 (1990).

7   Seiler, N. and Dezeure, F.: Polyamine transport in mammalian cells. Int. J. Biochem. *22*, 211–218 (1990).

8   Pegg, A.E.: Polyamine metabolism and its importance in neoplastic growth and as a target for chemotherapy. Cancer Res. *48*, 759–774 (1988).

9   Schuber, F.: Influence of polyamines on membrane functions. Biochem. J. *260*, 1–10 (1989).

10   Jänne, J., Alhonen, L., and Leinonen, P.: Polyamines: from molecular biology to clinical applications. Ann. Med. *23*, 241–259 (1991).

11   Scalabrino, G., Lorenzini, E.C., and Ferioli, M.E.: Polyamines and mammalian hormones. Part I: Biosynthesis, interconversion and hormone effects. Mol. Cell. Endocrinol. *77*, 1–35 (1991); and Scalabrino, G., and Lorenzini, E.C.: Polyamines and

mammalian hormones. Part II: Paracrine signals and intracellular regulators. Mol. Cell. Endocrinol. 77, 7–56 (1991).

12   Seiler, N.: Pharmacological próperties of the natural polyamines and their depletion by biosynthesis inhibitors as a therapeutic approach. Progr. Drug. Res. 37, 107–159 (1991).

13   Gilad, G.M., and Gilad, V.H.: Polyamines in neurotrauma. Ubiquitous molecules in search of a function. Biochem. Pharmacol. 44, 401–407 (1992).

14   Paschen, W.: Polyamine metabolism in different pathological states of the brain. Mol. Chem. Neuropathol. 16, 241–271 (1992).

15   Bardocz, S., Grant, G., Brown, D.S., Ralph, A. and Pusztai, A.: Polyamines in food. Implications for growth and health. J. Nutr. Biochem. 4, 66–71 (1993).

16   Matthews, H.R.: Polyamines, chromatin structure and transcription. BioEssays 15, 561–566 (1993).

17   Theoharides, T.C.: Polyamines spermidine and spermine as modulators of calcium dependent immune processes. Life Sci. 27, 703–713 (1980).

18   Alberts, B., Bray, D., Lewis, J., Raff, M., Roberts, K. and Watson, D.: The immune system. In: Molecular Biology of the Cell, pp. 952–1012, Garland Publishing Inc., New York (1983).

19   Roitt, I.M., Brostoff, J., and Male, D.K.: Immunology, Gower Medical Publishing Ltd., London (1985).

20   Paul, W.E. (ed.): Fundamental Immunology, 2nd ed., Raven Press, N.Y. (1989).

21   Klein, J.: Immunology, Blackwell, London (1991).

22   Seiler, N.: Polyamine catabolism and elimination in the vertebrate organism. In: Polyamines in the Gastrointestinal Tract (Dowling, R.H., Fölsch, U.R. and Löser, Chr., eds.), pp. 65–85, Kluwer, Dordrecht (1992).

23   Porter, C. and Sufrin, J.R.: Interference with polyamine biosynthesis and/or function by analogs of polyamines or methionine as a potential anticancer chemotherapeutic strategy. Anticancer Res. 6, 525–542 (1986).

24   McCann, P., Pegg, A.E. and Sjoerdsma, A. (eds.): Inhibition of Polyamine Metabolism. Academic Press, Orlando (1987).

25   Schechter, P.J., Barlow, J.L.R. and Sjoerdsma, A.: Clinical aspects of inhibition of ornithine decarboxylase with emphasis on therapeutic trials of Eflornithine (DFMO) in cancer and protozoan diseases. In: Inhibition of Polyamine Metabolism (McCann. P.P., Pegg, A.E. and Sjoerdsma, A., eds.), pp. 345–364, Academic Press, Orlando (1987).

26   Bey, P., Danzin, C. and Jung, M.: Inhibition of basic amino acid decarboxylases involved in polyamine biosynthesis. In: Inhibition of Polyamine Metabolism (McCann, P.P., Pegg, A.E. and Sjoerdsma, A., eds.), pp. 1–31, Academic Press, Orlando (1987).

27   Poulin, R., Lu, L., Ackermann, B., Bey, B. and Pegg, A.E.: Mechanism of irreversible inactivation of ornithine decarboxylase by α-difluoromethylornithine. J. Biol. Chem. 267, 150–158 (1992).

28   Rudkin, B.B., Mamont, P.S. and Seiler, N.: Decreased protein-synthetic activity is an early consequence of spermidine depletion in rat hepatoma tissue culture cells. Biochem. J. 217, 731–741 (1984).

29   Ackermann, D. and Wasmuth, W.: Zur Wirkungsweise des Histamins. Hoppe-Seyler's Z. Physiol. Chem. 259, 28–31 (1939).

30   Jadassohn, W., Fierz, H.E. and Vollenweider, H.: Untersuchungen über die Hemmung

der durch Histamin bewirkten Kontraktion und der anaphylaktischen Reaktion durch Iminokörper. Helv. Chim. Acta 27, 1384–1406 (1944).

31   Kovacs, A. and Juhasz, E.: Antihistaminic effects of suspended leukocytes, especially of eosinophils. Arch. Int. Pharmacodyn. 88, 383–392 (1952).

32   Amann, R. and Werle, E.: Über Komplexe von Heparin mit Histamin und anderen Di- und Polyaminen. Klin. Wschr. 34, 207–209 (1956).

33   Mamont, P.S., Duchesne, M.C., Joder-Ohlenbusch, A.M. and Grove, J.: Effects of ornithine decarboxylase inhibitors on cultured cells. In: Enzyme-Activated Irreversible Inhibitors (Seiler, N., Jung, M.J. and Koch-Weser, J., eds.), pp. 43–54. Elsevier/North-Holland Biomedical Press, Amsterdam (1978).

34   Seiler, N., Danzin, C., Prakash, N.J. and Koch-Weser, J.: Effects of ornithine decarboxylase inhibitors in vivo. In: Enzyme-Activated Irreversible Inhibitors (Seiler, N., Jung, M.J. and Koch-Weser, J., eds.), pp. 55–71. Elsevier/North-Holland Biomedical Press, Amsterdam (1978).

35   Ito, K. and Igarashi, K.: Polyamine regulation of the synthesis of thymidine kinase in bovine lymphocytes. Arch. Biochem. Biophys. 278, 277–283 (1990).

36   Netzker, R., Greiner, E., Eigenbrodt, E., Noguchi, T., Tanaka, T. and Brand, K.: Cell cycle-associated expression of M2-type isozyme of pyruvate kinase in proliferating rat thymocytes. J. Biol. Chem. 267, 6421–6424 (1992).

37   DeBenedette, M. and Snow, E.C.: Induction and regulation of casein kinase II during B lymphocyte activation. J. Immunol. 147, 2839–2845 (1991).

38   Colombatto, S., Fasulo, L., Fulgosi, B. and Grillo, M.A.: Regulation of lymphocyte carbohydrate metabolism by polyamines. Ital. J. Biochem. 38, 306A–307A (1989).

39   Bachrach, U., Menashe, M., Faber, J., Desser, H. and Seiler, N.: Polyamine biosynthesis and metabolism in transformed human lymphocytes. In: Advances in Polyamine Research (Caldarera, C.M., Zappia, V. and Bachrach, U., eds.), pp. 259–274, Raven Press, New York (1981).

40   Mustelin, T., Pessa, T., Lapinjoki. S., Gynther, J., Järvinen, T., Eloranta, T. and Andersson, L.C.: Two phases of ornithine decarboxylase activation during lymphocyte mitogenesis. In: Progress in Polyamine Research (Zappia, V. and Pegg, A.E., eds.) pp. 301–313, Plenum Press, New York (1988).

41   Scott, I.G., Pösö, H., Akerman, K.E.O. and Andersson, L.C.: Mitogens cause a rapid induction of ornithine decarboxylase activity in human T lymphocytes. Biochem. Soc. Trans. 13, 934–935 (1984).

42   Scott, I.G., Pösö, H., Akerman, K.E.O. and Andersson, L.C.: Rapid activation of ornithine decarboxylase activity by mitogenic (but not non-mitogenic) ligands to human T-lymphocytes. Eur. J. Immunol. 15, 783–787 (1985).

43   Kay, J.E. and Lindsay, V.J.: Polyamine synthesis during lymphocyte activation. Exp. Cell. Res. 77, 428–435 (1973).

44   Klimpel, G.R., Byus, C.V., Russell, D.H. and Lucas, D.O.: Cyclic AMP-dependent protein kinase activation and the induction of ornithine decarboxylase during lymphocyte mitogenesis. J. Immunol. 123, 817–824 (1979).

45   Kaczmarek, L. and Kaminska, B.: Molecular biology of cell activation. Exp. Cell Res. 183, 24–35 (1989).

46   Fillingame, R.H., Jorstad, C.M. and Morris, D.R.: Increased cellular levels of spermidine or spermine are required for optimal DNA synthesis in lymphocytes activated by concanavalin A. Proc. Natl. Acad. Sci. USA 72, 4042–4045 (1975).

47   DeBenedette, M., Olson, J.W. and Snow, E.C.: Expression of polyamine transporter activity during B lymphocyte cell cycle progression. J. Immunol. *150*, 4218–4224 (1993).

48   Seyfried, C.E. and Morris, D.R.: Relationship between inhibition of polyamine biosynthesis and DNA replication in activated lymphocytes. Cancer Res. *39*, 4861–4867 (1979).

49   Hölttä, E., Jänne, J. and Hovi, T.: Suppression of the formation of polyamines and macromolecules by D,L-α-difluoromethylornithine and methylglyoxal-bis(guanylhydrazone) in phytohemagglutinin-activated human lymphocytes. Biochem. J. *178*, 109–117 (1979).

50   Hölttä, E.: Polyamine requirement for polyribosome formation and protein synthesis in human lymphocytes. In: Recent Progress in Polyamine Research (Selmeci, L., Brosnan, M.E. and Seiler, N., eds.), pp. 137–150, Akademiai Kiado, Budapest (1985).

51   Elitsur, Y., Strom, J. and Luk, G.D.: Inhibition of ornithine decarboxylase activity decreases polyamines and suppresses DNA synthesis in human colonic *lamina propria* lymphocytes. Immunopharmacol. *25*, 253–260 (1993).

52   Sakamaki, Y., Terao, K., Ito, E., Kashiwagi, K. and Igarashi, K.: Swelling of the Golgi apparatus and decrease of galactosyltransferase in polyamine-deficient bovine lymphocytes and epithelium of mouse small intestine. Biochem. Pharmacol. *38*, 1083–1089 (1989).

53   Kay, J.E. and Pegg, A.E.: Effect of inhibition of spermidine formation on protein and nucleic acid synthesis during lymphocyte activation. FEBS Lett. *29*, 301–304 (1973).

54   Abdel-Monem, M.M., Newton, N.E. and Weeks, C.E.: Inhibitors of polyamine biosynthesis. 1. Alpha-methyl-(plus or minus)-ornithine, an inhibitor of ornithine decarboxylase. J. Med. Chem. *17*, 447–451 (1974).

55   Thomas, T.G., Gunnia, U.B., Yurkow, E.J., Seibold, J.R. and Thomas, T.J: Inhibition of calcium signalling in murine splenocytes by polyamines: differential effects on CD4 and CD8 T-cells. Biochem. J. *291*, 375–381 (1993).

56   Keightley, R.G., Cooper, M.D. and Lawton, A.R.: The T cell dependence of B cell differentiation induced by pokeweed mitogen. J. Immunol. *117*, 1538–1544 (1976).

57   Pollok, K.E., O'Brien, V., Marshall, L., Olson, J.W., Noelle, R.J. and Snow, E.C.: The development of competence in resting B cells. The induction of cyclic AMP and ornithine decarboxylase activity after direct contact between B and T helper cells. J. Immunol. *146*, 1633–1641 (1991).

58   Pasquali, J.L., Urlacher, A., Weryha, A., Storck, D. and Mamont, P.S.: Inhibition by D,L-α-difluoromethylornithine of the pokeweed mitogen-induced immunoglobulin production in cultured human lymphocytes. Immunopharmacol. *7*, 145–149 (1984).

59   Pasquali, J.L., Mamont, P.S., Weryha, A.M., Blervaque, A. and Siat, M.: Immunosuppressive effects of (2R,5R)-6-heptyne-2,5-diamine, an inhibitor of polyamine synthesis I. Effects on mitogen-induced immunoglobulin production in human cultured lymphocytes. Clin. Exp. Immunol. *72*, 141–144 (1988).

60   Nesher, G. and Moore, T.L.: The *in vitro* effects of methotrexate on peripheral blood mononuclear cells. Modulation by methyl donors and spermidine. Arthritis Rheum. *33*, 954–959 (1990).

61   Schuman, L.D., Baxter, C.S. and Petro, T.M.: Effect of the ornithine decarboxylase inhibitor, alpha-difluoromethylornithine on phorbol diester-induced inhibition of murine B lymphocyte differentiation. Cancer Lett. *47*, 11–19 (1989).

62   Aman, P., Oredsson, S.M. and Heby, O.: Inhibition of polyamine synthesis in human B lymphocytes during primary infection with Epstein-Barr virus (EBV) blocks cellular DNA synthesis but not the expression of EBV-encoded nuclear antigens (EBNA). Biochem. Biophys. Res. Commun. *159*, 945–952 (1989).

63   Altman, A., Coggeshall, K.M. and Mustelin, T.: Molecular events mediating T cell activation. Adv. Immunol. *48*, 227–360 (1990).

64   Brüne, B., Hartzell, P., Nicotera, P. and Orrenius, S.: Spermine prevents endonuclease activation and apoptosis in thymocytes. Exp. Cell Res. *195*, 323–329 (1991).

65   Schwartz, L.M. and Osborne, B.A.: Programmed cell death, apoptosis and killer genes. Immunol. Today *14*, 582–590 (1993).

66   Fesüs, L., Thomazy, V. and Falus, A.: Induction and activation of tissue transglutaminase during programmed cell death. FEBS Lett. *224*, 104–108 (1987).

67   Parchment, R.E.: The implications of a unified theory of programmed cell death, polyamines, oxyradicals and histogenesis in the embryo. Int. J. Dev. Biol. *37*, 75–83 (1993).

68   Grassilli, E., Bettuzzi, S., Monti, D., Ingletti, M.C., Franceschi, C. and Corti, A.: Studies on the relationship between cell proliferation and cell death: opposite patterns of SGP-2 and ornithine decarboxylase mRNA accumulation in PHA-stimulated human lymphocytes. Biochem. Biophys. Res. Commun. *180*, 59–63 (1991).

69   Häcker-Shahin, B. and Dröge, W.: Putrescine and its biosynthetic precursor L-ornithine augment the *in vivo* immunization against minor histocompatibility antigens and syngeneic tumors. Cell. Immunol. *99*, 434–443 (1986).

70   Allen, J.C., Smith, C.J., Hussain, J.I., Thomas, J.M. and Gaugas, J.M.: Inhibition of lymphocyte proliferation by polyamines requires ruminant plasma polyamine oxidase. Eur. J. Biochem. *102*, 153–158 (1979).

71   Novogrodsky, A., Quittner, S.. Rubin, A.L. and Stenzel, K.H.: Transglutaminase activity in human lymphocytes: early activation by phytomitogens. Proc. Natl. Acad. Sci. USA *75*, 1157–1161 (1978).

72   Folk, J.E., Park, M.H., Il Chung, S., Schrode, J., Lester, E.P. and Cooper, H.L.: Polyamines as physiological substrates for transglutaminases. J. Biol. Chem. *255*, 3695–3700 (1980).

73   Bowlin, T.L., McKown, B.J. and Sunkara, P.S.: Increased ornithine decarboxylase activity and polyamine biosynthesis are required for optimal cytolytic T lymphocyte induction. Cell. Immunol. *105*, 110–117 (1987).

74   Bowlin, T.L., Davis, G.F. and McKown, B.J.: Inhibition of alloantigen-induced cytolytic T lymphocytes *in vitro* with (2R,5R)-6-heptyne-2,5-diamine, an irreversible inhibitor of ornithine decarboxylase. Cell. Immunol. *111*, 443–450 (1988).

75   Schall, R.P., Sekar, J., Tandon, P.M. and Susskind, B.M.: Difluoromethylornithine (DFMO) arrests murine CTL development in the late pre-effector stage. Immunopharmacology *21*, 129–143 (1991).

76   Bowlin, T.L., Rosenberger, A.L. and McKown, B.J.: Alpha-difluoromethylornithine, an inhibitor of polyamine biosynthesis, augments cyclosporin A inhibition of cytolytic T lymphocyte induction. Clin. Exp. Immunol. *77*, 151–156 (1989).

77   Campbell, R.A., Kurtz, G.L., Bartos, F. and Bartos, D.: Allograft prolongation with polyamine enzyme-inhibitor, RMI 71.782A. Kidney Int. *19*, 264 (1981).

78   Ehrke, M.J., Porter, D.W., Eppolito, C. and Mihich, E.: Selective modulation by

α-difluoromethylornithine of T lymphocyte and antibody-mediated cytotoxic responses to mouse tumor allografts. Cancer Res. 46, 2798–2803 (1986).

79   Thomas, T.J., Gunnia, U.B. and Thomas, T.: Reversal of the abnormal development of T cell subpopulations in the thymus of autoimmune MRL-lpr/lpr mice by a polyamine biosynthesis inhibitor. Autoimmunity 13, 275–283 (1992).

80   Dröge, W., Männel, D., Falk, W., Lehmann, V., Schmidt, H., Nick, B., Häcker-Shahin, B. and Jänicke, R.: Suppression of cytotoxic T lymphocyte activation by L-ornithine. J. Immunol. 134, 3379–3383 (1985).

81   Susskind, B.M. and Chandrasekaran, J.: Inhibition of cytolytic T lymphocyte maturation with ornithine, arginine and putrescine. J. Immunol. 139, 905–912 (1987).

82   Daune-Anglard, G., Bonaventure, N. and Seiler, N.: Some biochemical and pathophysiological aspects of long-term elevation of brain ornithine concentrations. Pharmacol. Toxicol. 73, 29–34 (1993).

83   Sarhan, S., Knödgen, B. and Seiler, N.: The gastrointestinal tract as polyamine source for tumor growth. Anticancer Res. 9, 215–224 (1989).

84   Hessels, J., Kingma, A.W., Ferwerda, H., Keij, J., van den Berg, G.A. and Muskiet, F.J.: Microbial flora in the gastrointestinal tract abolishes cytostatic effects of α-difluoromethyl ornithine in vivo. Int. J. Cancer 43, 1155–1164 (1989).

85   Hessels, J., Kingma, A.W., Muskiet, F.A.J., Sarhan, S. and Seiler, N.: Growth inhibition of solid tumors in mice, caused by polyamine depletion, is not attended by alterations in cell-cycle phase distribution. Int. J. Cancer 48, 697–703 (1991).

86   Chamaillard, L., Quemener, V., Havouis, R. and Moulinoux, J.P.: Polyamine depletion stimulates natural killer cell activity in cancerous mice. Anticancer Res. 13, 1027–1033 (1993).

87   Bowlin, T.L., Rosenberger, A.L., McKown, B.J., Davis, G.F. and Sunkara, P.S.: The effect of alpha-difluoromethylornithine on natural killer cell and tumoricidal macrophage indution by interferon in vivo. Int. J. Immunopharmac. 8, 131–136 (1986).

88   Moulinoux, J.Ph., Quemener, V. and Khan, N.A.: Biological significance of circulating polyamines in oncology. Cell. Mol. Biol. 37, 773–783 (1991).

89   Dempsey, W.L., Hwu, P., Russell, D.H. and Morahan, P.S.: Bone marrow macrophages have polyamine and ectoenzyme phenotypes distinct from resident macrophages. Life Sci. 42, 2019–2027 (1988).

90   Segal, A.W. and Abo, A.: The biochemical basis of the NADPH oxidase of phagocytes. TIBS 18, 43–47 (1993).

91   Messina, L., Arcidiacono, A., Spampinato, G., Malaguarnera, L., Berton, G., Kaczmarek, L. and Messina, A.: Accumulation of ornithine decarboxylase mRNA accompanies activation of human and mouse monocytes/macrophages. FEBS Lett. 268, 32–34 (1990).

92   Messina, L., Spampinato, G., Arcidiacono, A., Malaguarnera, L., Pagano, M., Kaminska, B., Kaczmarek, L. and Messina, A.: Polyamine involvement in functional activation of human macrophages. J. Leukocyte Biol. 52, 585–587 (1992).

93   Taffet, S.M. and Haddox, M.K.: Bacterial lipopolysaccharide induction of ornithine decarboxylase in the macrophage-like cell line RAW 264: requirement of an inducible factor. J. Cell. Physiol. 122, 215–220 (1985).

94   Kierszenbaum, F., Wirth, J.J., McCann, P.P. and Sjoerdsma, A.: Impairment of macrophage function by inhibitors of ornithine decarboxylase activity. Infect. Immun. 55, 2461–2464 (1987).

95   Prosser, F.H. and Wahl, L.M.: Involvement of ornithine decarboxylase in macrophage collagenase production. Arch. Biochem. Biophys. *160*, 218–225 (1988).

96   Kaczmarek, L., Kaminska, B., Messina, L., Spampinato, G., Arcidiacono, A., Malaguernera, L., and Messina, A.: Inhibitors of polyamine biosynthesis block tumor necrosis factor-induced activation of macrophages. Cancer Res. *52*, 1891–1894 (1992).

97   Walters, J.D., Sorboro, D.M. and Chapman, K.J.: Polyamines enhance calcium mobilization in fMet-Leu-Phe-stimulated phagocytes. FEBS Lett. *304*, 37–40 (1992).

98   Flescher, E., Fossum, D. and Talal, N.: Polyamine-dependent production of lymphocytotoxic levels of ammonia by human peripheral blood monocytes. Immunol. Lett. *28*, 85–90 (1991).

99   Mozhenok, T.P., Bulychev, A.G. and Braun, A.D.: The effect of polyamines on lysosome fusion with phagosomes in mouse peritoneal macrophages. Tsitologia *32*, 882–887 (1990).

100   Bowlin, T.L., McKown, B.J., Davis, G.F. and Sunkara, P.S.: Effect of polyamine depletion *in vivo* by DL-alpha-difluoromethylornithine on functionally distinct populations of tumoricidal effector cells in normal and tumor-bearing mice. Cancer Res. *46*, 5494–5498 (1986).

101   Bowlin, T.L., Rosenberger, A.L. and Sunkara, P.S.: The effect of combination treatment with alpha-difluoromethylornithine and *Corynebacterium parvum* on B16 melanoma growth and tumoricidal effector cell generation *in vivo*. Cancer Immunol. Immunother. *20*, 214–218 (1985).

102   Bowlin, T.L., Hoeper, B.J., Rosenberger, A.L., Davis, G.F. and Sunkara, P.S.: Effects of three irreversible inhibitors of ornithine decarboxylase on macrophage-mediated tumoricidal activity and antitumor activity in B16F1 tumor-bearing mice. Cancer Res. *50*, 4510–4514 (1990).

103   Seiler, N., Sarhan, S. and Roth-Schechter, B.F.: Polyamines and the development of isolated neurons in cell culture. Neurochem. Res. *9*, 871–886 (1984).

104   Quemener, V., Moulinoux, J.P., Khan, N.A. and Seiler, N.: Effects of a series of homologous α,ω-dimethylaminoalkanes on cell proliferation: binding and uptake of putrescine by a human glioblastoma cell line (U251) in culture. Biol. Cell *70*, 133–137 (1991).

105   Mills, C.D., Shearer, J., Evans, R. and Caldwell, M.D.: Macrophage arginine metabolism and the inhibition or stimulation of cancer. J. Immunol. *149*, 2709–2714 (1992).

106   Hayashi, T., Shinki, T., Tanaka, H., Abe, E. and Suda, T.: Polyamines are involved in the 1-alpha,25-dihydroxyvitamin D3-induced fusion of mouse alveolar macrophages. J. Bone Miner. Res. *1*, 235–242 (1986).

107   Abe, E., Miyaura, C., Tanaka, H., Shiina, Y., Kuribayashi, T., Suda, S., Nishii, Y., DeLuca, H.F. and Suda, T.: 1α,25-Dihydroxyvitamin D3 promotes fusion of mouse alveolar macrophages both by a direct mechanism and by a spleen cell-mediated indirect mechanism. Proc. Natl. Acad. Sci. USA *80*, 5583–5587 (1983).

108   Tanaka, H., Shinki, T., Hayashi, T., Jin, C.H., Miyaura, C., Abe, E. and Suda, T.: Spermidine-dependent proteins are involved in the fusion of mouse alveolar macrophages induced by 1-alpha,25-dihydroxyvitamin D3 and interleukin-4. Exp. Cell. Res. *180*, 72–83 (1989).

109   Saunders, N.A., Ilett, K.F. and Minchin, R.F.: Pulmonary alveolar macrophages express a polyamine transport system. J. Cell. Physiol. *139*, 624–631 (1989).

110   Endo, Y., Kikuchi, T., Takeda, Y., Nitta, Y., Rikiishi, H. and Kumagai, K.: GM-CSF

and G-CSF stimulate the synthesis of histamine and putrescine in the hematopoietic organs *in vivo*. Immunol. Lett. *33*, 9–13 (1992).

111 Oppenheim, J.J., Kovacs, E.J., Matsushima, K. and Durum, S.K.: There is more than one interleukin 1. Immunol. Today *7*, 45–56 (1986).

112 Dinarello, C.A.: Biology of Interleukin 1. FASEB J. *2*, 108–115 (1988).

113 Endo, Y., Matsushima, K., Onozaki, K. and Oppenheim, J.J.: Role of ornithine decarboxylase in the regulation of cell growth by IL-1 and tumor necrosis factor. J. Immunol. *141*, 2342–2348 (1988).

114 Tahara, H., Otani, S., Matsui-Yuasa, I., Koyama, H., Nishizawa, Y., Morisawa, S. and Morii, H.: Role of putrescine in interleukin-1 beta production in human histiocytic lymphoma cell line U937. J. Cell. Physiol. *147*, 199–207 (1991).

115 Minami, Y., Kono, T., Miyazaki, T. and Taniguchi, T.: The IL-2 receptor complex: its structure, function and target genes. Annu. Rev. Immunol. *11*, 245–268 (1993).

116 Bowlin, T.L., McKown, B.J. and Sunkara, P.S.: Ornithine decarboxylase induction and polyamine biosynthesis are required for the growth of interleukin-2- and interleukin-3-dependent cell lines. Cell. Immunol. *98*, 341–350 (1986).

117 Bowlin, T.L., McKown, B.J., Babcock, G.F. and Sunkara, P.S.: Intracellular polyamine biosynthesis is required for interleukin-2 responsiveness during lymphocyte mitogenesis. Cell. Immunol. *106*, 260–272 (1987).

118 Bowlin, T.L., McKown, B.J. and Sunkara, P.S.: The effect of α-difluoromethylornithine, an inhibitor of polyamine biosynthesis, on mitogen-induced interleukin-2 production. Immunopharmacology *13*, 143–147 (1987).

119 Yukioka, K., Otani, S., Matsui-Yuasa, I., Shibata, T., Nishizawa, Y., Morii, H. and Morisawa, S.: Polyamine biosynthesis is necessary for interleukin-2-dependent proliferation but not for interleukin-2 production or high-affinity interleukin-2 receptor expression. J. Biochem. *102*, 1469–1476 (1987).

120 Mihm, S., Risso, A., Stohr, M., Oberdorfer, F. and Dröge, W.: Downregulation of T cell growth factor production by ornithine decarboxylase and its product putrescine: D,L-alpha-difluoromethylornithine suppresses general protein synthesis but augments simultaneously the production of interleukin-2. Exp. Cell. Res. *180*, 383–398 (1989).

121 McCarthy, M.A., Michalski, J.P., Sears, E.S. and McCombs, C.C.: Inhibition of polyamine synthesis suppresses human lymphocyte proliferation without decreasing cytokine production or interleukin 2 receptor expression. Immunopharmacology *20*, 11–20 (1990).

122 Sandler, S., Bendtzen, K., Eizirik, D.L., Sjöholm, A. and Welsh, N.: Decreased cell replication and polyamine content in insulin-producing cells after exposure to human interleukin-1β. Immunol. Lett. *22*, 267–272 (1989).

123 Donato, N.J., Rotbein, J. and Rosenblum, M.G.: Tumor necrosis factor stimulates ornithine decarboxylase activity in human fibroblasts and tumor target cells. J. Cell. Biochem. *46*, 69–77 (1991).

124 Manchester, K.M., Heston, W.D. and Donner, D.B.: Tumour necrosis factor-induced cytotoxicity is accompanied by intracellular mitogenic signals in ME-180 human cervical carcinoma cells. Biochem. J. *290*, 185–190 (1993).

125 Reid, K.B.M. and Porter, R.R.: The proteolytic activation systems of complement. Ann. Rev. Biochem. *50*, 433–464 (1981).

126 Lachmann, P.J.: Complement. In: Clinical Aspects of Immunology, 4th edition (Bachmann, P.J. and Peters, K., eds.), pp. 18–49, Blackwell, Oxford (1982).

127   Villiers, C.L., Arlaud, G.J. and Colomb, M.G.: Diamine-induced dissociation of the first component of human complement, C1. Eur. J. Biochem. *140*, 421–426 (1984).

128   Smith, C.J., Maschler, R., Maurer, H.R. and Allen, J.C.: Inhibition of cells in culture by polyamines does not depend on the presence of ruminant serum. Cell Tissue Kinet. *16*, 269–276 (1983).

129   Remacle-Bonnet, M., Culouscou, J.M., Pommier, G., Rance, R. and Depieds, R.: Immunoregulatory activities of human trophoblasts mediated by polyamine complexes. Am. J. Reprod. Immunol. *8*, 55–61 (1985).

130   Quan, C.P. Roux, C., Pillot, J. and Bouvet, J.P.: Delineation between T and B suppressive molecules from human seminal plasma. II. Spermine is the major suppressor of T-lymphocytes *in vitro*. Am. J. Reprod. Immunol. *22*, 64–69 (1990).

131   Vliagoftis, H., Boucher, W.S., Mak, L.L. and Theoharides, T.C.: Inhibition of mast cell secretion by oxidation products of natural polyamines. Biochem. Pharmacol. *43*, 2237–2245 (1992).

132   Talal, N. and Flescher, E.: Rheumatoid arthritis: An editorial perspective based on cytokine imbalance. J. Autoimmunity *1*, 309–317 (1988).

133   Melvin, M.A.L. and Keir, H.M.: Excretion of polyamines from mammalian cells in culture. In: Polyamines in Biomedical Research (Gaugas, J.M., ed.), pp. 363–381, Wiley, Chichester (1980).

134   Morgan, D.M.L., Ferulga, J. and Allison, A.C.: Polyamine oxidase and macrophage function. In: Polyamines in Biomedical Research (Gaugas, J.M., ed.), pp. 303–308, Wiley, Chichester (1980).

135   Flescher, E., Bowlin, T.L. and Talal, N.: Polyamine oxidation downregulates IL-2 production by human peripheral blood mononuclear cells. J. Immunol. *142*, 907–912 (1989).

136   Combe, B., Pope, R.M., Fischbach, M., Darnell, B., Baron, S. and Talal, N.: Interleukin-2 in rheumatoid arthritis: production of and response to interleukin-2 in rheumatoid synovial fluid, synovial tissue and peripheral blood. Clin. Exp. Immunol. *59*, 520–528 (1985).

137   Flescher, E., Bowlin, T.L., Ballester, A., Houk, R. and Talal, N.: Increased polyamine may downregulate Interleukin 2 production in rheumatoid arthritis. J. Clin. Invest. *83*, 1356–1362 (1989).

138   Yukioka, K., Wakitani, S., Yukioka, M., Furumitsu, Y., Shichikawa, K., Ochi, T., Goto, H., Matsui-Yuasa, I., Otani, S., Nishizawa, Y. and Morii, H.: Polyamine levels in synovial tissues and synovial fluids of patients with rheumatoid arthritis. J. Rheumatol. *19*, 689–692 (1992).

139   Ferrante, A., Storer, R.J. and Cleland. L.J.: Polyamine oxidase activity in rheumatoid arthritis synovial fluid. Clin. Exp. Immunol. *80*, 373–375 (1990).

140   Huang, Y.P., Miescher, P.A. and Zubler, R.H.: The interleukin 2 secretion defect *in vitro* in systemic lupus erythematosus is reversible in rested cultured T cells. J. Immunol. *137*, 3515–3520 (1986).

141   Morgan, D.M.L.: Polyamine oxidases. In: Polyamines in Biomedical Research (Gaugas, J.M., ed.), pp. 285–302, Wiley, Chichester (1980).

142   Schuler, W.: Zur Hemmung der Diaminoxydase (Histaminase). Experientia *7*, 230–232 (1952).

143   Seiler, N., Knödgen, B., Bink, G., Sarhan, S. and Bolkenius, F.N.: Diamine oxidase

and polyamine catabolism. In: Advances in Polyamine Research (Bachrach, U., Kaye, A. and Chayen, R., eds.), vol. 4, pp. 135–154, Raven Press, New York (1983).

144 Bolkenius, F.N. and Seiler, N.: Acetylderivatives as intermediates in polyamine catabolism. Int. J. Biochem. *13*, 287–292 (1981).

145 Quash, G. and Jonard, J.: Immunochimie des polyamines. C.R. Acad. Sci. Paris, Serie D, *265*, 934–936 (1967).

146 Jonard, J., Quash, G. and Wahl, R.: La spécificité des anticorps antipolyamines. C.R. Acad. Sc. Paris, Série D, *265*, 1099–1102 (1967).

147 Bartos, F. and Bartos, D.: Antipolyamine antibodies. In: Advances in Polyamine Research (Campbell, R.A., Morris, D.R., Bartos, D., Daves, G.D. and Bartos, F., eds.), Vol. 2, pp. 65–70, Raven Press, New York (1978).

148 Bartos, F., Bartos, D., Campbell, R.A., Grettie, D.P., McDaniel, P., Davis, M. and Smejtek, P.: Purification of rabbit antispermine antiserum by affinity chromatography. Res. Commun. Chem. Pathol. Pharmacol. *23*, 547–559 (1979).

149 Fujiwara, K., Asada, H., Kitagawa, T., Yamamoto, K., Ito, T., Tsuchiya, R., Sohda, M., Nakamura, N., Hara, K., Tomonaga, Y., Ichimaru, M. and Takahashi, S.: Preparation of polyamine antibody and its use in enzyme immunoassay of spermine and spermidine with β-D-galactosidase as a label. J. Immunol. Meth. *61*, 217–226 (1983).

150 Garthwaite, I., Stead, A.D. and Rider, C.C.: A monoclonal antibody-based immunoassay for the polyamines spermine and spermidine. Biochem. Soc. Trans. *17*, 1056–1057 (1989).

151 Schipper, R.G., Jonis, J.A., Rutten, R.G.J., Tesser, G.I. and Verhofstad, A.A.J.: Preparation and characterization of polyclonal and monoclonal antibodies to polyamines. J. Immunol. Meth. *136*, 23–30 (1991).

152 Bartos, F., Bartos, D., Grettie, D.P., Campbell, R.A., Marton, L.J., Smith, R.G. and Daves, G.D. Jr.: Polyamine levels in normal human serum. Comparison of analytical methods. Biochem. Biophys. Res. Commun. *75*, 915–919 (1977).

153 Atanassov, C.L., Delcros, J.G., Muller, S., Quash, G. and Van Regenmortel, M.H.V.: Immunization of rabbits with spermine induces antibodies to self antigens. Int. Arch. Allergy Immunol. *102*, 46–55 (1993).

154 Roch, A.M., Quash, G.A. and Huppert, J.: Mise en évidence dans les sérums humains d'anticorps (IgG) réagissant spécifiquement avec les polyamines. C.R. Acad. Sci. Paris, 287D, 1071–1074 (1978).

155 Furuichi, K., Ezoe, H., Obara, T. and Oka, T.: Evidence for a naturally occurring anti-spermine antibody in normal rabbit serum. Proc. Natl. Acad. Sci. USA *77*, 2904–2908 (1980).

156 Bartos, D., Bartos, F., Campbell, R.A., Grettie, D.P. and Smejtek, P.: Antibody to spermine: a natural biological constituent. Science *208*, 1178–1181 (1980).

157 Quash, G., Delain, E. and Huppert, J.: Effect of antipolyamine antibodies on mammalian cells in tissue culture. Exp. Cell Res. *66*, 426–432 (1971).

158 Feuerstein, B.G. and Marton, L.J.: Specificity and binding in polyamine/nucleic acid interactions. In: The Physiology of Polyamines (Bachrach, U. and Heimer, Y.M., eds.), vol. 1, pp. 109–124, CRC Press, Boca Raton (1988).

159 Schmid, N. and Behr, J.P.: Location of spermine and other polyamines on DNA as revealed by photoaffinity cleavage with polyaminobenzenediazonium salts. Biochemistry *30*, 4357–4361 (1991).

160   Behe, M. and Felsenfeld, G.: Effects of methylation on a synthetic polynucleotide: the B-Z transition in poly(dG-me^{5}dC). Proc. Natl. Acad. Sci. USA 78, 1619–1623 (1981).

161   Thomas, T.J. and Messner, R.P.: Beneficial effects of a polyamine biosynthesis inhibitor on lupus in MRL-lpr/lpr mice. Clin. Exp. Immunol. 78, 239–244 (1989).

162   Gunnia, U.B., Thomas, T. and Thomas, T.J.: The effects of polyamines on the immunogenicity of polynucleotides. Immunol. Invest. 20, 337–350 (1991).

163   Lafer, E.M., Valle, R.P.C., Möller, A., Nordheim, A., Schur, P.H., Rich, A. and Stollar, B.D.: Z-DNA-specific antibodies in human systemic lupus erythematosus. J. Clin. Invest. 71, 314–321 (1983).

164   Baeza, I.R., Abrego, A.R., Aviles, N.P. and Wong, C.: Effect of polyamines on the formation of DNA-immunoglobulin G complexes. Rev. Lat.-Amer. Microbiol. 22, 213–219 (1980).

165   Muckerheide, A., Apple, R.J., Pesce, A.J. and Michael, J.G.: Cationization of protein antigens. I. Alteration of immunogenic properties. J. Immunol. 138, 833–837 (1987).

166   Muckerheide, A., Domen, P.L. and Michael, J.G.: Cationization of protein antigens. II. Alteration of regulatory properties. J. Immunol. 138, 2800–2804 (1987).

167   Muckerheide, A., Pesce, A.J. and Michael, J.G.: Cationization of protein antigens. V. Effect of the degree of cationization on patterns of immune responsiveness. Cell. Immunol. 127, 67–77 (1990).

168   Domen, P.L., Muckerheide, A. and Michael, J.G.: Cationization of protein antigens. III. Abrogation of oral tolerance. J. Immunol. 139, 3195–3198 (1987).

169   Apple, R.J., Domen, P.L., Muckerheide, A. and Michael, J.G.: Cationization of protein antigens. IV. Increased antigen uptake by antigen-presenting cells. J. Immunol. 140, 3290–3295 (1988).

170   Piacentini, M., Cerú-Argento, M.P., Farrace, M.G. and Autuori, F.: Post-translational modifications of cellular proteins by polyamines and polyamine derivatives. In: Advances in Post-Translational Modifications of Proteins and Aging (Zappia, V., Galletti, P., Porta, R. and Wold, F., eds.), pp. 185–197. Plenum, New York (1988).

171   Davies, P.J.A., Chiocca, E.A., Basilion, J.P., Poddar, S. and Stein, J.P.: Transglutaminases and their regulation: Implications for polyamine metabolism. In: Progress in Polyamine Research (V. Zappia and A.E. Pegg. eds.), pp. 391–401. Plenum, New York (1988).

172   Gunzler, V., Schopf, R.E., Hanauske-Abel, H.M. and Schulte-Wissermann, H.: Transglutaminase and polyamine dependence of effector functions of human immunocompetent cells. The effect of specific inhibitors on lymphocyte proliferation and granulocyte chemiluminescence. FEBS Lett. 150, 390–396 (1982).

173   Ientile, R., Merendino, R.A., Fabiano, C., Di Giorgio, R.M. and Macaione, S.: Polyamines are involved in retinoic acid-mediated induction of tissue transglutaminase in human peripheral blood monocytes. Res. Commun. Chem. Pathol. Pharmacol. 77, 313–326 (1992).

174   Chan, W.Y., Seale, T.W., Shukla, J.B. and Rennert, O.M.: Polyamine conjugates and total polyamine concentrations in human amniotic fluid. Clin. Chim. Acta 91, 233–241 (1979).

175   Seale, T.W., Chan, W.Y., Shukla, J.B. and Rennert, O.M.: Isolation and characterization of a polyamine-peptide conjugate from human amniotic fluid. Clin. Chim. Acta 95, 461–472 (1979).

176 Seale, T.W., Chan, W.Y., Shukla, J.B. and Rennert, O.M.: A polyamine-conjugated peptide isolated from human plasma. Arch. Biochem. Biophys. *198*, 164–174 (1979).

177 Roch, A.M., Quash, G.A., Ripoll, H., Vigreux, B. and Niveleau, A.: Protein-bound polyamines and immune complexes containing polyamines in human plasma. Advances in Polyamine Research (Caldarera, C.M., Zappia, V. and Bachrach, U., eds.), Vol. 3, pp. 225–235, Raven Press, New York (1981).

178 Chan, W.Y., Griesmann, G., and Rennert, O.M.: Polyamine derivatives in growing cells. Advances in Polyamine Research (Caldarera, C.M., Zappia, V. and Bachrach, U. eds.) Vol. 3, pp. 213–223, Raven Press, New York.

179 Roch, A.M., Quash, G. and Huppert, J.: Mise en évidence immunochimique de l'attachement spécifique de la putrescine aux proteines plasmatiques dont la fibronectine. C.R. Acad. Sci. Paris 290D, 449–452 (1980).

180 Roch, A.M., Thomas, V., Quash, G., Moulinoux, J.P. and Delcros, J.G.: A quantitative and qualitative study of the transglutaminase-mediated insertion of polyamines into plasma proteins from patients with bronchopulmonary cancer. Int. J. Cancer *33*, 787–793 (1984).

181 Russell, D.H.: Increased polyamine concentrations in the urine of human cancer patients. Nature *233*, 144–145 (1971).

182 Bachrach, U.: Polyamines as markers of malignancy. Progr. Drug. Res. *39*, 9–33 (1992).

183 Rennert, O.M. and Shukla, J.B.: Polyamines in health and disease. In: Advances in Polyamine Research (Campbell, R.A., Morris, D.R., Bartos, D., Daves, G.D. and Bartos, F., eds.), Vol. 2, pp. 195–211, Raven Press, New York (1978).

184 Campbell, R.A., Gretti, D.P., Bartos, D. and Bartos, F.: Clinical polyamine analysis: Problems and promise. In: Advances in Polyamine Research (Caldarera, C.M., Zappia, V. and Bachrach, U., eds.), vol. 3, pp. 409–423, Raven, Press, New York (1981).

185 Puri, H., Campbell, R.A., Puri, V., Harner, M.H., Talwalkar, Y.B., Musgrave, J.E., Bartos, F., Bartos, D. and Loggan, B.: Serum-free polyamines in children with systemic lupus erythematosus. In: Advances in Polyamine Research (Campbell, R.A., Morris, D.R., Bartos, D., Daves, G.D. and Bartos, F., eds.), Vol. 2, pp. 359–367, Raven Press, New York (1978).

186 Furumitsu, Y., Yukioka, K., Kojima, A., Yukioka, M., Shichikawa, K., Ochi, T., Matsui-Yuasa, I., Otani, S., Nishizawa, Y., and Morii, H.: Levels of urinary polyamines in patients with rheumatoid arthritis. J. Rheumatol. *20*, 1661–1665 (1993).

187 Marton, L.J., Edwards, M.S., Levin, V.A., Lubich, W.P. and Wilson, C.B.: CSF polyamines: a new and important means of monitoring patients with medulloblastoma. Cancer *47*, 757–760 (1981).

188 Carrier, M., Copeland, J.G., Russell, D.H., Perrotta, N.J., Davis, T.P. and Emery, R.W.: Urinary polyamines are non-invasive markers of heart allograft rejection. J. Heart Transplant. *6*, 286–289 (1987).

189 Carrier, M., Russell, D.H., Davis, T.P., Emery, R.W. and Copeland, J.G.: Value of urinary polyamines as non-invasive markers of cardiac rejection in the dog. Ann. Thorac. Surg. *45*, 158–163 (1988).

190 Womble, J.R., Larson, D.F., Copeland, J.G. and Russell, D.H.: Urinary polyamine levels are markers of altered T lymphocyte proliferation/loss and rejection in heart transplant patients. Transplant Proc. *16*, 1573–1575 (1984).

191 Proctor, M.S., Fletcher, H.V., Jr., Shukla, J.B. and Rennert, O.M.: Elevated spermidine

and spermine levels in the blood of psoriasis patients. J. Invest. Dermatol. *65*, 409–411 (1975).

192   Thomas, T. and Kiang, D.T.: Structural alterations and stabilization of rabbit uterine estrogen receptor by natural polyamines. Cancer Res. *47*, 1799–1804 (1987).

193   Schalkwijk, J., van den Berg, W.B., van de Putte, L.B.A., Joosten, L.A.B. and van den Bersselaar, L.: Cationization of catalase, peroxidase, and superoxide dismutase. Effect of improved intraarticular retention on experimental arthritis in mice. J. Clin. Invest. *76*, 198–205 (1985).

194   Oite, T., Batsford, S.R., Mihatsch, M.J., Takamiyda, H. and Vogt, A.: Quantitative studies on *in situ* immune complex glomerulonephritis in the rat induced by planted cationized antigen. J. Exp. Med. *155*, 460–474 (1982).

195   Adler, S.G., Wang, H.J., Ward, H.J., Cohen, A.H. and Border, W.A.: Electrical charge: its role in the pathogenesis and prevention of experimental membranous nephropathy in the rabbit. J. Clin. Invest. *71*, 487–499 (1983).

196   Barnes, J.L. and Venkatachalam, M.A.: Enhancement of glomerular immune complex deposition by a circulating polycation. J. Exp. Med. *160*, 286–293 (1984).

197   Chan, L.K.L., Bord, N.H., Alexander, F., Barabas, A.Z. and Lannigan, R.: Effect of cationic proteins on the glomerular deposition of anionic proteins and immune complexes. Nephron *43*, 93–104 (1986).

198   Caulfield, J.P. and Farquhar, M.G.: Distribution of anionic sites in glomerular basement membranes: Their possible role in filtration and attachment. Proc. Natl. Acad. Sci. USA *737*, 1646–1650 (1976).

199   Gallo, G.R., Caulin-Glaser, T., Emancipator, S.N. and Lamm, M.E.: Nephrogenicity and differential distribution of glomerular immune complexes related to immunogen charge. Lab. Invest. *48*, 353–362 (1983).

200   Ford, P.M. and Kosatka, I.: Cationized IgM rheumatoid factor: *in vivo* glomerular localization and immunoabsorptive capacity in the mouse. Clin. Exp. Immunol. *62*, 150–158 (1985).

201   Livneh, A., Halpern, A., Perkins, D., Lazo, A., Halpern, R. and Diamond, B.: A monoclonal antibody to a cross-reactive idiotype on cationic human anti-DNA antibodies expressing λ light chains: A new reagent to identify a potentially different pathogenic subset. J. Immunol. *138*, 123–127 (1987).

202   Cavalot, F., Miyata, M., Vladutiu, A., Terranova, V., Dubiski, S., Burlingame, R., Tan, E., Brentjens, J., Milgrom, F. and Andres, G.: Glomerular lesions induced in the rabbit by physicochemically altered homologous IgG. Am. J. Pathol. *140*, 581–600 (1992).

203   Kirschbaum, B.B.: Interactions between renal brush border membranes and polyamines. J. Pharmacol. Exp. Ther. *228*, 409–416 (1984).

204   Delcros, J.G., Roch, A.M., Thomas, V., El Alaoui, J.P., Moulinoux, J.P. and Quash, G.: Protein-bound polyamines in the plasma of mice grafted with Lewis lung carcinoma. FEBS Lett. *220*, 236–242 (1987).

205   Rosenthal, S.M., Fisher, E.R. and Stohlmann, E.F.: Nephrotoxic action of spermine. Proc. Soc. Exp. Biol. Med. *80*, 432–434 (1952).

206   Rosenthal, S.M. and Tabor, C.W.: The pharmacology of spermine and spermidine. Distribution and excretion. J. Pharmacol. Exp. Ther. *116*, 1 31–138 (1956).

207   Schmiedeke, T.M.J., Stöckl, F., Weber, R., Sugisaki, Y., Batsford, S.R. and Vogt, A.: Histones have high affinity for the glomerular basement membrane: relevance for immune complex formation in lupus nephritis. J. Exp. Med. *169*, 1879–1894 (1989).

208 Thomas, T.J. and Messner, R.P.: Structural specificity of polyamines in left-handed Z-DNA formation. J. Mol. Biol. *201*, 463–467 (1988).

209 Thomas, T.J. and Messner, R.P.: Difluoromethylornithine therapy of female NZB/W mice. J. Rheumatol. *18*, 215–222 (1991).

210 Faaber, P., Rijke, T.P.M., van de Putte, L.B.A., Capel, P.J.A. and Berden, J.H.M.: Cross-reactivity of human and murine anti-DNA antibodies with heparin sulfate. J. Clin. Invest. *77*, 1824–1830 (1986).

211 Suzuki, T., Burlingame, R.W., Cavalot, F., Andres, G., Kashiwazaki, S. and Tan, E.: Antibodies in rabbits immunized with cationized IgG react with histones H3 and H4. Arthr. Rheum. *35*, 1218–1226 (1992).

212 Thomas, T.J., Meryhew, N.L. and Messner, R.P.: DNA sequence and conformational specificity of lupus antibodies. Preferential binding to the left-handed Z-DNA form of polynucleotides. Arthr. Rheum. *31*, 367–377 (1988).

213 Thomas, T.J., Meryhew, N.L. and Messner, R.P.: Enhanced binding of lupus sera to polyamine-induced Z-DNA form of polynucleotides. Arthr. Rheum. *33*, 356–365 (1990).

214 Thomas, T.J., Gunnia, U. and Thomas, T.: Genetic variations of polyamine biosynthesis in autoimmune mice. Arthr. Rheum. *33*, S80 (Abstract B 51) (1990).

215 Shivakumar, S., Tsokos, G.C. and Datta, S.K.: T cell helper α/β expressing double-negative (CD4-/CD8-) and CD4+ helper cells in humans augment the production of pathogenic anti-DNA autoantibodies associated with lupus nephritis. J. Immunol. *143*, 103–112 (1989).

216 Claverie, N., Pasquali, J.L., Mamont, P.S., Danzin, C., Weil-Bousson, M. and Siat, M.: Effects of (2R-5R)-6-heptyne-2,5-diamine, an inhibitor of polyamine synthesis: II. Beneficial effects on the development of a lupus-like disease in MRL-lpr/lpr mice. Clin. Exp. Immunol. *72*, 293–298 (1988).

217 Gunnia, U.B., Amenta, P.S., Seibold, J.R. and Thomas, T.J.: Successful treatment of lupus nephritis in MRL-lpr/lpr mice by inhibiting ornithine decarboxylase. Kidney Int. *39*, 1–9 (1991).

218 Wolos, J.A., Logan, D.E. and Bowlin, T.: Methylacetylenic putrescine (MAP), an inhibitor of polyamine biosynthesis, prevents the development of collagen-induced arthritis. Cell. Immunol. *125*, 498–507 (1990).

219 Hsu, H.C., Thomas, T., Seibold, J.R. and Thomas, T.J.: Studies on the effects of an ornithine decarboxylase inhibitor on lupus nephritis reveal a post-translational modification of the enzyme. Agents & Actions *39*, Suppl. C, C204–C206 (1993).

220 Singh, A.B., Thomas, T.J., Thomas, T., Singh, M. and Mann, R.A.: Differential effects of polyamine homologues on the prevention of D,L-α-difluoromethylornithine-mediated cell growth and normal immune response. Cancer Res. *52*, 1840–1847 (1992).

221 Boggust, W.A. and O'Connell, S.: Increased production of antibody-forming spleen cells induced by polyamine administration and elevated spleen polyamine oxidase activity in mice antigenically stimulated with sheep red blood cells and in mice with tumours. IRCS Med. Sci. *12*, 265–266 (1984).

222 Calvert, J.E., Duggan-Ken, M.F.. Smith, S.W.G., Givan, A.L. and Bird, P.: The CD5$^+$ B cell: A B cell lineage with a central role in autoimmune disease? Autoimmunity *1*, 223–240 (1988).

223 Wickstrom, K.: Polyamine and histopathological changes after unilateral endotoxin-induced uveitis and its contralateral effects. Acta Ophthalmol. *70*, 506–514 (1992).

224   Wickstrom, K., Lundgren, B., Torngren, L. and Ostberg, C.: Aqueous humor poly-
      amines and alkaline phosphatase activity in endotoxin-induced uveitis: correlations to
      diverse leukocyte subsets. Ophthalmic Res. *24*, 175–180 (1992).
225   Lamster, I.B., Mandella, R.D., Zove, S.M. and Harper, D.S.: The polyamines
      putrescine, spermidine and spermine in human gingival crevicular fluid. Arch. Oral
      Biol. *32*, 329–333 (1987).
226   Bartholeyns, J., Fozard, J., Prakash, N.: Dexamethasone inhibition of carrageenan paw
      oedema in the rat requires *de novo* synthesis of putrescine. Br. J. Pharmacol. *72*,
      182P–183P (1981).
227   Bartholeyns, J., Fozard, J., Prakash, N.: Blockade of the antiinflammatory action of
      dexamethasone by DL-alpha-difluoromethylornithine: comparison with actinomycin
      D and cycloheximide. Br. J. Pharmacol. *73*, 212P. (1981).
228   Oyanagui, Y.: Anti-inflammatory effects of polyamines in serotonin and carrageenan
      paw edemata. Possible mechanism to increase vascular permeability inhibitory protein
      level which is regulated by glucocorticoids and superoxide radical. Agents & Actions
      14, 228–237 (1984).
229   Rennert, O.M., Buehler, B., Miale, T. and Lawson, D.: Polyamines and platelet
      aggregation. Life Sci. *19*, 257–264 (1976).
230   Subbarao, K. and Foster, F.: Inhibitory effect of diamines and polyamines on human
      platelet aggregation and (^{14}C)-serotonin release. Thromb. Haemostasis *38*, 313 (1977).
231   Scalabrino, G., Ferioli, M.D., Piccoletti, R. and Bernelli-Zazzera, A.: Activation of
      polyamine biosynthetic decarboxylases during the acute phase response of rat liver.
      Biochem. Biophys. Res. Commun. *143*, 856–862 (1987).
232   Colombatto, S., Fasulo, L. and Grillo, M.: Polyamines in rat liver during experimental
      inflammation. Agents & Actions *24*, 326–330 (1988).
233   Dowling, R.H.: Polyamines in intestinal adaptation and disease. Digestion, *46* (Suppl.
      2), 331–344 (1990).
234   Mennigen, R., Kusche, J., Streffer, C. and Krakamp, B.: Diamine oxidase activities in
      the large bowel mucosa of ulcerative colitis patients. Agents & Actions *30*, 264–266
      (1990).
235   Thompson, J.S., Burnett, D.A.. Markin, R.S. and Vaughan, W.P.: Intestinal mucosa
      diamine oxidase activity reflects involvement in Crohn's disease. Am. J. Gastroenterol.
      83, 756–760 (1988).
236   Schmidt, W.U., Sattler, J., Hesterberg, R., Röher, H.D., Zoedler, Th., Sitter, H. and
      Lorenz, W.: Human intestinal diamine oxidase (DAO) activity in Crohn's disease: A
      new marker for disease assessment? Agents & Actions *30*, 267–270 (1990).
237   Kanof, M.E., Rance, N.E., Hamilton, S.R., Luk, G.D. and Lake, A.M.: Congenital
      diarrhea with intestinal inflammation and epithelial immaturity. J. Pediatr. Gastroen-
      terol. Nutr. *6*, 141–146 (1987).
238   Luk, G.D. and Canellakis, Z.N.: Diacetylputrescine and its analog suppress c-myc
      expression and activation of human B-lymphocytes. Biochem. Int. *20*, 169–176 (1990).
239   Ryan, J.L., Bondy, P.K., Gobran, L. and Canellakis, Z.N.: Acetylated diamines inhibit
      endotoxin-induced lymphocyte activation. J. Immunol. *132*, 1888–1891 (1984).
240   Canellakis, Z.N., Marsh, L.L. and Bondy, P.K.: Polyamines and their derivatives as
      modulators in growth and differentiation. Yale J. Biol. Med. *62*, 481–491 (1989).
241   Porter, C.W., McManis, J., Casero, R.A. and Bergeron, R.J.: Relative abilities of
      bis(ethyl) derivatives of putrescine, spermidine and spermine to regulate polyamine

biosynthesis and inhibit L1210 leukemia cell growth. Cancer Res. *47*, 2821–2875 (1987).

242   Igarashi, K., Kashiwagi, K., Fukuchi, J., Isobe, Y., Otomo, S. and Shirahata, A.: Spermine-like functions of N1,N12-bis(ethyl) spermine: stimulation of protein synthesis and cell growth, and inhibition of gastric ulceration. Biochem. Biophys. Res. Commun. *172*, 715–720 (1990).

243   Komori, T. and Ohsugi, Y.: Norspermidine inhibits LPS-induced immunoglobulin production in an FCS-independent mechanism different from spermidine and spermine. Int. J. Immunopharmacol. *13*, 67–73 (1991).

244   Singh, A.B., Thomas, T.J., Singh, M. and Mann, R.A.: Attenuation of murine acute graft-versus-host disease by the administration of DL-alpha-difluoromethylornithine. Clin. Immunol. Immunopathol. *65*, 242–246 (1992).

245   Bernacki, R.J., Bergeron, R.J. and Porter, C.: Antitumor activity of N,N'-bis(ethyl)spermine homologues against human MALME-3 melanoma xenografts. Cancer Res. *52*, 2424–2430 (1992).

246   Prakash, N.J., Bowlin, T.L., Edwards, M.L., Sunkara, P.S. and Sjoerdsma, A.: Antitumor activity of a novel synthetic polyamine analogue, N,N'bis[3-(ethylamino)propyl]-1,7-heptane diamine: Potentiation by polyamine oxidase inhibitors. Anticancer Res. *10*, 1281–1288 (1990).

247   Bowlin, T.L., Prakash, N.J., Edwards, M.L. and Sjoerdsma, A.: Participation of T-lymphocytes in the curative effect of a novel synthetic polyamine analogue, N,N'-bis[3-(ethylamino)propyl]1,7-heptanediamine against L1210 leukemia *in vivo*. Cancer Res *51*, 62–66 (1991).

248   Seiler, N., Sarhan, S., Mamont, P., Casara, P. and Danzin, C.: Some biological consequences of S-adenosylmethionine decarboxylase inhibition by MDL 73,811. Life Chem. Rep. *9*, 151–162 (1991).

249   Regennass, U., Caravatti, G., Mett, H., Stanek, J., Schneider, P., Mueller, M., Matter, A., Vertino, P. and Porter, C.W.: New S-adenosylmethionine decarboxylase inhibitors with potent antitumor activity. Cancer Res. *52*, 4712–4718 (1992).

250   Seiler, N., Koch-Weser, J., Knödgen, B., Richards, W., Tardif, C., Bolkenius, F.N., Schechter, P., Tell, G., Mamont, P., Fozard, J., Bachrach, U. and Grosshans, E.: The significance of acetylation in urinary excretion of polyamines. In: Advances in Polyamine Research (Caldarera, C.M., Zappia, V. and Bachrach, U., eds.), vol. 3, pp. 197–211, Raven Press, New York (1981).

251   Sarhan, S., Quemener, V., Moulinoux, J.P., Knödgen, B. and Seiler, N.: On the degradation and elimination of spermine by the vertebrate organism. Int. J. Biochem. *23*, 617–626 (1991).

252   Corti, A., Dave, C., Williams-Ashman, H.G., Mihich, E. and Schenone, A.: Specific inhibition of the enzymic decarboxylation of S-adenosyl-methionine by methylglyoxal bis(guanylhydrazone) and related substances. Biochem. J. *139*, 351–356 (1974).

253   Seiler, N.: Inhibition of enzymes oxidizing polyamines. In: Inhibition of Polyamine Metabolism (McCann, P.P., Pegg, A.E. and Sjoerdsma, A., eds.), pp. 49–77, Academic Press, Orlando (1987).

254   Bolkenius, F.N. and Seiler, N.: Polyamine oxidase inhibitors. In: Design of enzyme inhibitors as drugs (Sandler, M. and Smith, H.J., eds.), pp. 245–256. Oxford University Press, Oxford (1989).

Progress in Drug Research, Vol. 43 (E. Jucker, Ed.)
© 1994 Birkhäuser Verlag, Basel (Switzerland)

Biologically active quinazolones

By Shradha Sinha and Mukta Srivastava

Division of Medicinal Chemistry, Central Drug Research Institute, Lucknow 226 001, India

Introduction

Quinazolinones form a large group among the pharmacologically active chemical moieties and are generally of little toxicity without serious side effects to the human body. Quinazolinones are versatile nitrogen hetero-cyclic compounds, displaying a broad spectrum of biological and phar-macological activities in animal as well as in human systems. The chemistry and pharmacology of quinazolinones have been of great interest to medicinal chemists. In 1885, Weddige synthesized the first quinazolone and named it anhydroformylorthoamidobenzamide. Later on, extensive work on this nucleus was done for the amelioration of human suffering from various diseases and many drugs incorporating this nucleus were developed.

Quinazolones were thoroughly reviewed by Amim et al. [A] in 1970, after that by Gupta et al. [B] in 1971 and later on by Yakhontov [C] in 1977 and Johne [D, E] in 1981 and 1982. This review is intended to provide an account of developments in pharmaceutically interesting quinazolone derivatives, described during the last thirteen years, and the review is concerned mainly with the biologically active 4(3H)-quinazolinones cited in the chemical abstracts up to 1993.

2   Anthelmintic activity

Helminthiasis comprises a group of ailments that are produced by parasitic worms in various parts of the body, predominantly in the gastrointestinal tract. The therapeutic compounds that are used to bring about either death or expulsion of the helminths from the infected hosts are termed as Anthel-mintics. Although many types of compounds have been synthesized as anthelmintics, not much research has yet been carried out on quinazolinone derivatives.

Several compounds containing a quinazolone nucleus have been introduced in therapy for the treatment of infections caused by different intestinal nematodes and cestodes [1]. Alaimo et al. [2] reported the anthelmintic activity of 2-(5-nitro-2-thienyl)-4-(substituted amino) quinazolines against *H. nana*, *S. obvelata* and *A. suum*. The most active compounds are those bearing a hydroxy alkylamino substituent at position 4. A series of 2-(2-benzimidazolyl methyl thio)-3-aryl or cyclo-4-quinazolones **I** and N-(3-aryl-4-quinazolon-2-yl mercaptoacetyl) hydrazones **II** was synthesized by

Husain et al. [3] with a view to ascertaining whether the presence of a quinazolone nucleus can induce anthelmintic activity.

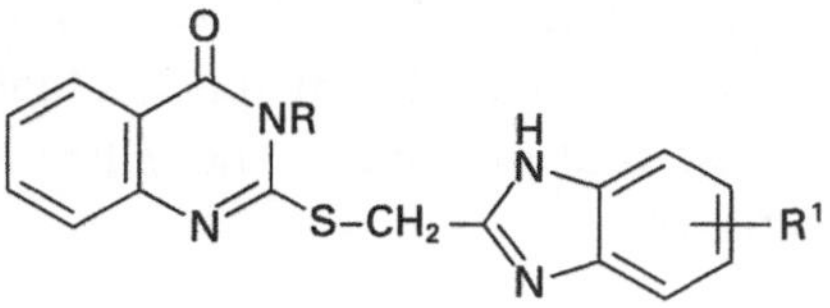

I
R = Ph, 4-ClPh, 4-BrPh, α-naphthyl,
2-tolyl, 3-anisyl
R^1 = H & 5-Cl

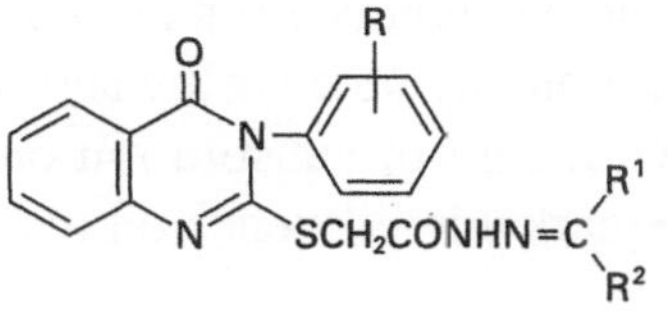

II
R = H, 2-Me, 4-Me
R^1 = Ph, 2-ClPh, 4-OHPh, 2-furyl,
R^2 = H & Me

Tewari et al. [4] synthesized quinazolin-4(3H)-one-2-yl thioacetyl ureas and α-hydroxybenzylquinazolin-4(3H)-ones **III** and found that N^3-[3-(p-chlorophenyl)-quinazol(3H)-4-one-2yl mercapto acetyl] N^2-O-tolyl urea **IIIa** and 2-mandelyl-3-(p-tolyl)quinazol-(3H)-4-one **IIIb** were not active at a single oral dose of 250 mg/kg against *H. nana* and *N. brasiliensis* infections in mice. 3-(3-Amino-2-hydroxypropyl)-4(3H) quinazolones **IVa** and 3-(3-amino acetonyl)-4(3H) quinazolones **IVb** were synthesized and evaluated for anthelmintic activity. Some derivatives of **IVa** and **IVb** exhibited coccidostatic and anthelmintic activity [5], while compound **V** was comparable to Zoalen (275 mg/kg/os) and showed low toxicity [6].

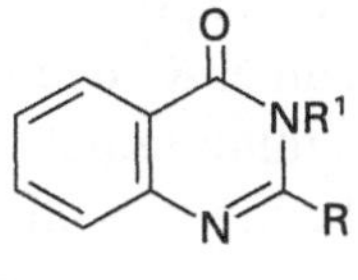

IIIa R =
2-MeC$_6$H$_4$NHCONHCOCH$_2$S,
R^1 = 4-ClC$_6$H$_4$
IIIb R = PhCHOH,
R^1 = 4-MeC$_6$H$_4$

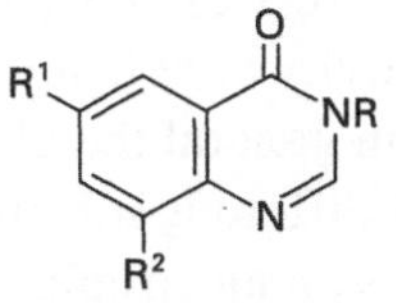

IVa R = CH$_2$CH(OH)CH$_2$R$_3$R$_4$,
R^1R^2 = H, Cl, Br, R^3 = H, R^4 = cyclohexyl
IVb R = CH$_2$COCH$_2$NR^{3}R^4,
R^1, R^2 = H, Cl, Br
NR^3R^4 = morpholino, pyrrolidino,
piperidino

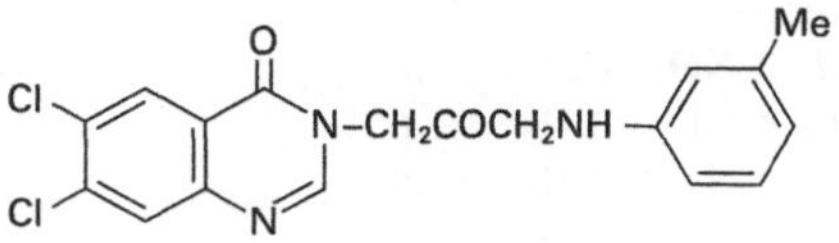

V

Bhaduri et al. reported the synthesis and anthelmintic activity of imidazoquinazolines **VI**. Findings of the activity indicate that compounds **VIa–VIg** cause 100% clearance of *H. nana* at a dose of 100 mg/kg, while **VIf** is inactive against both *H. nana* and *A. ceylanicum* and **VIg** and **VIe** do not exhibit any noteworthy activity against *A. ceylanicum*. Thus it appears that the nature of substitution on the nitrogen atom at position 3 and 7 has a remarkable influence on the biological activity.

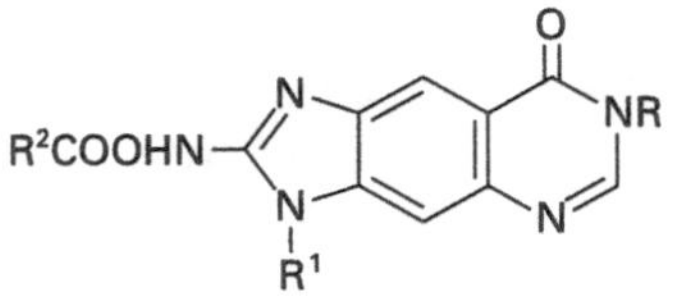

VI

	R	R^1	R^2
VIa	CH_3	H	CH_3
VIb	CH_3	H	C_2H_5
VIc	n-C_4H_9	H	CH_3
VId	n-C_4H_9	H	C_2H_5
VIe	CH_3	$CH_2CH_2OHC_2H_5$	
VIf	CH_3	$(CH_3)_2C_6H_5$	C_2H_5

A series of 2-(0-arylidene amino phenyl) 3-(5-alkyl-1,3,4-thiadiazol-2-yl) quinazolin-4-ones **VII** has been synthesized by Shukla et al. [8] and screened for its cestocidal activity against *H. nana* infection in rats to ascertain whether the presence of the arylidene amino phenyl group at position 2 and the 1,3,4-thiadizolyl group at position 3 showed any effect on anthelmintic activity. Compound **VIIa** showed maximum (77.2%) clearance of infection in rats at a dose of 250 mg/kg. Compounds **VIIb–VIIk** also exhibited appreciable activity showing reduction of worm load from 20.5–56.4%, the rest of the compounds were either inactive or showed insignificant activity at 500 and 400 mg/kg dose levels. It is apparent from the results that in general the elongation of the alkyl chain at R^1 decreases the activity and different substituents (R) in arylidene amino moiety alter the activity; R as an electrophile reduces the cestocidal activity while as a nucleophile it increases the activity.

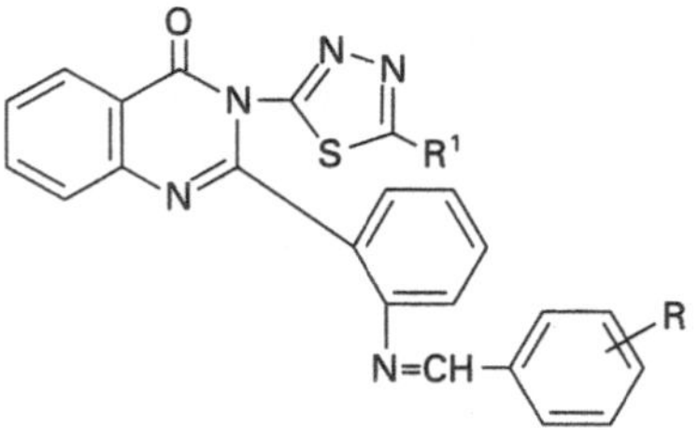

VII

	R	R^1	Gestocidal activity %
VIIa	4-NO_2	H	77.2
VIIb	2-NO_2	H	56.4
VIIc	3-NO_2	H	48.0
VIId	4-Cl	CH_3	50.0
VIIe	3-NO_2	CH_3	35.2
VIIf	2-NO_2	CH_3	35.0
VIIg	4-Cl	C_2H_5	25.6
VIIh	3-NO_2	C_2H_5	38.8
VIIi	4-Cl	C_3H_7	30.2
VIIj	3-NO_2	C_3H_7	28.0
VIIk	2-NO_2	C_3H_7	20.5

Compounds with a (benzylidene amino) phenyl group at position 3 were also synthesized by Shukla et al. [9]. They demonstrated that compound **VIII** exhibited the maximum activity in this series, which caused 100% elimination of *H. nana* in mice; the rest of the compounds were found to be inactive against *H. nana*. In the case of *N. brasiliensis*, the activity ranged from 20–42%. Compound **VIII** showed maximum 42% while compound **IX** with Br at positions 6 and 8, exhibited only 20% anthelmintic activity. Shukla et al. [10] synthesized 2-methyl-phenyl-3-aminoacetoxy-6,8-substi-tuted-1,3(4H)-quinazolin-4-ones **X** and reported their anthelmintic activity against *H. nana* in mice at 250, 400 and 500 mg/kg oral doses. The activity ranged from 15–70% and maximum activity (70%) was exhibited by 2-phenyl-3-piperazino-acetoxy-6,8-dibromo-1,3-quinazolin-4-one **Xa** at a dose of 250 mg/kg.

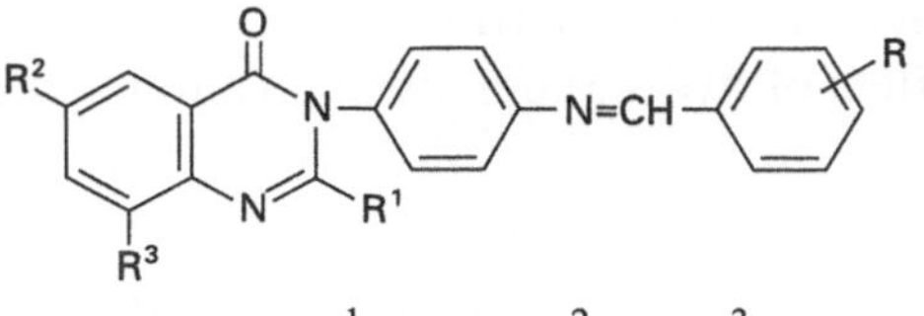

VIII $R = 3\text{-}NO_2$, $R^1 = C_6H_5$, $R^2 = H$, $R^3 = I$
IX $R = 2\text{-}OH$, $R^1 = C_6H_5$, $R^2R^3 = Br$

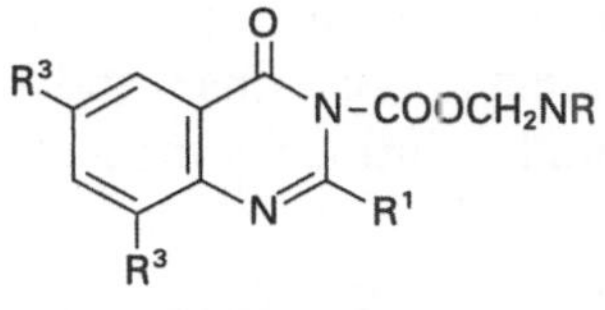

Xa $R = \text{piperazino}$,
       $R^1 = C_6H_5$, $R^2R^3 = Br$

Shukla et al. [11] demonstrated that substitution of the 4-(3-phthalimido, acetamido and propionamido) phenyl group at position 3 in the quinazolone nucleus **XI** also exhibited anthelmintic activity against *N. brasiliensis* and *A. ceylanicum* in rats and hamsters respectively, but these compounds were found to be inactive against *H. nana*. Compound **XI** showed 15.2–43.0% and 16–17% anthelmintic activity against *N. brasiliensis* and *A. ceylanicum* respectively, at a dose of 250 mg/kg for 3 days. The maximum activity of 43% was shown by 2-phenyl-3[4-(3-phthalimido propionamido)] phenyl-6,8-dibromo-quinazolin-4-one **XIa** against *N. brasiliensis* while 2-methyl-3[4-(3-phthalimido propionamido)] phenyl quinazolin-4-one **XIb** exhibited a maximum 70% clearance against *A. ceylanicum*. It is evident from the results that introduction of the propionamido group enhances the activity against both types of parasites.

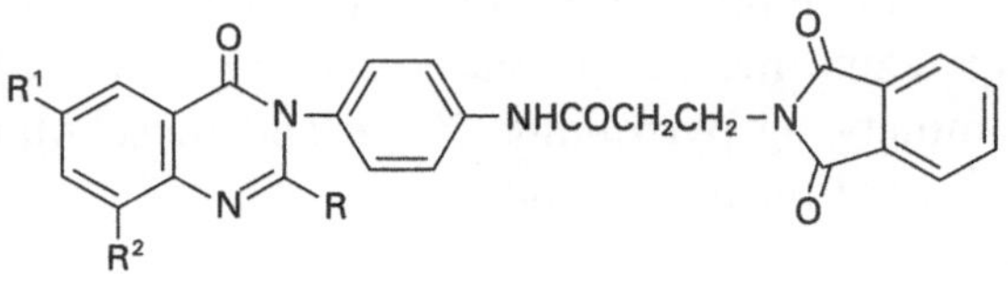

XI
XIa $R = C_6H_5$, R^1, $R^2 = Br$
XIb $R = CH_3$, R^1, $R^2 = H$

6,8-Disubstituted-3-aryl-2-[mercapto-4-aryl-1,3,4-triazol-5-ylmethylthio]-
1,3-quinazolin-4-ones **XII** and 2-methyl/phenyl-3-(4-substituted phenyl
imino-4-oxothiazolidine-3-yl phenyl)-6,8-disubstituted-1,3-quinazolin-4-
ones **XIII** have been synthesized by Shukla et al. [12] and evaluated for
their anthelmintic activity against *H. nana* in mice, *A. ceylanicum* in
hamsters and *N. brasiliensis* in rats. None of these compounds showed
activity against *H. nana*. Compound **XIIa** exhibited 78% activity against
N. brasiliensis infection while **XIIb** exhibited 72% clearance of *A. ceylanicum*. The activity against *N. brasiliensis* and *A. ceylanicum* ranged from
15–78% and 10–72%, respectively. Compound **XIII** showed only 15–55%
activity against *A. ceylanicum* and 20–85% clearance against *N. brasiliensis*. It is evident from these results that substitution by an electrophile
decreased the anthelmintic activity while a nucleophile enhanced it. QSAR
studies of **XII** and **XIII** have been carried out in terms of structural and
physico-chemical parameters, where positive contribution of substituents
present at positions 6 and 8 and effect of hydrophobicity at position 3 were
found to influence the activity.

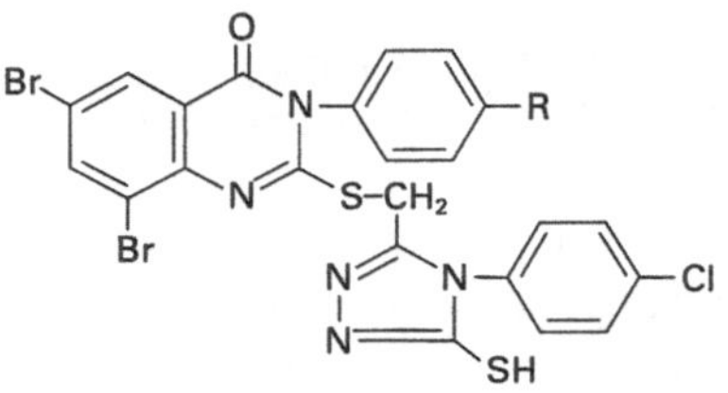

XII
XIIa R = Cl
XIIb R = Br

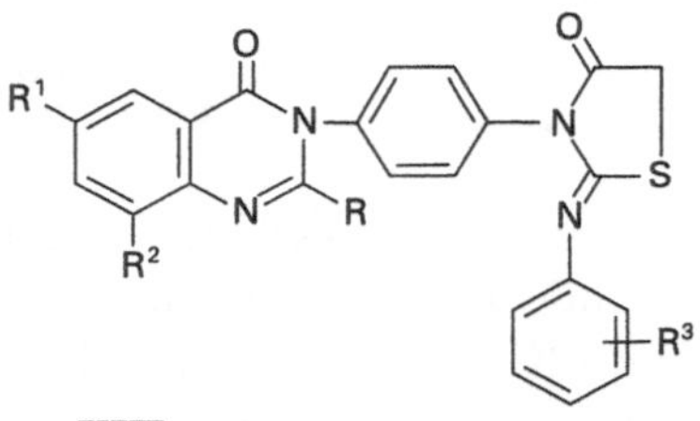

XIII
R = CH_3, C_6H_5, R^1, R^2 = H, Br,
R = Cl, Br, CH_3

Synthesis and anthelmintic activity of 2-substituted 3-[p-N^1-arylsulphonyl-
biguanidophenyl] quinazolin-4-one hydrochlorides **XIV** were reported by
Shukla et al. [13]. Compound **XIVa** was found to be the most active of the
series showing 81.0% clearance of infection against *H. nana* at a dose of
250 mg/kg for 3 days. The cestodicidal activity reported here clearly
demonstrates that the presence of a methyl group as in compound **XIVa** and
a substituted phenyl group as in compound **XIVb** at R position alters the
activity. Introduction of piperazine residue increased the activity, while
replacement of piperazine moiety by pyrrolidine **XIVc** and morpholine
XIVd residue showed inactivity of the compounds.

Misra et al. [14] reported the anthelmintic activity of N-(2-alkyl-1,3-quina-zolin-4-yloxymethyl)-N4-(p-substituted phenyl)thiosemicarbazides against *H. nana* and *N. brasiliensis*. None of the compounds of the series were found to be active against *H. nana* while the percentage clearance against *N. brasiliensis* ranged from 21.8–7.4% in rats.

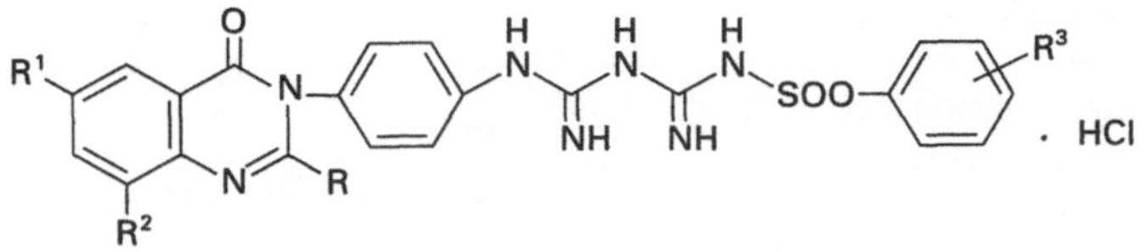

XIV
XIVa R = CH3, R^1, R^2 = H, Br, I, R^3 = OMe
XIVb R = 3-Nitro-4(4'-methylpiperazino)phenyl, R^1, R^2, R^3 = H
XIVc R = 3-Nitro-4-(pyrrolidino)phenyl, R^1, R^2, R^3 = H
XIVd R = 3-Nitro-4-(morpholino)phenyl, R^1, R^2, R^3 = H

The macrofilaricidal activity exhibited by amodiaquin, though weak, prompted Shukla et al. [15] to synthesize some of its structural analogs bearing a quinazolone nucleus viz. 2-[N(3'-substituted aminomethyl-4'-hy-droxyphenyl) carbamoyl] quinazolin-4(3H)ones **XV** and to evaluate their anthelmintic activity against *Brugia pahanqi* and *H. nana* in jirds and rats, respectively. Compound **XVa** at a dose of 250 mg/kg for 3 days induced 60–62% worm expulsion in rats while **XVb–XVf** also exhibited activity, showing inhibition of worm load from 27–55%; the rest of the compounds were either inactive or showed insignificant activity at 500 and 400 mg/kg dose levels.

Pandey et al. [16] reported the synthesis of quinazolin triazine derivatives **XVI**. Among which compound **XVIa** exhibited significant anthelmintic activity (85.2, 62.0 and 68.2%) against *A. ceylanicum, N. brasiliensis* and *H. nana,* respectively.

2-Methyl-3-(substituted) amino-4-quinazolinones **XVII** were synthesized and screened for anthelmintic activity by Gupta et al. [17]. Compounds **XVIIa** and **XVIIe** were found to effect 100% clearance of worms while 80% clearance was observed for **XVIII**.

Several 3-[4-[3-(2,3,4-substituted) phenyl-1-oxo(2,3-substituted propane)] phenyl]-2-phenyl/methyl-6,8-substituted-4(3H)-quinazolinones **XIX** were synthesized to evaluate their cestodicidal activity *in vivo* against *H. nana* infection in rats [18]; the activity ranged from 20–75% and the maximum

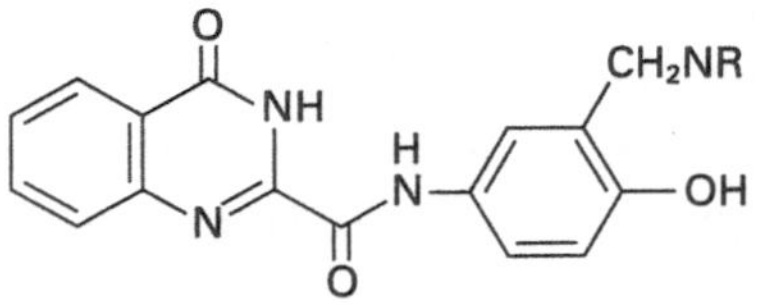

XV
XVa 4-(4-chlorophenyl)-1-piperazinyl
XVb Piperidino
XVc 4-Methyl-1-piperazinyl
XVd 4-Phenyl-1-piperazinyl
XVe 4-Phenyl piperidino
XVf 4-Hydroxy-4-phenylpiperidino

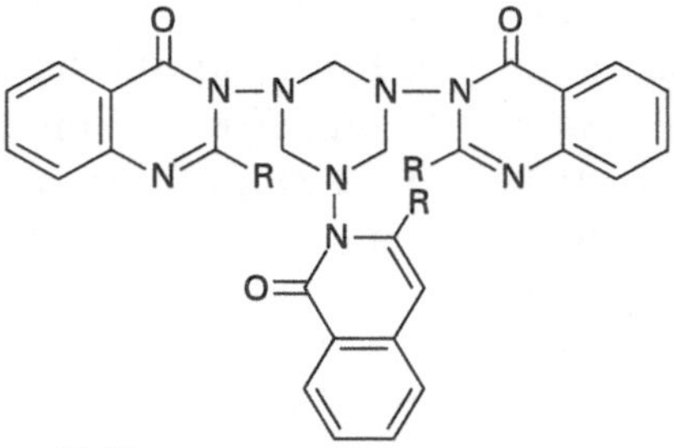

XVI
XVIa R = Benzoyl

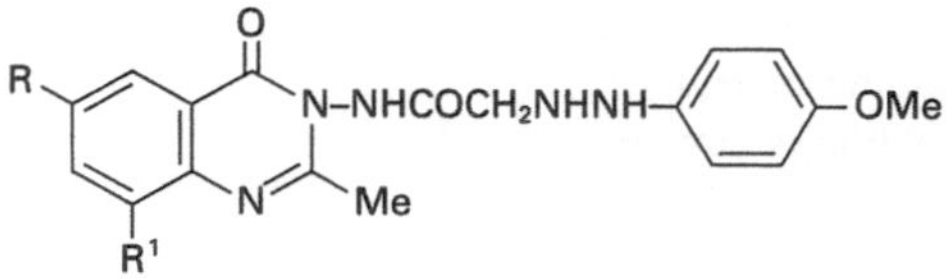

XVII
XVIIa R, R^1 = H
XVIIb R, R^1 = Br

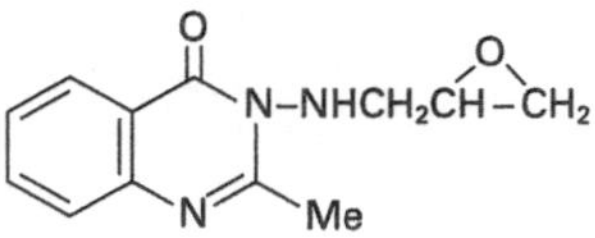

XVIII

clearance (75%) was shown by compound **XIXa** at a 250 mg/kg dose while minimum clearance (20%) was exhibited by **XIXb**.

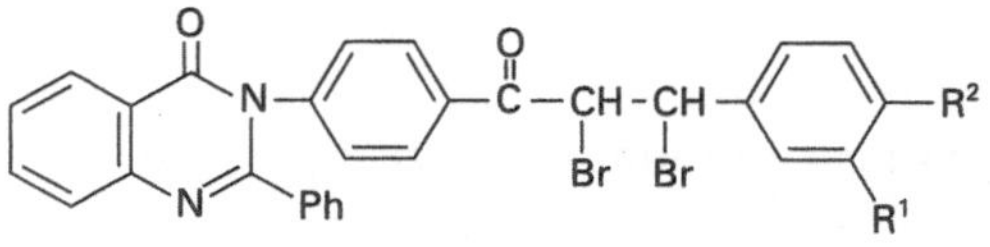

XIX
XIXa R^1 = H, R^2 = OH
XIXb R^1, R^2 = OMe

3   Effects on the central nervous system

3.1   Introduction

The importance of the central nervous system (CNS) as the key regulator of various activities of different organs of the human body is well known. The slightest abberration in the functioning of CNS may produce serious disorders, either hyperkinetic or hypokinetic. The hyperkinetic disorders are characterized by the stimulation of the central nervous system in which enormous energy is wasted in the form of hyperactions of limbs and sense organs, whereas in hypokinetic disorders, depression of CNS is the characteristic feature.

Extensive and intensive work has been done on quinazolinone moiety, and brought forth several compounds; only one compound, Methaqualone, has found a firm place in therapeutic practice and is being successfully used. It is still believed that structural modifications in methaqualone may produce better drugs; the 2nd and 3rd positions of the quinazolones have been the target for substitution with other moieties.

The drugs, administered to overcome CNS disorders, have been shown to produce effects on three aspects of cerebral biochemistry, i.e. energy metabolism, general aspects of membrane function and change in the concentration of neurotransmitters. Because of the very diverse fields of action of neurotransmitters, their enzymes and other CNS active chemical entities, it is rather difficult to define completely and concisely the effect of CNS active drugs in terms of specific transmitter activity. Owing to the multiplicity of action of neurotropic and psychotropic drugs acting on various central neurons simultaneously, it is essential to classify these drugs according to their major type of action on the CNS. The CNS active agents may be classified on the basis of their effects on gross behaviour:

1. CNS depressants, 2. CNS stimulants, 3. selective modifiers of specific CNS functions, (a) anticonvulsant, (b) antiparkinsonian, (c) hypnotic, muscle relaxant, (d) analgesic and antipyretic.

3.2   Behavioural activity

Several 2-substituted 1-aryl substituted-4-quinazolones **XX** were synthesized and tested for different biological activities. All of them were found to possess CNS depressant and analgesic activities [19–26].

Some derivatives of 2-(N^4-arylpiperazinocarbonyl methyl thio) 3-aryl-6-bromo-4(3H)-quinazolinones **XXI** have also been reported as psychotropic agents [27].

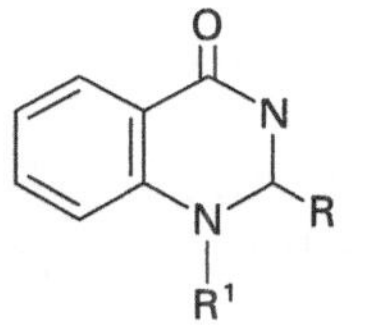

XX
R = Me, CH$_2$COOH, CONH$_2$, CF$_3$, CHMe$_2$, CH(CH$_2$)$_n$
n = 2, 3, 4, 6, R^1 = Substituted phenyl

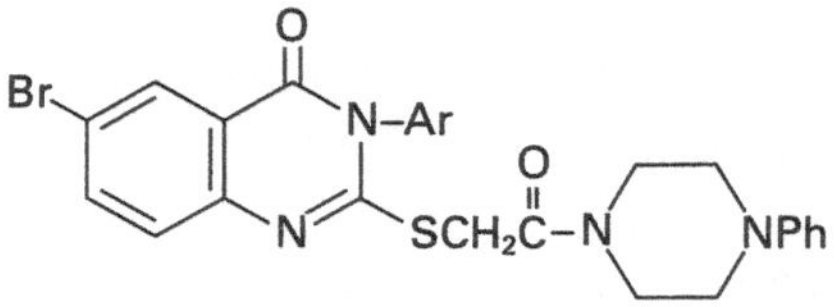

XXI

A number of 2-mercapto-3-arylsubstituted-4(3H)-quinazolinones are known to be potent CNS active agents [28]. S-substituted 2-mercapto-3-aryl (or aralkyl)-4(3H)-quinazolinones showed CNS stimulant activity at dose levels of 600 mg/kg and above [29].

Bhargava and Singh [30] synthesized and screened fourteen derivatives of 3-aryl-6-bromo-2-substituted thio-4(3H)-quinazolinones out of which only 6-bromo-2-(N,N-diisobutylcarboxamidomethylthio)-3-phenyl   and   6-bromo-2-(N,N-dibenzylcarboxamidomethylthio)-3-(4-methoxyphenyl-4 (3H)-quinazolinones exhibited CNS depressant activity.

Tewari et al. [31] reported that 2-aryl-3-(2'hydroxyethyl) 6,8-disubstituted-4(3H)-quinazolinones **XXII** at doses of 200, 464 and 100 mg/kg showed CNS depressant activity. ALD50 of these compounds was quite high which showed their relative nontoxicity, while 2-phenyl-3(benzothiazol-2'-yl alkyl/aryl) quinazolin-4-ones **XXIII** increased the spontaneous motor activity in albino mice of either sex. ALD50 of **XXIIIa–XXIIIg** were found to be >1000 >1000 >825, 562, 825, 825 and 681 mg/kg i.p., respectively [32]. These compounds exhibited no antitremorine effect.

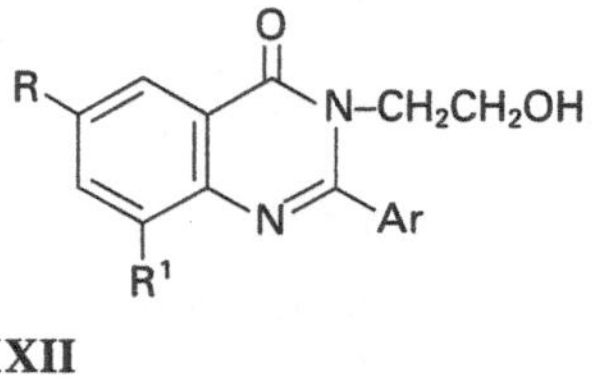

XXII
Ar = C_6H_5, $CH_2NHCOC_6H_5$,
R^1, R^2 = H, Br, Cl, I

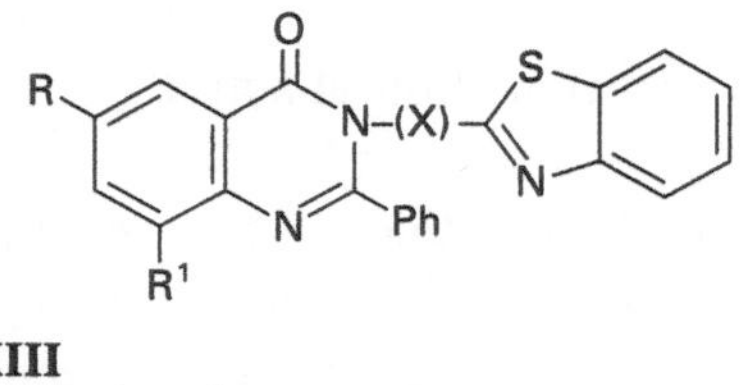

XXIII
XXIIIa R, R^1 = H, X = –CH_2–
XXIIIb R, R^1 = H, X = –$\overset{|}{C}H$–CH_2–$CHMe_2$
XXIIIc R, R^1 = H, X = –C_6H_4–(o)
XXIIId R = Br, R^1 = H, X = –CH_2–CH_2–
XXIIIe R = Br, R^1 = H, X = –$\overset{|}{C}H$–
                                          $\quad\quad$ Me
XXIIIf R, R^1 = Br, X = –$\overset{|}{C}H$–
                                   CH_2–$CHMe_2$
XXIIIg R, R^1 = Br, X = –C_6H_4–(o)

Some 2-methyl-3-(substituted phenyl)-6-substituted-4(3H)-quinazolinone derivatives **XXIV** had potent tranquilizing, antidepressant and anticonvulsant effects. Substitution of the bromo group at position 6 did not produce any effect, but iodo substituted derivatives showed tranquilizing and antidepressant activities and were devoid of anticonvulsant activity [33].

Agarwal et al. [34] reported that 1-(2-arylindol-3-yl)-2-[4-morpholinophenyl)-6,8-disubstituted-quinazolin-4(3H)-on-2-yl] ethanes were psychotropic and rather non toxic, while 1-(2-alkyl-6-substituted quinazolin-4-one-3-yl)-2-methyl-4'-(3,4-benzylidene)-5-oxoimidazoles **XXV** were non toxic and CNS depressant [35].

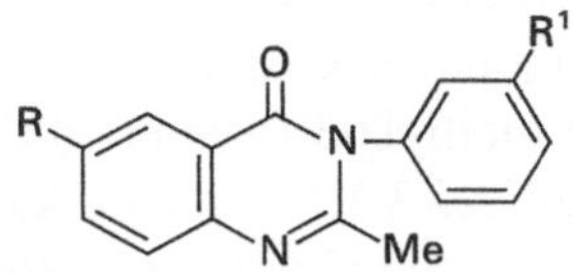

XXIV
R = H, Br, I, R^1 = Ac, COCH$_2$CH$_2$NR^2,
R^2 = C$_6$H$_5$, piperazinyl

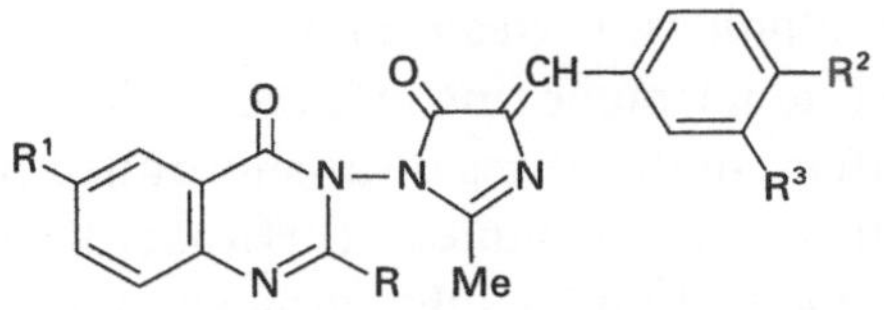

XXV
R = CH$_3$, C$_2$H$_5$, R^1 = H, I, R^2 = H, CH$_3$,
R^3 = H, OMe

2-Phenyl-3[4-(N,N-disubstituted carbamoyl)phenylamino]-8-substituted-4(3H)-quinazolinones **XXVI** were synthesized by Nigam et al. [36]. They reported that compounds where R^2 was H possessed both stimulant and depressant activities while compounds where R^2 was Br **XXVIa** exhibited stimulant action only.

It was concluded that presence of the bromo group might increase the stimulant activity. However 2-phenyl/3-[4-N,N-disubstituted aminocarbonyl)phenyl]-8-substituted-4(3H)-quinazolones **XXVII** were found to be non toxic with ALD50 values of 1000 or more. Compounds with R as Ph and CH$_2$Cl and R^3 as H (**XXVIIa**, **XXVIIb**) were found to be weakly stimulating [37].

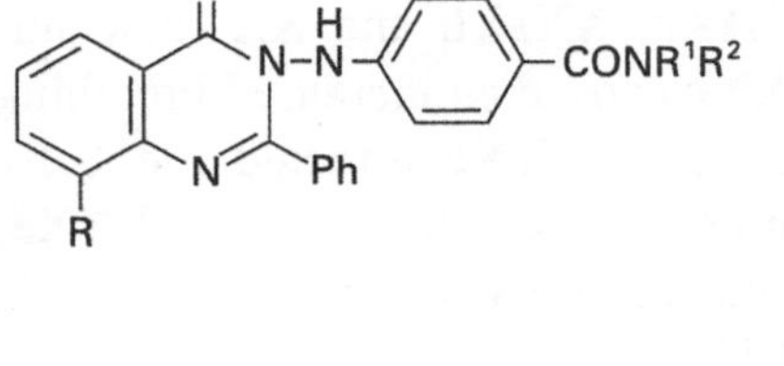

XXVI   R = H, Br, NR^{1}R^2 = Morpholino,
           piperidino, N-methyl piperazino
XXVIa R = Br, NR^{1}R^2 = Morpholino

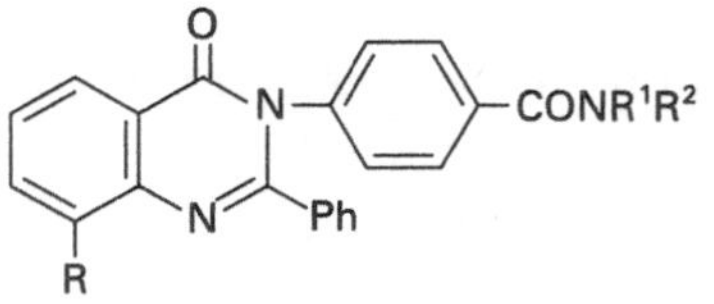

XXVII R = H, Br, NR^1R^2 = Morphino, piperidino, N-phenylpiperazino, diethylamino
XXVIIa R = Br, NR^1R^2 = N-Phenylpiperazino
XXVIIb R = H, NR^1R^2 = Morpholino

Saxena et al. [38] reported the synthesis of some new bis(4-oxo-3-phenyl-6,8-disubstituted-quinazolin-2yl) disulphides, sulphides, sulfones and alkylene disulphides and their CNS activities. All compounds showed CNS depressant activity. Results indicated that the sulphides and sulphones were better CNS depressants than their corresponding disulphides and alkylene disulphides. It was also observed that bromination at positions 6 and 8 of the quinazolone ring induced a relatively more pronounced CNS depressant effect. In the series of 2-(substituted phthalimido methyl)-3-(4-substituted phenyl)-6-substituted-4(3H)-oxo-3,1-quinazolines **XXVIII**, introduction of the thalimidomethyl group at position 2 in place of the phenyl or methyl group resulted in a loss of activity [39]; only compound **XXVIIIa** showed a CNS depressant effect while **XXVIIIb** showed a stimulant effect. No significant activity was observed against supramaximal electroconvulsion in mice.

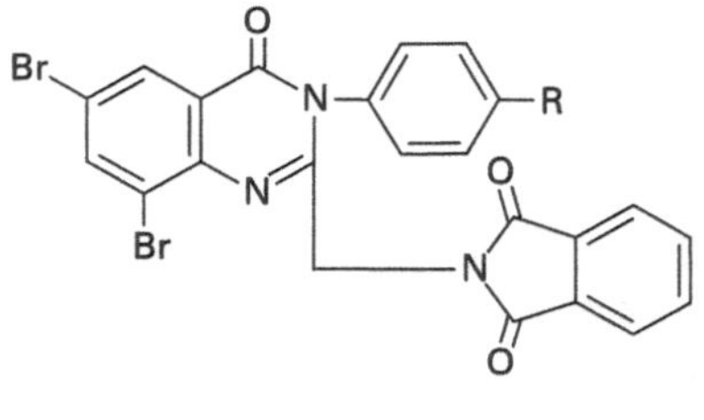

XXVIIIa R = OH
XXVIIIb R = NO_2

A number of 3-(benzylidene amino phenyl)- and 3-(2'-aryl-4'-oxothia-zolidin-3'-yl)-2-phenyl quinazolin-4(3H)-ones **XXIX, XXX** have been synthesized with the presumption that the union of two heterocyclic moieties would produce more potent compounds [40]. All the compounds showed a stimulatory effect except **XXIXa, XXIXb** and **XXXa**. Compounds **XXIXc, XXIXd, XXXb** and **XXXc** caused an increased breathing rate, while **XXIXg, XXXa, XXXc, XXXd, XXXe** affected the belly muscles as they induced writhing. Compounds **XXIXg, XXIXf, XXXa, XXXc, XXXe** also induced hypothermia, the most potent being **XXXe** which decreased body temperature by 1.8° C.

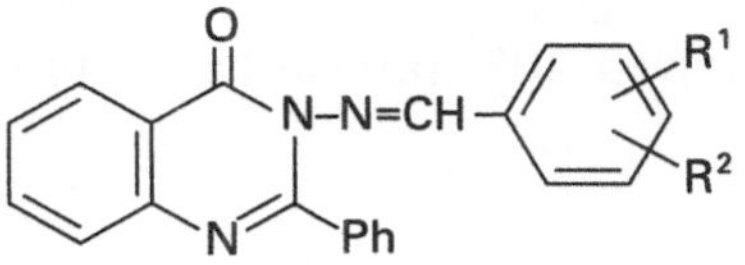

XXIX
XXIXa R^1 = H, R^2 = 4-OMe
XXIXb R^1 = OH, R^2 = 3-OMe
XXIXc R^1 = H, R^2 = 4-OH
XXIXd R^1 = H, R^2 = 3-OH
XXIXe R^1 = OH, R^2 = 4-OH

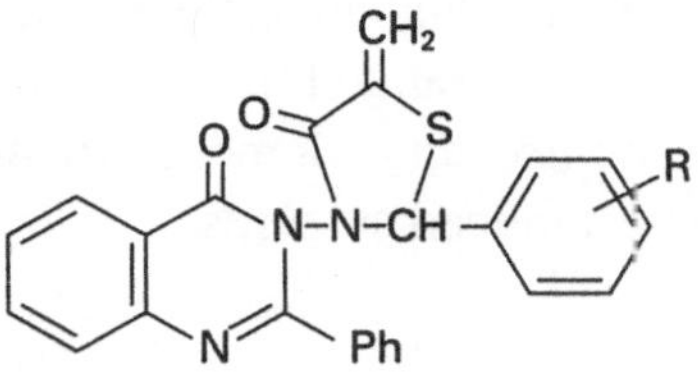

XXX
XXXa R = 3-OH
XXXb R = 2-Cl
XXXc R = 4-OMe
XXXd R = 3-OMe
XXXe R = 3-NO_2

Saxena et al. [41] synthesized 2-alkyl/aryl-3(arylhydrazino)quinazolin-4(3H)-ones as CNS active agents. CNS stimulant activity in 2-carbamoyl-methylthio and 2[(ω-dimethylaminoalkyl)thio]-3-alkyl/aryl-4(3H)-quina-zolinones **XXXI** was reported by Lakhan et al. [42], and it was observed that at higher dose levels the survival rate of the animals is rather low. Further they reported that compounds **XXXIa–XXXIc** showed CNS depressant activity [43].

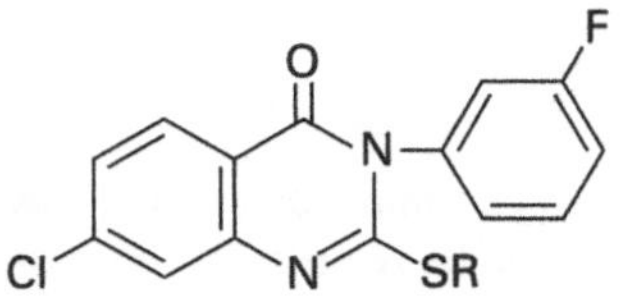

XXXI
XXXIa R = CH_2CONH_2
XXXIb R = $CH_2CH_2NMe_2$

In order to improve the CNS depressant effect of quinazolones some new quinazolones incorporating morpholine, malonyl urea and piperazines moieties were synthesized by Mukerji et al. [44]. These N'-[4(3H)-quina-zolon-3-yl]-N-methyl-4N-alkyl and aryl piperazines **XXXIIa**, morpho-lines **XXXIIb** and malonyl ureas **XXXIIc** showed depressant effects and also decreased the percent average of motor activity in albino mice. These compounds showed little protection (43.0–60.0%) against the chemical seizures induced by metrazole. Results indicate that **XXXIIb** containing morpholine moiety at position 3 showed only 14% protection while introduction of malonyl urea moiety made it lose its anticonvulsant activity.

Mukerjee et al. [45] synthesized a series of 3-alkyl/aryliminomethyl-4(3H)-quinazolones **XXXIII** and 3-alkyl/aryl (bis-iminomethylene)-4(3H)-quinazolones **XXXI** and investigated their CNS depressant activity in albino mice; the LD50 ranged from 400 mg/kg to 800 mg/kg i.p. and showed their relative nontoxicity. Some of them also showed 80% protection against pentylene-induced seizures.

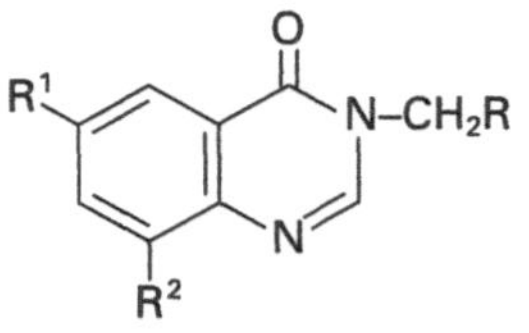

XXXII $R^1, R^2 = H, Cl, Br, I$
XXXIIa R = Substituted piperazines
XXXIIb R = Morpholinyl
XXXIIc R = Malonylurea

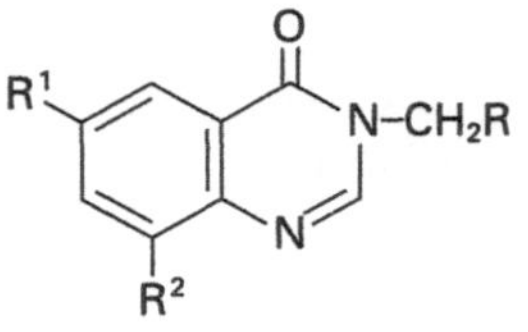

XXIII
R = OH, NH_2, Cl, NHCOMe, $NHCH_2$, NMe_2, NEt_2, N-methylpiperazino, phthalimido, NHC_6H_5, NHC_6H_4 (substituted) etc, $R^1, R^2 = H, Br, Cl, NO_2$

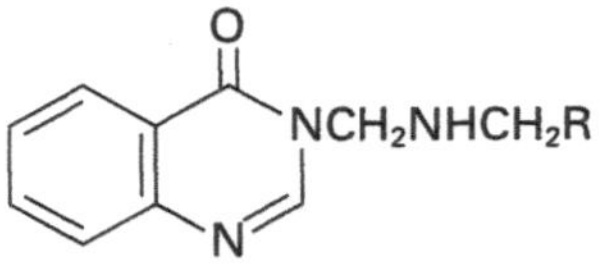

XXXIV
R = NHMe, $NHCHMe_2$, NMe_2, NEt_2, NHPh, N-methyl piperazino, phthalimido, NHPh (substituted)

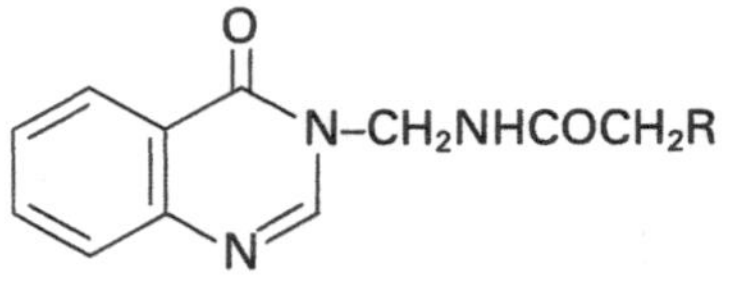

XXXV
R = Morpholino, pyrrolidino, piperidino, N-Me piperazino, phthalimido, N-methylanilino, N-ethyl anilino

New amides and carbamido methyl-4(3H)-quinazolones **XXXV** displayed CNS depressant effects shown by loss of righting reflex and ataxia [46]. Decreased percentage of motor activity was also observed and the average percentage decrease was 43 to 55%. Mukerjee et al. [47] also synthesized 3-(4'-aryl substituted carbamido) acetyl amino methyl-4(3H)-quinazolones **XXXVI** and evaluated their CNS and anticonvulsant activities. In general all compounds showed CNS depressant effects and little protection against the chemical-induced seizures by metrazole at one fifth of their ALD50. Compounds **XXXVIa–XXXVIc** showed maximum 40% protection and mortality up to 20% to 80% while compounds **XXXVId–XXXVIf** exhibited a 20% protection and mortality up to 60–100%. The rest of the compounds did not exhibit any anticonvulsant activity and have shown mortality nil to 100%. Results indicate that presence of a nitro group enhanced the toxicity.

Nautiyal et al. [48] synthesized a new series of 1-deoxy-1(4-quinazolon-3-yl) amino/methyl amino-D-fructose **XXXVII** with a view to observing the effect of aldose and amines linkage on CNS. Gross behaviour studies showed a decrease in motor activity. Some of them showed the effect of ptosis. These compounds were found to possess a maximum protection of 20% and mortality from 40% to 100% against metrazole-induced seizures.

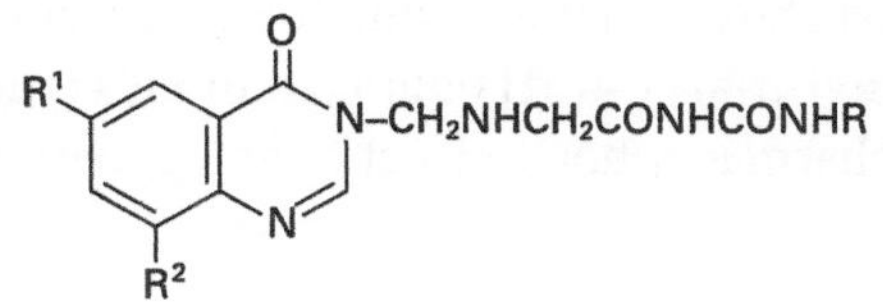

XXXVI			
	R	R^1	R^2
XXXVIa	Ph	H	H
XXXVIb	4-MePh	H	H
XXXVIc	2-MePh	Br	H
XXXVId	Ph	NO_2	H
XXXVIe	Ph	Br	Br
XXXVIf	4-MePh	Br	H
XXXVIg	4-OMePh	NO_2	H

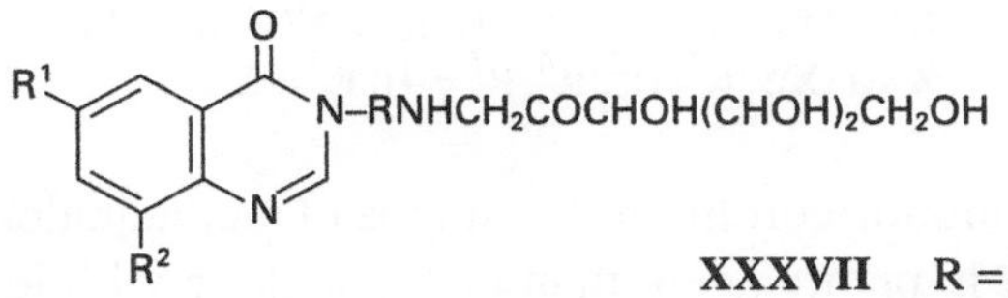

R^1—[quinazolone ring]—N–CH$_2$NHCH$_2$CONHCONHR, R^2

R^1—[quinazolone ring]—N–RNHCH$_2$COCHOH(CHOH)$_2$CH$_2$OH, R^2

XXXVII R = NHCO, NHCS, CH$_2$NHCO and CH$_2$NHCS, R^1, R^2 = H, Br, NO_2, Cl

Mukerjee et al. [49, 50] demonstrated the effect of thiazoline moiety at N'-3-position by the synthesis of 3-(2'-arylimino-4-oxo-thiazolin-3-yl) methyl quinazolones **XXXVIII**. They reported the CNS depressant effect by decreased spontaneous motor activity, slow respiration and loss of righting reflexes. Compounds **XXXVIIIa–XXXVIIIc** afforded 20% protection against metrazole-induced seizures, whereas most of the compounds were able to counteract metrazole toxicity to varying degrees. Introduction of bromo and nitro groups at position 6 or a bromo group at position 6 and 8 of the quinazolone nucleus seemed to lead to the complete disappearance of anticonvulsant effects.

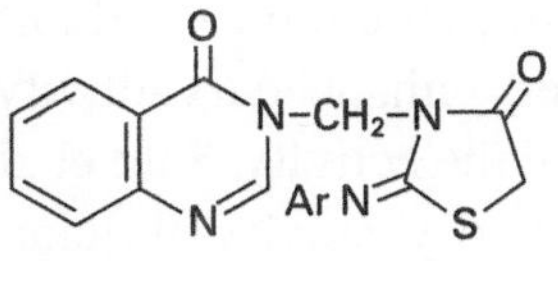

XXXVIIIa Ar = 4-MePh
XXXVIIIb Ar = Ph
XXXVIIIc Ar = 4-OMePh

Several 2-(fluoromethyl)-3-aryl-4H-quinazolinones **XXXIX** were synthesized by Junichi et al. [51] and were found to possess significant antidepressant activity. These compounds were compared to methaqualone and 2-(fluoromethyl)-3(3-chloro-2-tolyl)-4(3H)-quinazolinone **XXXIXa** was found to be more potent in regard to antidepressant activity and less toxic than methaqualone.

Compound **XXXIXa** was more potent in CNS depressant activity and less toxic than methaqualone while **XXXIXb** exhibited potent central muscle-relaxing activity and markedly reduced toxicity as compared with 6-aminomethaqualone. In conclusion it was shown that introduction of a fluoro group in the 2-methyl group of 2-methyl-3-aryl-4(3H)-quinazolinones is an effective step toward exploiting the pharmacophoric effect of halogenation [52].

XXXIX R^1 = H, Cl, R^2 = H, Cl, NO_2, NH_2NHAc,
R^3 = H, Me, Cl, R^4, R^5 = H, Cl
XXXIXa R^1, R^2, R^5 = H, R^3 = Me, R^4 = Cl
XXXIXb R^1, R^4, R^5 = H, R^2 = NH_2, R^3 = Me
XXXIXc R^1, R^2, R^4, R^5 = H, R^3 = Me

Ochiai et al. [53] reported a 2-monofluoromethyl analogue of methaqualone **XXXIXc** to be a more potent hypnotic agent than methaqualone with less toxicity. A large number of fluorinated 2-alkyl-3-aryl-4(3H)-quinazolinones and their corresponding 4-thioanalogs **XL** were synthesized and screened for their hypnotic, analgesic and behavioural activities as well as acute toxicity, spontaneous motor activity [54]. 6-Fluoro-2-methyl-3(p-bromophenyl)-4(3H)-quinazolinone exhibited pronounced spontaneous motor activity, hypnotic activity, behavioural activity and acute toxicity.

Further work on fluorinated 2-alkyl/phenyl-3-aryl-4(3H)-quinazolones, 2-thio/alkylthio-3-aryl-4(3H)-quinazolones and thioquinazolones **XLIa–XLId**) for CNS depressant activity was also reported by Joshi et al. [55]. Compound **XLIb** is the most potent one. Compounds **XLIa** and **XLIb** showed 60% and 100% protection against pentylene tetrazole induced seizures while most of the compounds showed only 20% protection. Condition avoidance test in rats showed that **XLIb–XLId** were equally potent exhibiting 80% response. Results suggested that introduction of a fluoro group at the different positions of quinazolone moiety enhanced its activity. Presence of a thio group at position 2 also increased the activity. Sato et al. [56] reported the CNS depressant and anti-inflammatory activity of quinazolinone acetamides **XLII** demonstrating that 2-fluoromethyl-3-(2-methyl-phenyl)-6-amino-4(3H)-quinazolinone **XLIII** was a more potent muscle relaxant than mephenesin in mice [57].

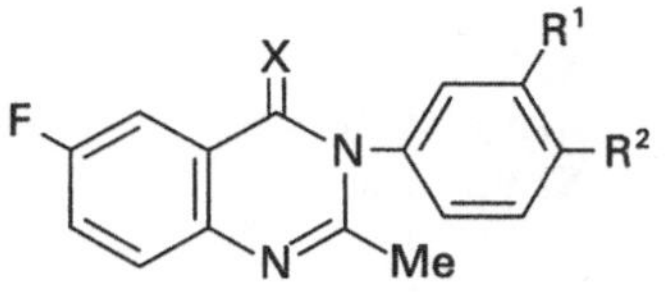

XL
X = O, S, R^1, R^2 = H, Me

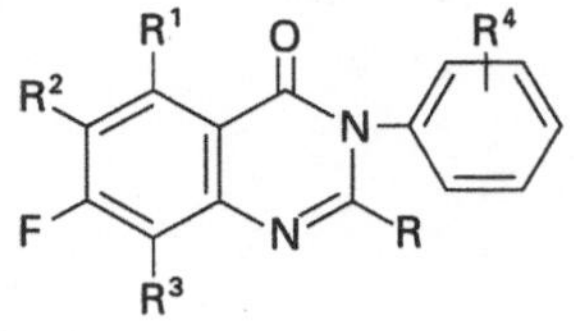

XLI

	R	R^1	R^2	R^3	R^4
XLIa	Me	H	H	H	2-Me
XLIb	SH	F	F	F	4-F
XLIc	n–C_3H_7S	F	F	F	4-F
XLId	C_6H_5	H	H	H	H

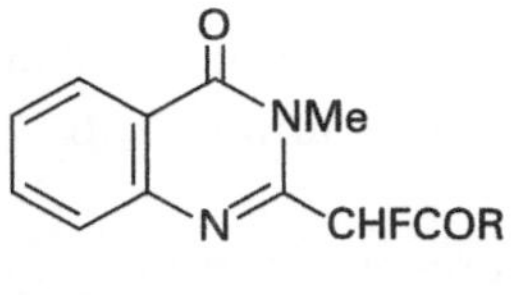

XLII
R = Heterocyclic amines

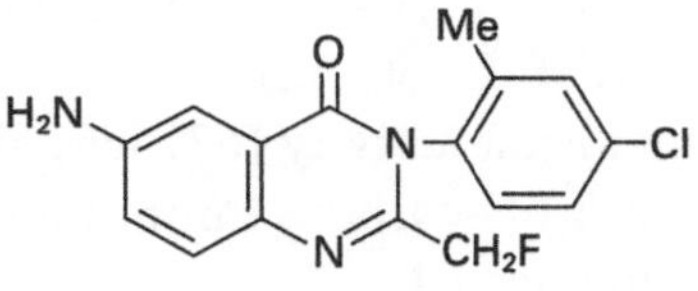

XLIII

3.3 Anticonvulsant activity

Numerous compounds **XLIV** related to methaqualone exhibited anticonvulsant activity [58]. 2-Methyl-3-(2-methyl-4-aminophenyl)quinazolin-(3H)-4-one **XLIVa** showed greater activity than methaqualone against maximal electroshock seizures. Compound **XLIVb** exhibited pronounced anticonvulsant activity but showed greater toxicity than **XLIVa**. Examination of forty-two different quinazolinone derivatives [59] revealed that 2-methyl-3-(p-bromophenyl)-4(3H)-quinazolinone **XLVa** was the most potent compound, fourteen times more active than troxidone **XLVI**, but its 4-thio analog **XLVb** had less anticonvulsant activity. Substitution of 4-bromophenyl group at position 2 instead of position 3 in the quinazolinone nucleus resulted in decreased anticonvulsant activity.

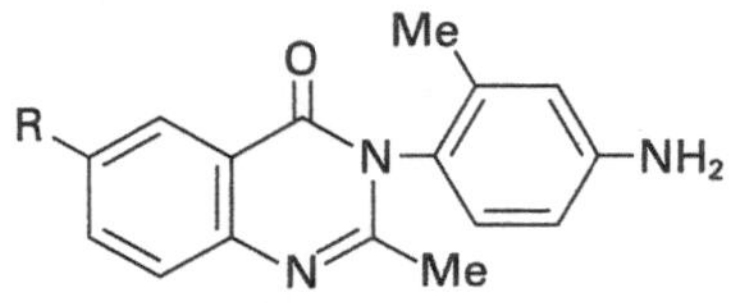

XLIV
XLIVa R = H
XLIVb R = Cl

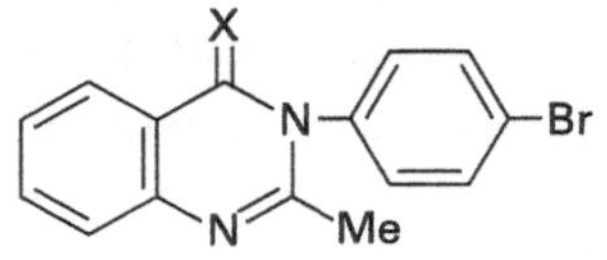

XLV
XLVa X = O
XLVb X = S

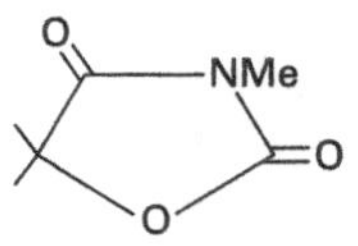

XLVI

Sedative and anticonvulsant activities were also shown in a large number of 2-methyl-3-aryl-4(3H)-quinazolinones substituted at positions 5, 6, 7 and 8 **XLVII–L** [60–62].

Anticonvulsant activity [63] was also shown by 2-mercapto-3-anilino-'2-mercapto-3-(4'-carboxyanilino) and 2-mercapto-3-dimethylamino-4(3H)-quinazolinones **LI**.

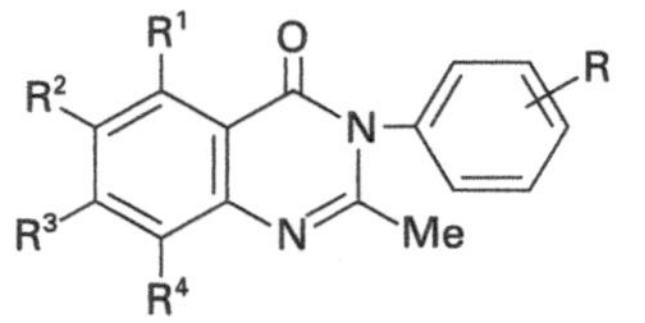

XLVII
R = 2-Me, 2-Et, $R^1R^2R^3R^4$ = H, Cl, NO_2, NH_2

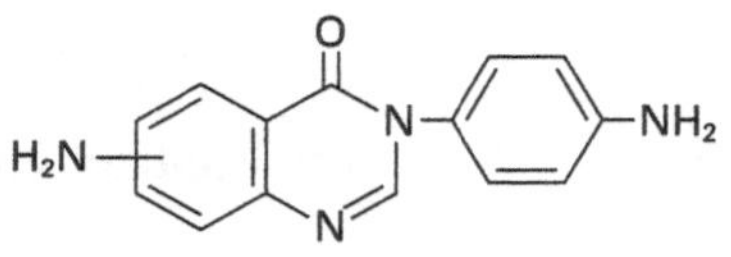

XVIII

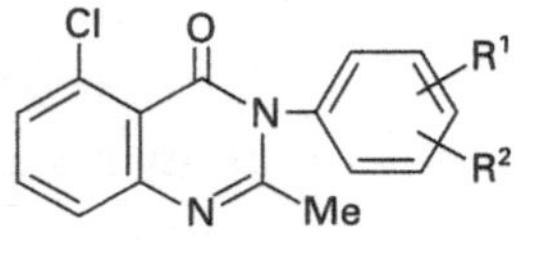

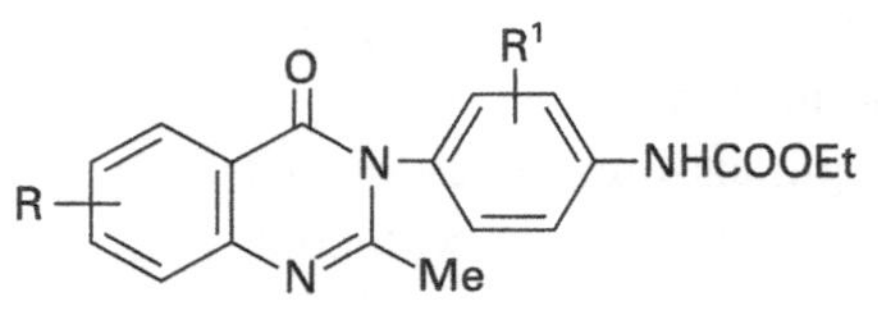

XLIX
R = H, 7-NH_2, 7-Me, R^1 = 6-Me, 4, 5-Me$_2$,
4-OMe, 4-Cl, 2-Me

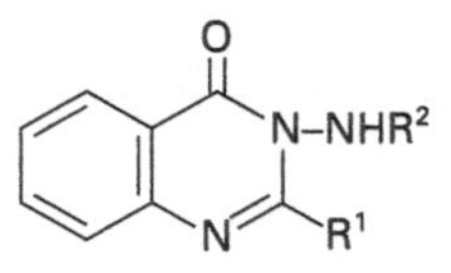

L
R^1 = H, 2-Me, R^2 = 2-Cl, 4-Cl, 3-Cl,
3-OMe, 4-OMe

LI
R^1 = H, SH, R^2 = H, C_6H_5, C_6H_4COOH, NMe_2

Philips [64] reported that 3-alkyl or aryl-4-quinazolinones with electron donating groups at position 8, such as halogen amino or substituted amino **LII** exhibited long-lasting sedative and anticonvulsant effects.

Glasser et al. [65] synthesized and screened a series of 2-thio quinazoline-4-ones **LIII** and **LIV** for CNS activity in mice with a dosage ranging from 10–600 mg/kg. Full protection against electroshock was observed in the case of 2-ethylthio-3-(2-phenyl) ethyl-quinazolin-4-one **LIIIa** and 2-carboxymethyl thio-3-(2-phenyl)ethyl-quinazolin-4-one **LIIIb** at doses of 100 mg/kg and 600 mg/kg, respectively.

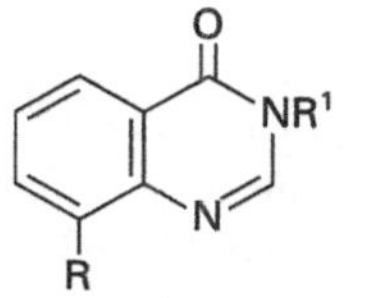

LII
R = Cl, NH$_2$, Br, R^1 = Alkyl

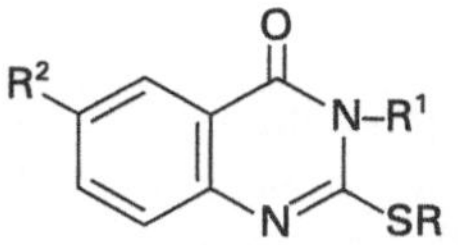

LIII
LIIIa   R = C$_2$H$_5$, R^1 = CH$_2$CH$_2$C$_6$H$_5$, R^2 = H
LIIIb   R = CH$_2$COOH, R^1 = CH$_2$CH$_2$C$_6$H$_5$, R^2 = H

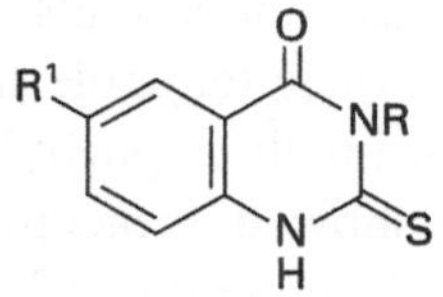

LIV
R = C$_6$H$_5$, CH$_2$CH$_2$C$_6$H$_5$, R^1 = H, Cl

Shukla et al. [66] reported the CNS and anticonvulsant activity of 2-(substituted) phenoxymethyl-3-heterocyclic substituted-4(3H)-quinazolones **LV**. All of them showed CNS depressant activity. The protection against pentylene tetrazole induced seizures was ranged from 10–60%. 2-(2-methoxyphenoxymethyl) 3-(2'-thiazolyl)-4-quinazolone (**LVa**) was found to exhibit maximum protection (60%) while 2-(2-chlorophenoxymethyl)3-(2'-thiazolyl)-6,8-dibromo-4-quinazolone **LVb** exhibited no protection and 100% mortality was observed during 24 hours.

These results showed that introduction of a nucleophile at R, R^1, R^2 positions reduced the protective ability. Substitution of the pyridyl group at position 3 also reduced the ability of protection in comparison to thiazolyl group as in compounds **LVc** and **LVd**. Further, 2-phenoxymethyl-3-N-substituted amino carbonyl methyl-8-substituted-4(3H)-quinazolones **LVI** was synthesized and evaluated for anticonvulsant activity [67]. The protective ability ranged from 20–70% against pentylene tetrazole induced seizures. Maximum protection was observed in compounds **LVIa–LVIc** while **LVId** showed minimum protection. These results possibly indicate that introduction of a nucleophile in phenyl ring at position 2 reduced the protective ability while an electrophile enhanced it.

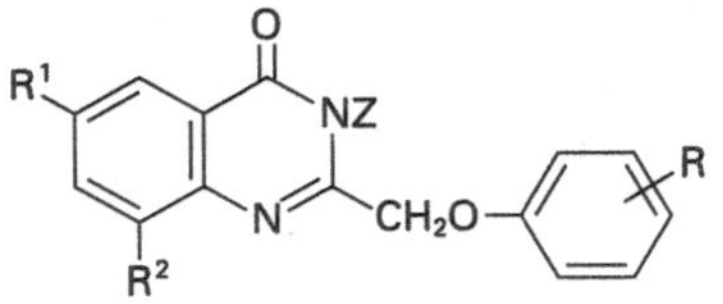

LV
LVa R = 4-Me, R^1, R^2 = H, Z = 2-thiazolyl
LVb R = 2-Cl, R^1, R^2 = Br, Z = 2-thiazolyl
LVc R = 4-NO2, R^1, R^2 = H, Z = 2-pyridyl
LVd R = 2-Cl, R^1, R^2 = H, Z = 2-pyridyl

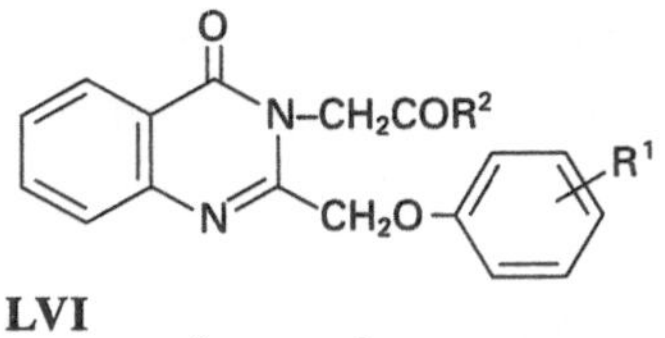

LVI
LVIa R^1 = H, R^2 = morpholinyl
LVIb R^1 = 2-Me, R^2 = thiazolyl
LVIc R^1 = 2-Me, R^2 = morpholinyl
LVId R^1 = 2-Cl, R^2 = piperidinyl

Husain et al. [68] synthesized some 2-aryloxymethyl-3-α-substituted carboxymethyl-6,8-disubstituted-4(3H)-quinazolones as anticonvulsant agents, which showed 20–60% protection against pentylene tetrazole induced seizures in mice. 2-Alkyl-2[4(3H)-oxo-2-(3,4,5-trimethoxyphenyl)-3-quinazolyl]ethanoic acids and amides **LVII** also showed protection against pentylene tetrazole induced seizures in mice. Compound **LVII** exhibited 40% protection [69].

Barthwal et al. [70] reported some quinazolone 1,3,4-oxadiazoles which showed anticonvulsant activity with maximum protection (70%) by compound **LVIII**.

A series of 2,3-disubstituted-4(3H)-quinazolinones **LIX** was synthesized by Ossmon et al. [71] as potential anticonvulsants.

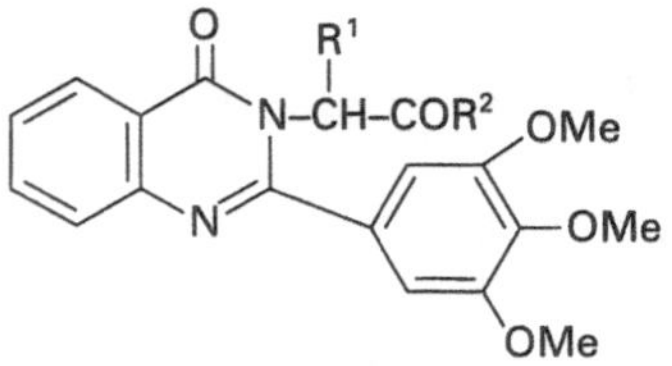

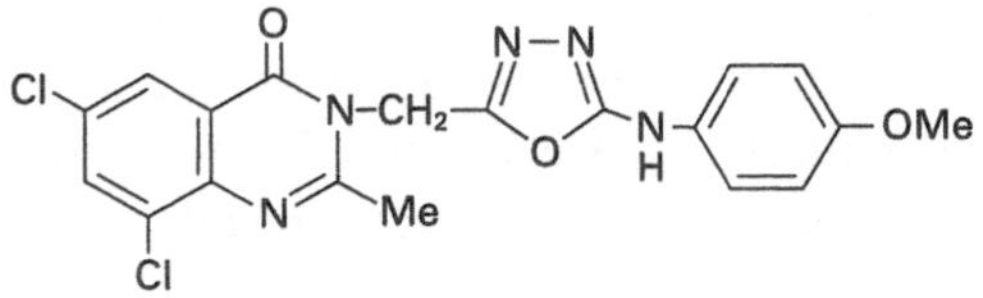

LVII
R^1 = isobutyl, R^2 = morpholinyl

LVIII

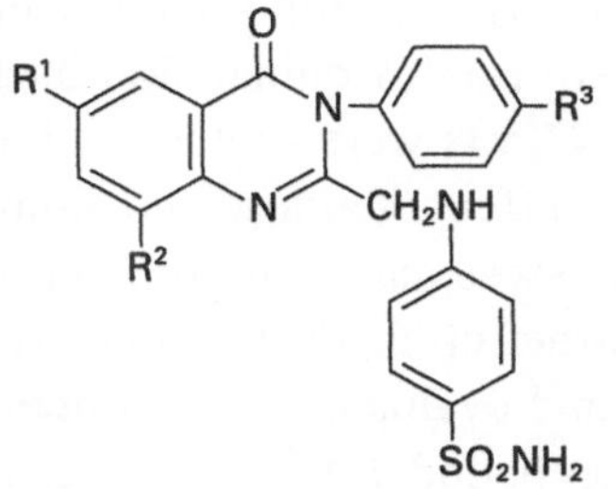

LIX
R^1, R^2 = H, Br, R^3 = H, Br, Cl, NO2

Misra et al. [72, 73] reported that 2-phenyl/methyl-3-0, 3 or 4-(benzimida-zol-2'-yl)phenyl-6,8-substituted/unsubstituted quinazolin (3H)-4-ones at 100 mg/kg protected mice against convulsion. Compounds **LXa** and **LXb** showed 80% protection against pentylene tetrazole seizures in mice.

2-Methyl-3-(3,5-dialkyl-4-hydroxyphenyl)-4-quinazolones **LXI** were syn-thesized as anticonvulsant agents by Rastogi et al. [74] which provided 40% protection against pentylene tetrazole induced convulsions. Several substi-tuted styryl quinazolones possessed anticonvulsant activity against penty-lene tetrazole induced seizures in mice [75]. Vizgunova et al. [76] synthe-sized 1,2-disubstituted 4-quinazolinones **LXII–LXIV** which were shown to exhibit anticonvulsant activity in mice.

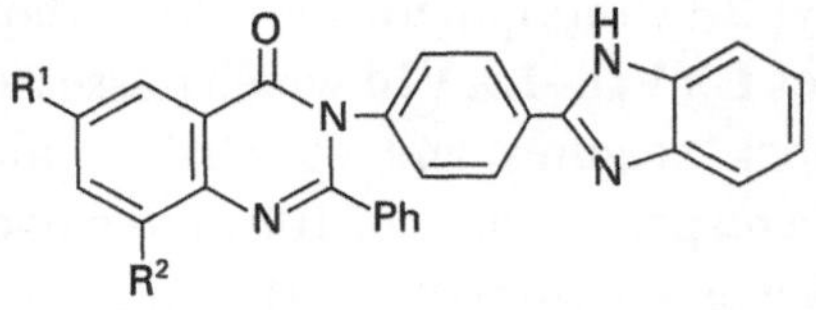

LX
LXa R, R^1 = Br
LXb R = I, R^1 = H

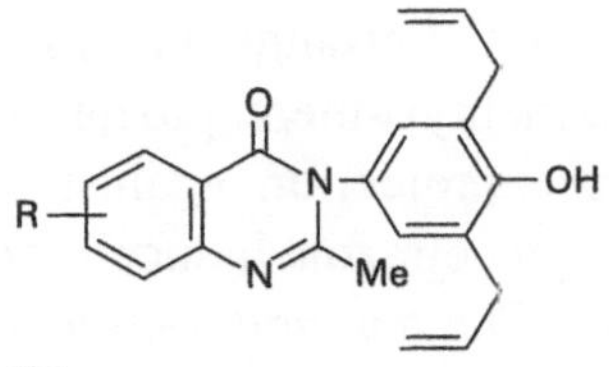

LXI
R = H, Cl, Br, I

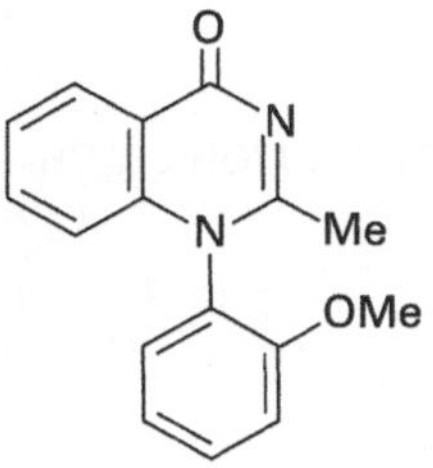

LXII

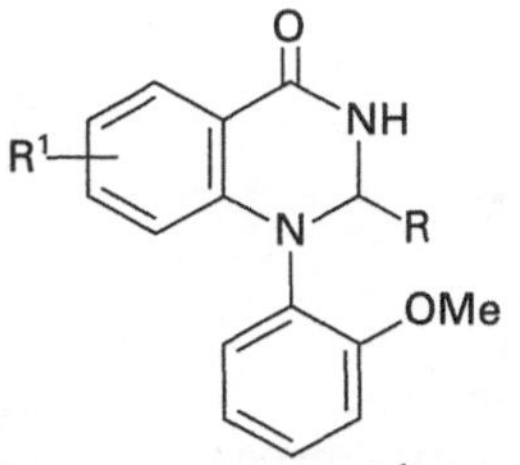

LXIII R = 2-furyl, R^1 = H
LXIV R = Me, R^1 = Br

3-(chloroacylamino)-2-methyl-4(3H)-quinazolones were reported as anticonvulsant agents [77]. A new series of 1-deoxy-1-[(4-quinazolon-3-yl) amino/methyl amino-D-fructose derivatives **XXXVII** were synthesized by Nautiyal et al. [48] with a view to observing the effect of aldose and amine linkage on CNS activity. They were found to possess maximum protection up to 20% and mortality up to 40–100%. Kornet et al. [78] synthesized 2-alkyl-3-amino-4(3H)-quinazolinones **LXV** and evaluated their anticonvulsant effect and neurotoxicity in mice. Compound **LXVa** was active against maximal electroshock seizures at 300 mg/kg and had no toxicity at this dose, while **LXVb** was active at 300 mg/kg against both the maximal electroshock and pentylene tetrazole seizures. This drug, however, exhibited neurotoxicity in all tested animals. Dwivedi et al. [79] reported that 2-methyl-3-(3-methyl-2-pyridyl)-4-quinazolone **LXVc** at 100 mg/kg i.p. dose showed 100% protection against pentylene tetrazol-induced convulsions in mice. The LD50 of **LXVc** was 1000 mg/kg i.p. In mice it shows its relative nontoxicity. A number of 6,8-disubstituted-3-[5-(2-hydroxy-3[substituted   phenyl]amino)propyl]thio(1,3,4-thiadizol-2-yl]-2-methyl-4(3H)-quinazolinones **LXVI** were synthesized to observe the effect of a 2-thiadiazolyl group at position 3 for anticonvulsant activity [80].

Presence of piperazine moiety at position 2 enhanced the anticonvulsant activity against electroshock seizures and pentylene tetrazole seizures as reported by Satsangi et al. [81] in 3-aryl-2-(1'-arylpiperazin-4'-yl-carboxamido methyl)-mercapto quinazolinones **LXVIb–LXVId** which possessed 20–60% protection against electroshock seizures and 49–80% against pentylene tetrazole induced seizures at a respective dose of 100 mg/kg body weight. The maximum protection 60% was shown by **LXVIb** and **LXVIc** while 80% protection was exhibited by **LXVId** with R^1 as 4-Cl and R^2 as 3-F. These compounds also potentiated the pentobarbital sleeping time in a range of 7.81 ± 4 to 54.65 ± 7 min.

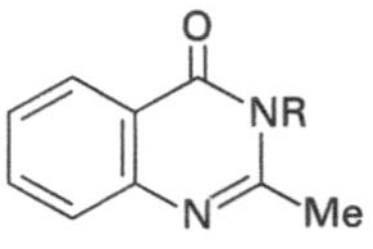

LXV
LXVa R = NMe$_2$
LXVb R = Morpholino
LXVc R = 3-Methyl-2-pyrido

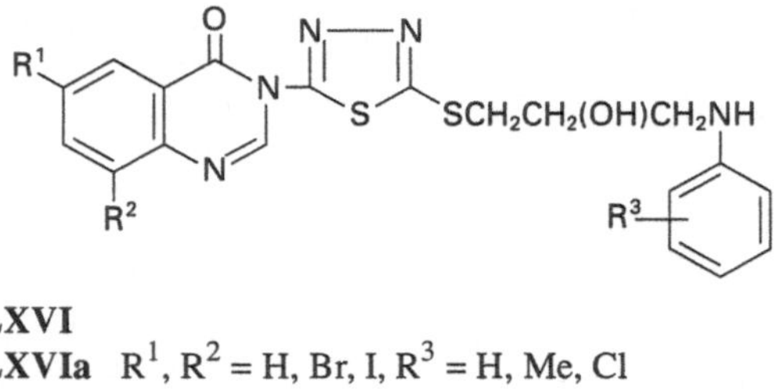

LXVI
LXVIa R^1, R^2 = H, Br, I, R^3 = H, Me, Cl

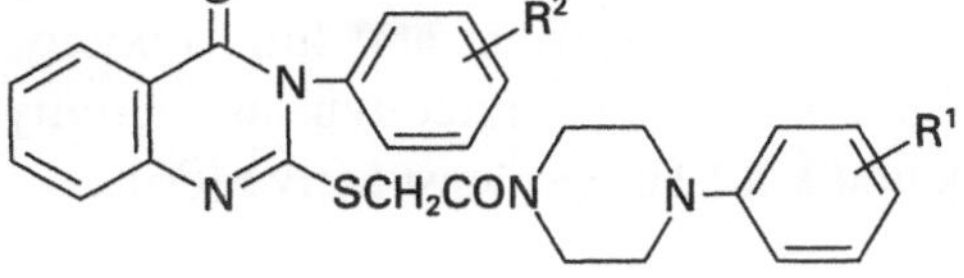

LXVIb R^1 = 3-Me, H, R^2 = H
LXVIc R^1 = 4-Me, R^2 = H
LXVId R^1 = 4-Cl, R^2 = 3-F

Wolfe et al. [82] synthesized some new 2-substituted-3-aryl-4(3H)-quina-zolinones and observed that compound **LXVII** with a single orthosubstit-uent at 3-aryl had the most promising anticonvulsant activity. Khalil and El-Din [83] reported the anticonvulsant activity of triazinylquinazolinones **LXVIII** and observed that **LXVIIIa** showed anticonvulsant activity; how-ever **LXVIIIb** was inactive.

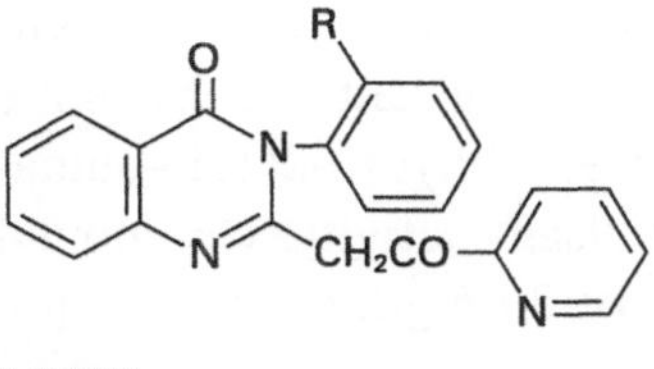

LXVII
R = Cl, Br, I, OMe, Me, F

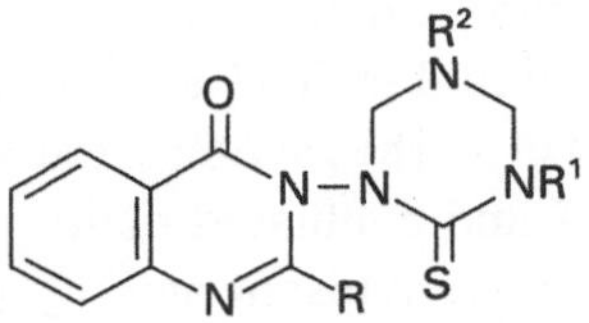

LXVIII
LXVIIIa R = Me, R^1 = 4-ClPh, R^2 = 4-ClPh, 4-MePh
LXVIIIb R = Ph, R^1 = 4-ClPh, Ph, R^2 = 4-ClPh

Anticonvulsant activity of 2-methyl-3-(heterocyclic)-6,8-disubstituted qui-nazolinones **LXIX** was tested in mice [84]. The compound **LXIXa** with no substitution was most active (i.p. LD50 = 1200 mg/kg), while the least active compound was **LXIXb** with a bromo group at positions 6 and 8.

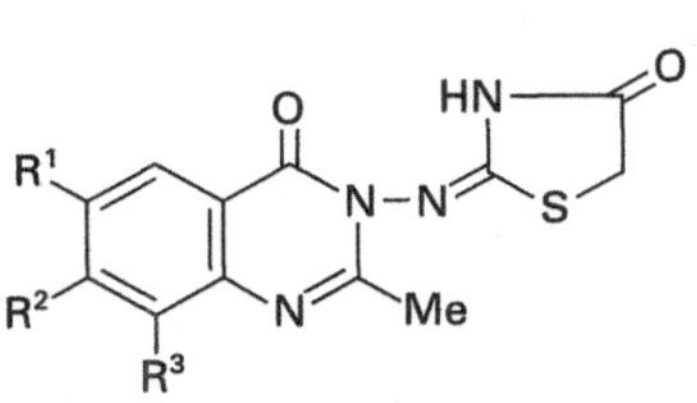

LXIX R^1 = H, Cl, Br, Me, R^2 = H, NO2,
R^3 = H, Cl, Br
LXIXa R^1, R^2, R^3 = H
LXIXb R^1, R^3 = Br, R^2 = H

Desh Pande et al. [85] studied the anticonvulsant activity of 6,8-dibromo-3-[(5-aryl-1,3,4-oxadiazol-2-yl)methyl]-2-methyl-4(3H)-quinazolinones **LXX** against supramaximal electroshock seizures in rats and metrazole-in-duced seizures (MES) in mice and reported that compounds **LXXa** and **LXXb** possessed anticonvulsant activity against MES. The hydroxyphenyl compound appeared to be promising as it possessed anticonvulsant activity without any central nervous system depressant effect and little toxicity. While the compound **LXXIa** exhibited significant anticonvulsant activity at LD50 800 mg/kg, i.p., the compound **LXXIb** was least active [86].

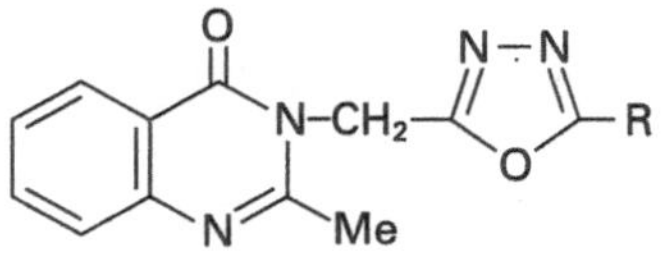

LXX
LXXa R = 2-ClPh
LXXb R = 4-OHPh

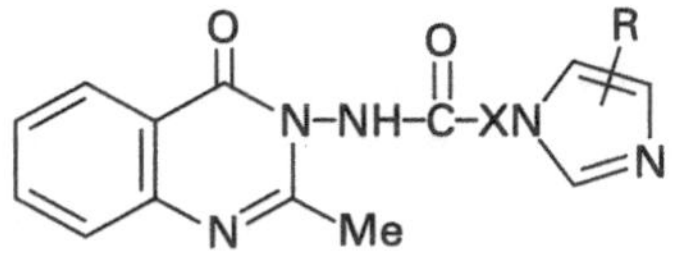

LXXI
LXXIa R = Me, X = (CH2)2
LXXIb R = H, X = CHMe

3-(Chloroacylamino)-2-methyl-4(3H)-quinazolinone derivatives were synthesized by Buyuktimkia [87] and showed anticonvulsant and hypnotic activities. Kornet et al. [88] synthesized 3 amino-3,4-dihydro-2(1H)-quinazolinones **LXXII** and evaluated their anticonvulsant activity. Compound **LXXII** showed anticonvulsant activity (ED50 of 30 mg/kg in mice) in a maximal electroshock seizure test.

Some 3-alkyl-3,4-dihydro-2(1H)-quinazolinones **LXXIII** were synthesized for testing anticonvulsant agents against maximal electroshock seizures [89].

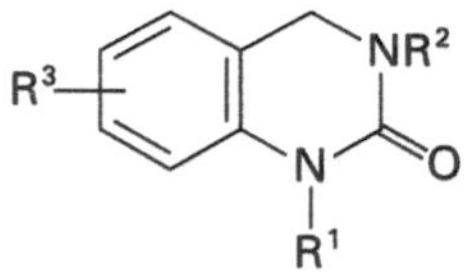

LXXII R^1 = H, R^2 = NMe2, R^3 = H
LXXIII R^1 = H, 2-FPh, R^2 = alkyl, cycloalkyl,
          R^3 = H, 8-Me, 6-Me

3.4   Hypnotic activity

Methaqualone (2-methyl-3-(O-tolyl)-4-(3H)-quinazolone) possesses the optimal hypnotic activity, and even relatively minor structural changes in the molecular formula greatly diminish or even abolish the hypnotic activity. The hypnotic activity of methaqualone was first reported in 1955 [90], and this compound is now extensively used clinically as a non-barbiturate hypnotic. It also depresses polysynaptic spinal reflexes [91].

Rastogi et al. [92] synthesized some dimethyl quinazolone derivatives and reported that dimethyl quinazolone is more potent than methaqualone and mephenesin in producing ataxia, hind limb paralysis, loss of righting and pineal reflexes and abolishing painful stimuli. It does not affect straub tail response in smaller doses like methaqualone and mephenesin while higher doses abolished the response indicating thereby the presence of a central muscle relaxant component in smaller doses and peripheral muscle relaxant activity in higher doses. Gorduchwk et al. [92] reported that sedative activity of 4-phenylquinazolin-2-ones **LXXIV** increased in the order of **LXXIVa** < **LXXIVb** < **LXXIVc** < **LXXIVd**

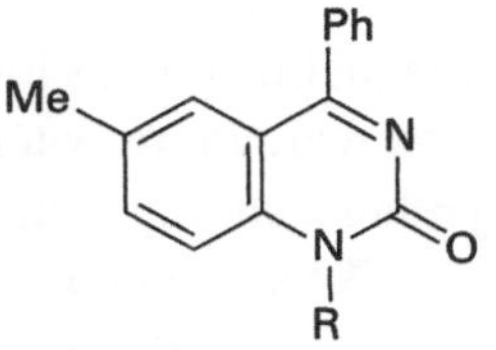

LXXIV
LXXIVa R = CHF$_2$O
LXXIVb R = CF$_3$SO$_2$
LXXIVc R = CF$_3$S

3-Amino-2-(heteroaryl)amino-4(3H)-quinazolinones **LXXV** potentially useful as sedatives, cardiotonics and antihistaminics, were synthesized [94]. 2-Methyl-3-disubstituted aryl-5-chloro-4(3H)-quinazolinones **LXXVI** were reported to exhibit sedative action and were found to be highly selective psychotropic agents and tranquilizers [95].

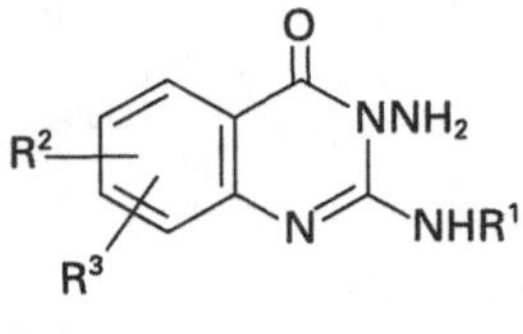

LXXV
R^1 = Heteroaryl, R^2, R^3 = H, alkyl, alkoxy, halo

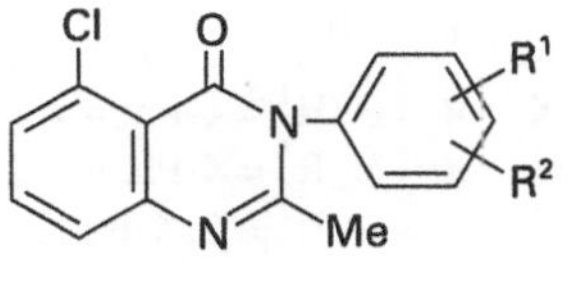

LXXVI
R^1 = H, 2-Me, R^2 = Cl, OMe

Among the therapeutically used quinazolones are centazolone **LXXVII** and lonetill **LXXVIII**. Compound **LXXVII** proved to be a potent tranquilizer, sedative and muscle relaxant, whilst **LXXVIII** has been reported as a potent tranquilizer with excellent resorption [96, 97].

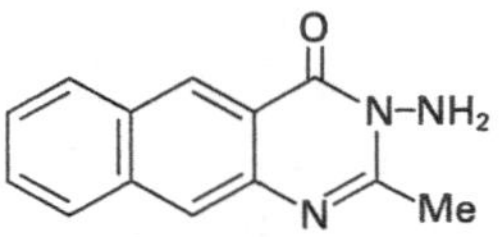

LXXVII 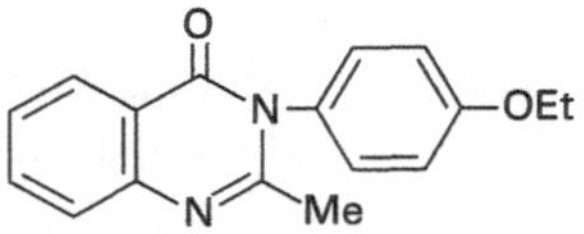   **LXXVIII**

3.5   Analgesic and muscle relaxant activity

Methaqualone and dimethyl quinazolone both showed central and peripheral muscle relaxant activity. In low doses both induce ataxia and hind limb weakness, but in higher doses a peripheral neuromuscular action comes into play. Both selectively inhibited polysynaptic reflexes and were more potent than mephenesin [98]. Fisnerova et al. [99, 100] synthesized some keto derivatives of 4-(3H)-quinazolinone and reported that **LXXIX** showed oral analgesic activity comparable to that of aminophenazone in mice with lower toxicity. A significant analgesic activity was exhibited by compounds **LXXXa** and **LXXXb**. A series of alkyl thio-4-(3H)-quinazolinones **LXXXI** were synthesized and some of them showed analgesic activity [101].

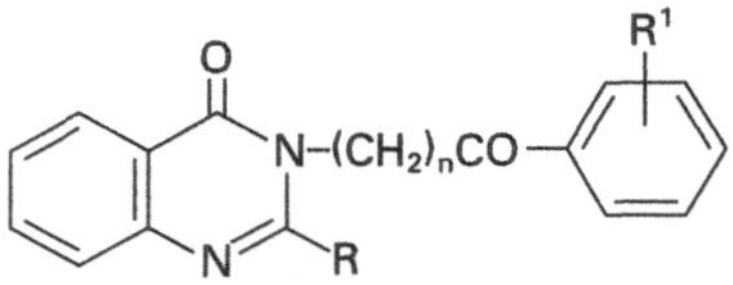

LXXIX   R = H, R^1 = 4-Ph, n = 1
LXXXa   R = H, R^1 = 4-Ph, n = 2
LXXXb   R = H, R^1 = 2, 4-F Ph, n = 2

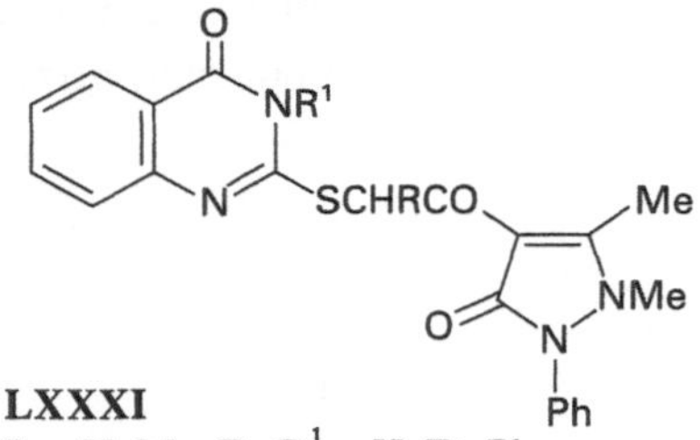

LXXXI
R = H, Me, Et, R^1 = H, Et, Ph

Gordiichuk et al. [93] reported that analgesic activity of 4-phenyl quinazolin-2-ones **LXXXII** increased symbatically with the value of Hammett substituent constant. Compound **LXXXIIa** showed little activity, but **LXXXIId, LXXXIIe, LXXXIIh** and **LXXXIIj** exhibited significant activity. The activity increased in the order of **LXXXIIa << LXXXIIb = LXXXIIc < LXXXIId = LXXXIIe** and **LXXXIIf < LXXXIIg < LXXXIIh < LXXXIIL = LXXXIIj**.
3-(5-Aryl-1,3,4-oxadiazol-2-yl-methyl)-2-methyl-4(3H)-quinazolinones **LXXXIII** demonstrated moderate analgesic activity, whereby compound **LXXXIIIa** was the most active.

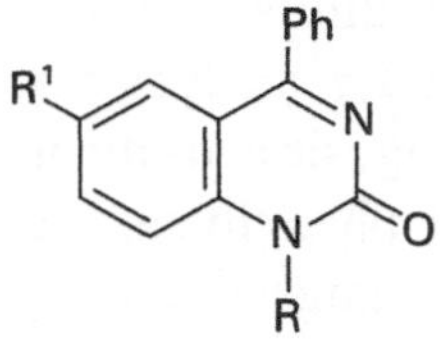

LXXXII
LXXXIIa R = CHF$_2$SO$_2$, R^1 = H
LXXXIIb R = CF$_3$S, R^1 = H
LXXXIIc R = CF$_3$O, R^1 = H
LXXXIId R = CHF$_2$S, R^1 = H
LXXXIIe R = CHF$_2$O, R^1 = H
LXXXIIf R = CHF$_2$SO$_2$, R^1 = Me
LXXXIIg R = CF$_3$SO$_2$, R^1 = Me
LXXXIIh R = CHF$_2$O, R^1 = Me
LXXXIIi R = CF$_3$O, R^1 = Me
LXXXIIj R = CF$_3$S, R^1 = Me

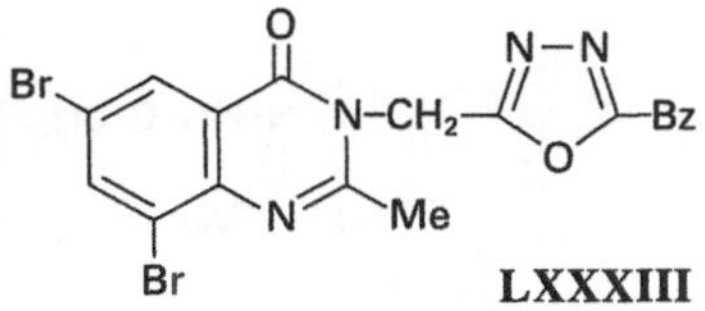

LXXXIII

Sadanandam et al. [103] reported the synthesis and analgesic activity of 2,
3-dihydro-1-(β-phenylethyl)-2-aryl- and 2,3-diaryl-4(1H)-quinazolinones
LXXIV. Compounds **LXXXIVa** and **LXXXIVb** showed potent analgesic
activity.

A number of 1,2,3,4-tetrahydro-4-quinazolinone derivatives were screened
for analgesic activity, among them compound **LXXXV** had the highest
analgesic activity at LD50 2500–3100 mg/kg i.p. in mice [104].

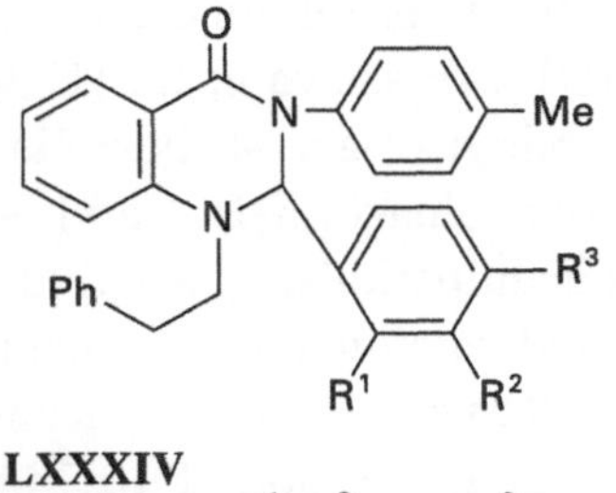

LXXXIV
LXXXIVa R^1, R^3 = Cl, R^2 = H
LXXXIVb R^1 = H, R^{2}R^3 = –OCH$_2$O–

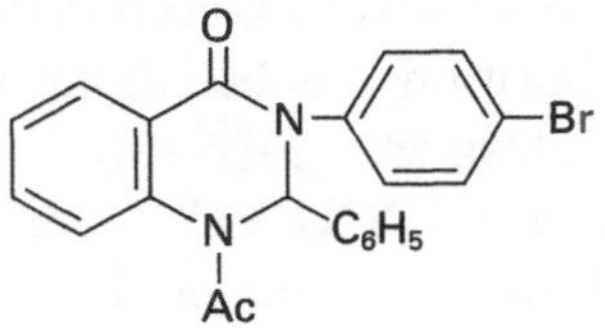

LXXXV

Shanker et al. [105] reported the analgesic activity of N^4 [N-(6,8-dibromo-
2-methyl-3-quinazolin-4(3H)-onyl)acetamido]N'-substituted   sulfanilamides **LXXXVI**. Compound **LXXXVIa** followed by **LXXXVIb** was
found to be almost on a par with aspirin in its analgesic activity, while
LXXXVIc was moderate in its activity, and **LXXXVId** showed a weak
analgesic activity.

Further, a series of 3-α-(S-substituted mercaptoacetamido) **LXXXVII** and

3-α-(N,N-disubstitutedaminoacetamido)-6,8-dibromo-2-methyl-quinazo-lin-4-ones were synthesized and evaluated for analgesic activity. Compound **LXXXVIIa** exhibited remarkable analgesic activity; its potency was shown to be higher than that of standard phenylbutazone and aspirin; compound **LXXXIIb** exhibited a very mild analgesic activity while others were inactive [106].

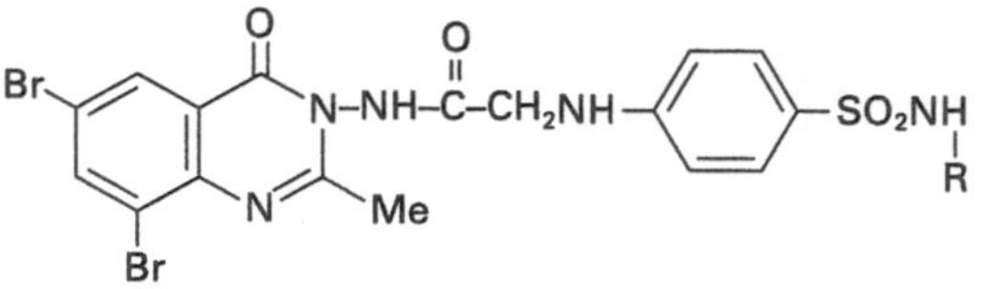

LXXXVI
LXXXVIa R = 5-Methoxy isoxazolyl
LXXXVIb R = 2, 6-Dimethoxy-4-pyrimidyl
LXXXVIc R = 5-Methyl-2(1, 3, 4-thiadiazolyl)
LXXXVId R = H

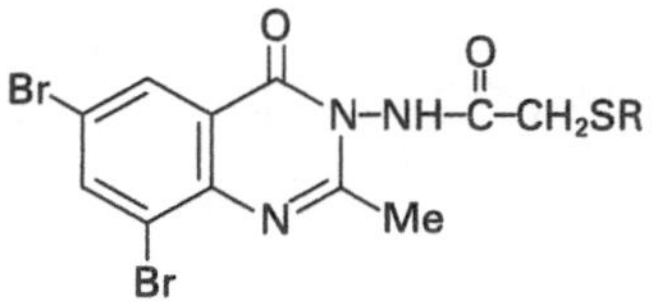

LXXXVII
LXXXVIIa R = ter-Butyl
LXXXVIIb R = 2-Carboxyphenyl
LXXXVIIc R = sec-Butyl

3.6   Antiparkinsonian activity

Quinazolinones possess antiparkinsonian activity [107]. Earlier reports have shown that incorporation of bulky groups in the quinazolinone nucleus at position 2 is beneficial for activity [108, 109]. Srivastava et al. [110] synthesized 3-[2-alkyl 4(3H)-oxo-3-quinazolinyl]-2-aryl-4-thiazolid-inones **LXXXVIII** and 3-(2-alkyl-4(3H)-oxoquinazolinyl)-4-aryl-3-chloro-2-azetidinones **LXXXIX** and studied their antiparkinsonian activity against tremor or rigidity, ptosis, hypokinesia and catatonia. Compounds **LXXXVIIIa, LXXXVIIIb** and **LXXXIXa, LXXXIXb** showed significant antiparkinsonian activity. These compounds at a concentration of 10^{-4} M have also been evaluated for their effect on dopamine receptor binding, and they significantly inhibit the binding *in vivo*.

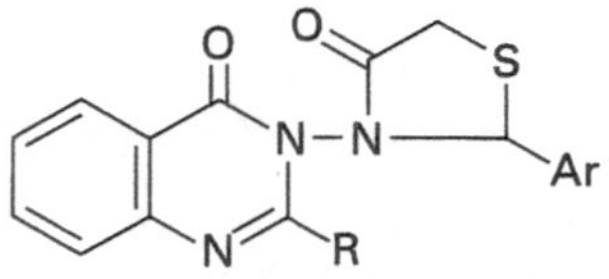

LXXXVIII
LXXXVIIIa R = Me, Ar = 4-N(Me)$_2$C$_6$H$_4$
LXXXVIIIb R = Et, Ar = C$_6$H$_5$

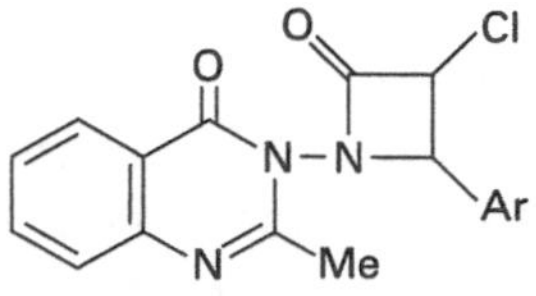

LXXXIX
LXXXIXa Ar = C$_6$H$_5$
LXXXIXb Ar = 2-Furyl

Tewari et al. [111] reported that 3-hydroxyquinazolinone derivatives **XC** when tested for antitremorine activity in mice, did not exhibit significant activity. A series of 3-(2-hydroxyethyl)-2-methyl quinazolinones **XCI** and **XCII** was synthesized by Khanna et al. [112]. Compounds **XCIa**, **XCIb**, **XCIc** and **XCII** showed maximum antiparkinsonian activity in albino rats with no toxicity (ALD50>1000 mg/kg).

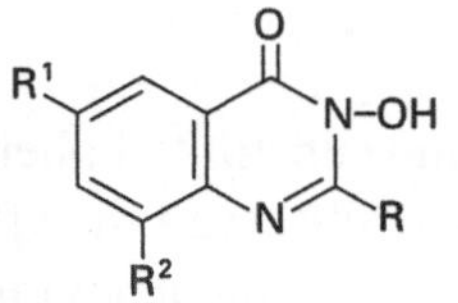

XC
R = $C_6H_5CONHCH_2$, $C_6H_5CH(OH)$,
$C_6H_5CH = CH$, R^1, R^2 = H, Br

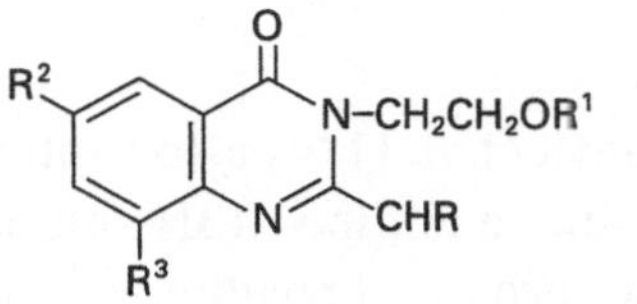

XCI
XCIa R = H_2, R^1 = H, R^2, R^3 = Br
XCIb R = $CHC_6H_3(OMe)_2$,
R^1 = $COCH_2NHC_6H_4Me$-2, R^2, R^3 = Br
XCIc R = H_2, R^1 = $CH_2CH(OH)CH_2R^4$, R^2,
R^3 = Br, R^4 = morpholinyl

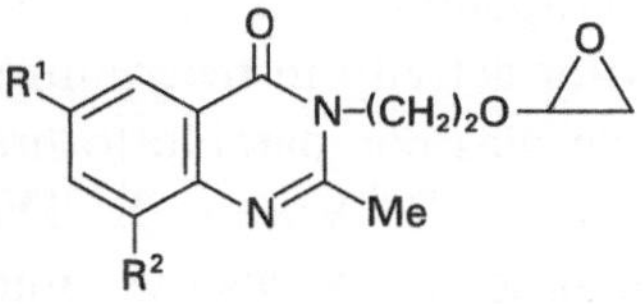

XCII
R^1, R^2 = H, Br

Srivastava et al. [113] reported the synthesis of α-arylazo-N-(quinazolinyl)benzylidenimines incorporating a formazan moiety and evaluated them against antiparkinsonian activity. Oxotremorine-induced tremors were antagonized by nine compounds **XCIIIa–XCIIIi**, out of which **XCIIIa**, **XCIIIe**, **XCIIIf**, **XCIIIg** and **XCIIIi** exhibited significant tremor, rigidity, hypokinesia and catatonia activity when compared to l-dopa. Compounds **XCIIIa** and **XCIIIe** exhibited significant antiparkinsonian activity against all parameters. In general, the ALD50 value was found to be greater than 1000 mg/kg, i.p. It is concluded that the presence of mono- and dichloro groups along with furyl substituents is beneficial for antiparkinsonian activity.

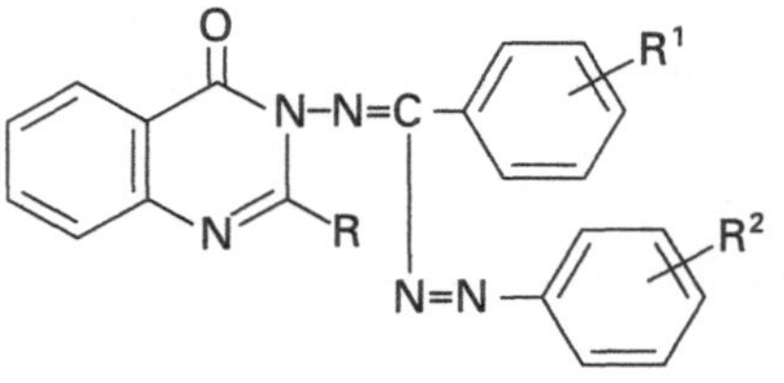

XCIII
XCIIIa R = Me, R^1 = H, R^2 = 4-Cl
XCIIIb R = Me, R^1 = H, R^2 = 2, 5-Cl$_2$
XCIIIc R = Me, R^1 = 2-Cl, R^2 = 3-Cl
XCIIId R = Me, R^1, R^2 = 2-Cl
XCIIIe R = Me, R^1 = 3-Furyl, R^2 = 2, 5-Cl$_2$
XCIIIf R = Me, R^1 = 3-Furyl, R^2 = 4-Cl
XCIIIg R = Me, R^1 = 4-NMe$_2$, R^2 = 2, 5-Cl$_2$
XCIIIh R = Me, R^1 = 4-NMe$_2$, R^2 = 4-Cl
XCIIIi R = Et, R^1 = 2-Cl, R^2 = 4-Cl

Srivastava et al. [114] also synthesized 2-methylamino substituted phenyl-3-substituted anilino-4(3H)-quinazolinones **XCIV** and observed the effect of bulky groups at position 2 on antiparkinsonian as well as on behavioural activities. Their antiparkinsonian activity was compared with bromocriptine. Compound **XCIVa** showed significant inhibition of oxotremorine-induced tremors. Compounds **XCIVa–XCIVe** showed significant antirigidity activity which was better than bromocriptine. Compounds **XCIVb, XCIVd** and **XCIVe** increased significantly the locomotor activity in reserpinized rats. A significant reduction in catatonia which was comparable to bromocriptine was observed with compounds **XCIVa, XCIVd** and **XCIVe**. Compounds **XCIVf–XCIVh** also showed a decrease in spontaneous motor activity. *In vitro*, these quinazolones **XCIVa, XCIVb** and **XCIVe** showed on dopamine (DA) receptor binding a significant inhibition of 3H-spiroperidol at a concentration ranging from 0.1 m mole to 0.1 μ mole. These observations suggest that compounds **XCIVa** and **XCIVb** bind with DA receptor; a possibility exists that these may also bind to 5HT$_2$ receptor.

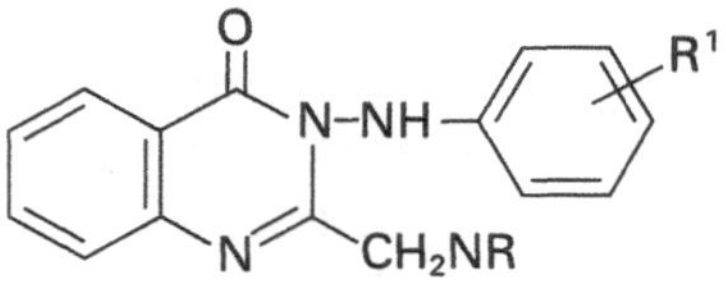

XCIV
XCIVa R = (CH$_2$)$_2$Ph, R^1 = H
XCIVb R = 2-ClC$_6$H$_4$, R^1 = H
XCIVc R = 2-ClC$_6$H$_4$, R^1 = H
XCIVd R = 2, 4-Cl$_2$–C$_6$H$_3$, R^1 = 4-NO$_2$
XCIVe R = CH$_2$C$_6$H$_5$, R^1 = H
XCIVf R = 3-ClC$_6$H$_4$, R^1 = H
XCIVg R = 2, 4-Cl$_2$C$_6$H$_3$, R^1 = H
XCIVh R = 4-OMeC$_6$H$_4$, R^1 = H

2-[2-(4-Substituted phenyl)-1,2-disubstituted ethyl]-3-substituted phenyl) 4(3H)-quinazolinones **XCV** were evaluated for antiparkinsonian profile, that is, tremor, rigidity hypokinesia and catatonia. Compounds **XCVa, XCVb** and **XCVc** showed inhibition of oxotremorine-induced tremors, and the activity of the former two compounds was comparable to that of l-dopa. Compounds **XCVb**, **XCVc** and **XCVd** 4 showed significant antifrigidity activity which was better than that of l-dopa, while **XCVa**, **XCVe** and **XCVf** showed antirigidity activity similar to l-dopa, and compound **XCVf** also exhibited anticatatonic effects greater than l-dopa [115]. Srivastava et al. [116] further reported that 6,8-dibromo-3-(4-chlorophenyl)-2-{3-[4-(dimethylamino)phenyl]-1,2,3,4-tetrahydro-2-quinoxalinyl})-4(3H)-quinazolinone **XCVI** showed maximum antiparkinsonian activity with no toxicity.

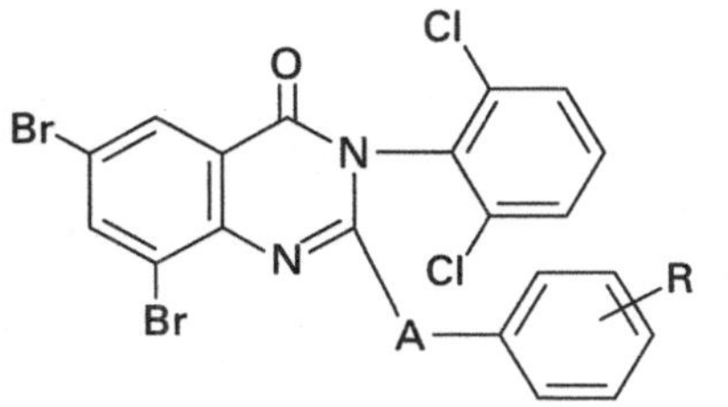

XCV
XCVa R = 4-OMe, A = CH–CH, R^1 = C_5H_{10}
              | |
             NR^1 NR^1

XCVb R = 4-OMe, A = CH–CH, R^1 = $C_{12}H_{10}$
              | |
             NR^1 NR^1

XCVc R = 4-OMe, A = CH–CH, R^1 = C_4H_8O
              | |
             R^1 R^1

XCVd R = 4-OMe, A = CH–CH
              | \
             Br– O_2H_4Cl

XCVe R = 4-NMe_2, A = CH–CH
              | \
             Br– OC_2H_4Cl

XCVf R = 4-NMe_2, A = CH–CH, R^1 = C_4H_8O
              | \
             NR^1 NR^1

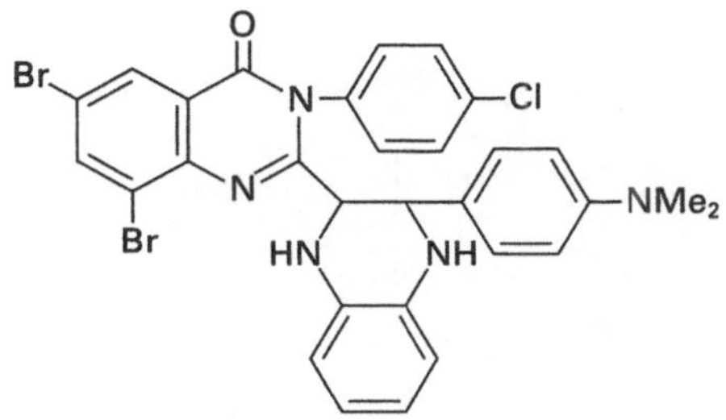

XCVI

3.7   Enzyme inhibitory activity

Central nervous system acting properties of quinazolinones are mediated through action on various enzymes involved in the synthesis and degradation of biogenic amines in CNS. Several derivatives of quinazolinones have been reported as the inhibitors of enzyme monoamine oxidase which is chiefly responsible for the breakdown of these neurotransmitter amines in CNS [117, 118].

Parmar et al. [119, 120] reported that 2-methyl-3-(2-furfurylmethyl)-4-qui-
nazolones inhibited pyruvic acid oxidation, and it was the highest in the
case of 2-methyl-3-furfuryl methyl)-4-quinazolone. Considerable inhibition (17–83%) of pyruvic acid oxidation was observed in case of substituted
2-methyl-3-(2,4-dimethylphenyl)4-quinazolones [121]. The maximum inhibition was exhibited by compound **XCVII** whereas the compounds with
a nucleophile at positions 6 and 8 showed minimum inhibition. 6-Fluoro-
2-methyl-3-phenyl-4(3H)-quinazolinones also showed significant inhibition of pyruvic acid oxidation by rat brain homogenate [54].

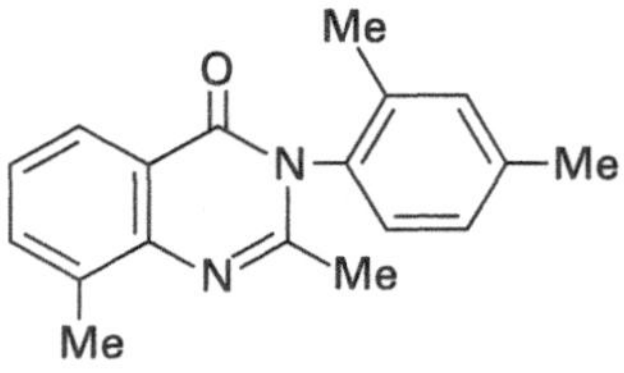

XCVII

Selective NAD-dependent oxidation of substituents of tricarboxylic acid
cycle L-glutamate and β-hydroxybutyrate were inhibited by quinazolone
allyl ethers and allylphenones [122, 123]. Joshi et al. [124] reported that
substituted   2-methyl-3-(γ-dialkylaminopropyl)-4-quinazolones   and   2-
methyl-3-(γ-morpholino aminopropyl)-4-quinazolones **XCVIII** showed
anti-acetylcholine-esterase activity in rat brain homogenate. An increase in
the inhibitory activity was observed with halogen substitution at position
6, but introduction of an additional substituent at position 8 was found to
decrease the inhibitory effect. The degree of inhibition was found to be
dependent on the length of the alkyl chain and an increase in enzyme
inhibition was found to be in the order of dimethyl < diethyl < dibutyl.
Compound **XCVIIIa** showed 74.5 and 100.0% inhibition at the concentrations of 1.0×10^{-3} M and 1.5×10^{-3} M respectively, while **XCVIIIb** exhibited only 38.8 and 44.8% inhibition.

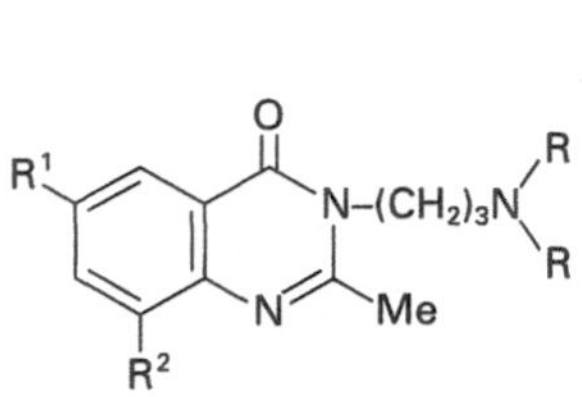

XCVIII
XCVIIIa R = Butyl, R^1 = Cl, R^2 = H
XCVIIIb R = Butyl, R^1, R^2 = Br

Parmar et al. [125] synthesized several substituted piperazino quinazolones and investigated their ability to affect respiratory activity of rat brain homogenate. Several 2,3-substituted quinazolones with 2-bromo-4-methyl phenyl or 2-methyl-4-bromophenyl substituent at position 3 of the quinazolone nucleus were synthesifed by Nagar et al. [126] and evaluated for their ability to inhibit oxidation of pyruvic acid. Significant inhibition of oxidation of pyruvic acid, as reflected by decrease in oxygen uptake, was observed with 2,3-disubstituted and 2, 3, 6 and 2, 3, 8-trisubstituted quinazolones, whereas 2,3,6,8-tetrasubstituted quinazolones were devoid of inhibitory effects. Rastogi et al. [127] have investigated the MAO inhibitory action in 2-methyl-3(4'-hydrazinocarbonyl methylene-oxyphenyl)-4-quinazolones XCIX using rat liver homogenate and observed that all the quinazolones XCIXa–XCIXe inhibited monoamine oxidase at a final concentration of 3×10^{-4} M, and compound XCIXa showed low inhibitory effects. Enzyme inhibition was significantly enhanced by the introduction of halogen substituent at position 6 of the quinazolone nucleus XCIXb and XCIXc; however, the electronegativity of the halogen substitutent was found to be in no way related to the enzyme inhibitory property.

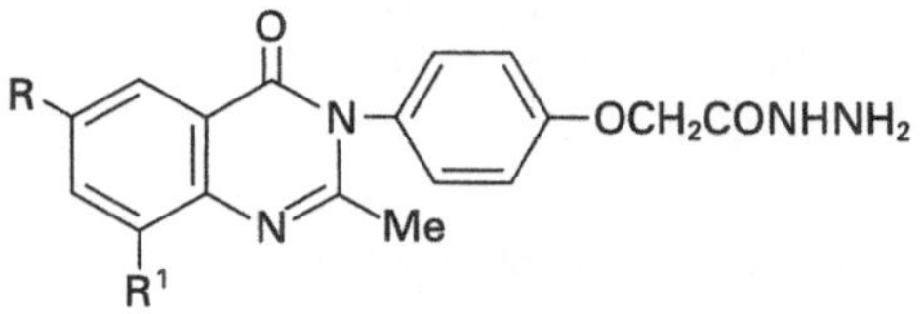

XCIX
XCIXa R, R^1 = H
XCIXb R, R^1 = Cl
XCIXc R, R^1 = Br

Several substituted styryl quinazolones were synthesized and tested for their ability to inhibit the oxidative deamination of kynuramine by monoamine oxidase from the rat brain [75]. Quinazolones with a hydrazide group were better inhibitors than the corresponding precursor esters. Among hydrazides, 2-(3-methoxy-4-hydroxystyryl)-3-benzhydrazide)-4-quinazolone C showed the maximum (76%) inhibition.

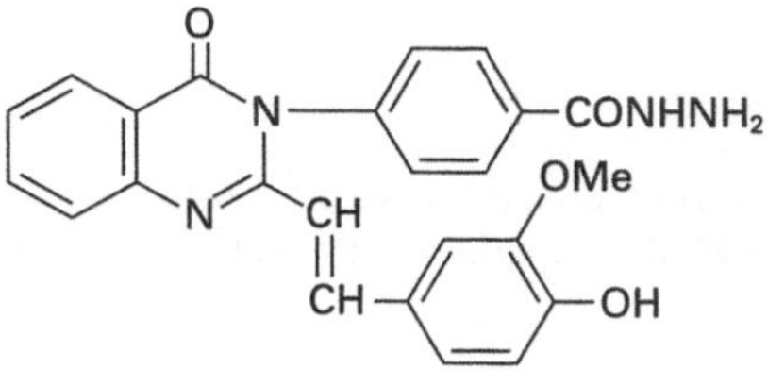

C

Barthwal [70] reported that acetylcholinesterase inhibitory properties of substituted hydrazides were weaker than those of their corresponding esters. Conversion of hydrazides into semicarbazides resulted in increased MAO and acetylcholinesterase inhibitory potency. Oxadiazoles also possessed weaker inhibitory activity than their corresponding thiosemicarbazides.

Gupta et al. [128] investigated the MAO activity of substituted quinazolone series **CI** and observed that all quinazolones inhibited MAO to a considerable extent. The degree of enzyme inhibition was found to be significantly enhanced by introduction of a substituent at the 6 or 8 position, and presence of carbethoxy alkyl moiety or β-alanine at position 3 showed stronger inhibition 77.33, 72.33, 74.52% by **CIa**, **CIb**, **CIc**, respectively, than α-alanine and valine. Results indicated that lengthy chains at position 3 decreased the inhibition (50.38 and 51.30%), as shown by compounds **CId** and **CIe**, respectively.

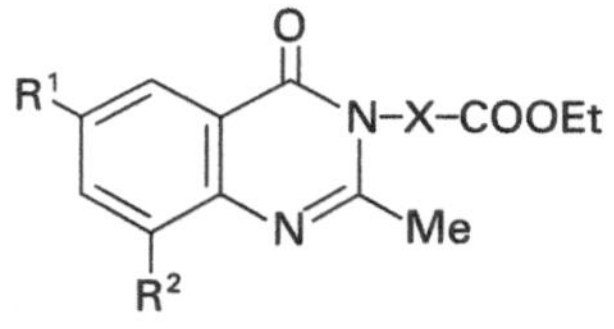

CI
CIa R = Cl, R^1 = H, X = –CH$_2$CH$_2$–
CIb R = Br, R^1 = H, X = –CH$_2$CH$_2$–
CIc R, R^1 = Br, X = –CH$_2$CH$_2$–
CId R, R^1 = H, X = CH(Me)CH(Me)
CIe R = Br, R^1 = H, X = CH(Me)CH(Me)

2-Piperidino/morpholino methyl-3-(substituted phenyl)-4(3H)-quinazolones **CII** were synthesized by Shanker et al. [129] and screened for their *in vitro* as well as *in vivo* MAO inhibitory activity. The maximum inhibition (59.2%) of MAO was observed by compound **CIIa**, and the minimum inhibition (42.0%) was exhibited by **CIIb** at the concentration of 1×10^{-4} M. An examination of enzyme inhibitory activity in relation to the chemical structure showed that the compounds with a piperidino or methyl piperidino group at position 2 showed a greater increase of MAO activity than 7 morpholinomethyl substitution at the same position.

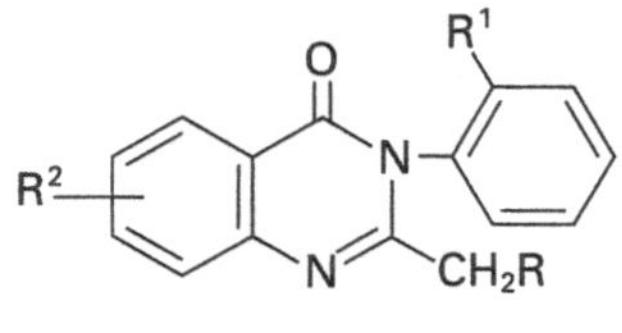

CII
CIIa R = Morpholinyl, R^1 = Me, R^2 = 6-Br
CIIb R = 3-Methyl piperidinyl, R^1 = H, R^2 = 6, 8-Br$_2$

A series of 2-mercaptoacetyl-N-(4-aryloxy)phenyl ureido-3-aryl-4(3H)-quinazolinones **CIII** have been evaluated for MAO inhibitory activity [130]. The enzyme inhibition ranged from 73.6%–82.8%. Maximum inhibition was shown by the compound **CIIIa** with a 4-methoxy group at the N^3-phenyl ring, while the introduction of bromine at positions 6 and 8 decreased the inhibition **CIIIb**, **CIIIc**.

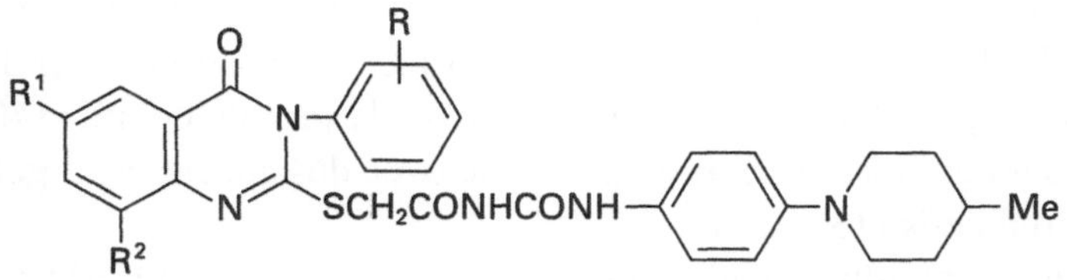

CIII
CIIIa R = 4-OMe, R^1, R^2 = H
CIIIb R = 4-Cl, R^1 = Br, R^2 = H
CIIIc R = 4-Me, R^1, R^2 = Br

Nautiyal et al. [48] synthesized a new series of 1-deoxy-1-[(4-quinazolon-3yl) amino/methylamino-D-fructose] **XXXVII** and showed that compounds with R^1, R^2 = Br, R^1, R^2 = Cl, R^1, R^2 = H and R = NHCO, NHCS, CH NHCO and CH NHCS groups exhibited MAO inhibitory activity over a period of three hours, but over a period of 24 hours none of the compounds exhibited antagonism to the reserpine-induced syndrome.

3.8   Methaqualone

Methaqualone is a nonbarbiturate, high-melting lipophilic solid, insoluble in neutral or alkaline aqueous solution but readily soluble in acids due to weak basicity of the N(1)atom. Methaqualone base is sufficiently soluble in propylene glycol for the preparation of an intravenous solution [131]. It is both a cyclic amide and a pyrimidine derivative and as such has a formal structural resemblance to the piperidone hypnotics and the barbiturates. The N(3)-substituent however prevents tautomerism and it is therefore stable enough to be gas-chromatographed satisfactorily on a variety of stationary phases [132–134].
Although there is substantial clinical literature on methaqualone by Christenson [135], there is yet little basic pharmacological information. The drug has been shown to alter thermoregulatory processes [136]. However,

according to the few reports available in literature [137] it antagonized tremorine-induced tremors.

Physiologic disposition and metabolism
It has been possible to establish the therapeutic plasma level of meth-aqualone in man after a single oral dose [132] or after chronic dosage [138] by the development of sensitive methods of assay. In normal fasting subjects absorption is rapid and peak levels are reached within 2 hours, but in a controlled trial [139] a preparation of hydrochloride was absorbed signifi-cantly faster than one of the base. The drug is strongly protein bound [140] at plasma levels up to those seen in severe acute over-dosage and is largely excluded from red cells [132].

In rats and mice it is rapidly absorbed in the gastrointestinal tract [141] and chiefly metabolized in liver to SKF 525 A (β-diethylaminoethyl-2,2-diphenylpenanoate) which blocked drug-metabolizing enzymes in liver microsomes, prolonged sleeping time and loss of righting reflex caused by methaqualone. It does not block the effect of methaqualone on temperature regulation [137]. Further, increased chronic pretreatment with phenobarbi-tone markedly reduced sleeping time and enhanced the rate of urinary elimination of the drug metabolites [142]. It is relevant that chronic admin-istration of methaqualone to rats has been found to induce microsomal protein synthesis and to increase the activity of microsomal drug metabo-lizing enzymes [143].

It was also shown that acid hydrolyzable conjugates were present in mouse urine but the proportion of unchanged drug was found to be considerably higher than that in rat or human urine [144]. Eberhardt et al. [145] found four unidentified urinary metabolites after oral administration of therapeu-tic doses of unchanged drug in man. This was confirmed by Akagi et al. [146, 147] who identified the major urinary metabolite in rabbit as glu-curonide of benzyl alcohol.

Nowak et al. [148] were not able to detect unchanged methaqualone in the urine of rabbit, dogs or monkeys, but small quantities in relation to the dose, were found in rat urine.

These data suggest that the major route of metabolism of methaqualone in man involves relatively nonspecific hydroxylation of the tolyl substituent and that little unchanged drug is excreted [149–152]. However, Murata et al. indicate the possibility of a different oxidative route of metabolism of methaqualone [153–155].

Mechanism

The mechanism of the CNS depressant action of methaqualone is not known. It is relevant, however, that the drug competitively inhibits the NAD-linked oxidation of tricarboxylic acid cycle intermediates in preparations of rat brain and in isolated mitochondria [156, 157].

Several attempts have been made to identify the neurologic site of action of methaqualone and to characterize its electroencephalographic (EEG) effects [158].

Early experiments indicated that methaqualone was depressant at the cortical level but it is not certain whether it also depresses the activity of brain stem reticular formation [159, 160]. The mechanism underlying the anticonvulsant effectiveness of methaqualone is unknown. It seems possible that the anticonvulsant properties of methaqualone might be secondary to its disruptive effects on temperature regulation or its stimulation of pituitary adrenal activity [136]. Clinical studies [159–161] have revealed qualitative differences between the EEG sleep pattern produced by methaqualone and those produced by other hypnotic drugs such as meprobamate, glutethimide and pentobarbitone.

Clinical pharmacology, abuse and overdosage

Etzler and Joswig [162] and Barcelo [163] reported the first controlled clinical trials of the hypnotic effects of methaqualone. Double-blind assessments with medical patients with the use of placebo controls showed that methaqualone hydrochloride (150 mg orally) was as effective as cyclobarbitone (200 mg) or sodium quinalbarbitone (100 mg). These findings in respect to cyclobarbitone were confirmed by Baird and Buckler [164]. Some patent literature suggests that improved hypnotic or sedative effects may be obtained by combining therapeutic doses of methaqualone and phenothiazines or histamines but few well-planned trials have been carried out [165, 166].

In Britain several cases of methaqualone abuse have been reported. Madden [167] described dependency of the barbiturate type in subjects taking methaqualone hydrochloride, although no abstinence syndrome was apparent upon withdrawal of the drug. The first cases of poisoning were recognized in Germany [168, 169] where methaqualone was available initially without prescription and where it was the key agent [170] in a high proportion of completed suicides. It is notable moreover that marked respiratory depression is rarely seen, in comparison with barbiturate intoxication [171, 172].

3.9   Structure-activity relationship

Substitutions in the quinazolone nucleus at various positions have profound influence on the pharmacological activity of quinazolone.

Substition at position 2

The presence of a methyl group at position 2 of the quinazolone nucleus is essential for establishing appreciable hypnotic and anticonvulsant properties [95, 97]. Compounds with a methyl group at this position also showed antiparkinsonian activity [112] but when this group is replaced by CH NHCOC H or other bulky groups, the compounds become inactive [111]. It was also observed that introduction of a phthalimidomethyl group resulted in a loss of activity [39]; contrary to these findings [27], compounds containing an aryl piperazine methyl thio and 2-mercapto group [28, 65] showed potent CNS and anticonvulsant activity. However, introduction of a phenoxymethyl group also led to significant activity [66, 67]. Compounds with a 2-flouro-methyl group were found to be more potent, and possessed hypnotic and antidepressant effects linked with less toxicity than methaqualone [51, 52].

Substitution at N^3 position

The CNS depressant activity seemingly incipient in 3-phenyl-4-quinazolone moiety was found to attain substantial levels in the 2-methyl and 2-ethyl analogs. Introduction of morpholinyl 2-thiazolyl and 2-pyrrolodinyl groups led to significant anticonvulsant activity [66]. Compounds with a carbamido acetyl amino methyl group showed a CNS depressant effect but little protection against chemical-induced seizures by metrazole [47]. Introduction of a flouro group at the phenyl ring at position 3 enhanced the anticonvulsant activity [54]. It has been postulated that increase in the electron density around the position of 1' N^3-phenyl ring by methyl at the 2' position increases the CNS activity [174, 175].

Substitution at C^4 position

The presence of a C=O group has been shown to be essential for CNS activity. The corresponding thio compounds were found to be less active.

Substitution at C^6 and C^8 positions

Compounds with fluorine at these positions exhibited strong anticonvulsant activity [52]. Substitution of less electronegative atoms imparts more MAO inhibitory activity. Further substitution at position 8 by bromine increases the MAO inhibitory activity [176].

4   Antiinflammatory activity

Quinazolones have been found to possess antiinflammatory activity. The structure-activity relationship in these compounds has revealed that variation in the substitution at positions 2,3,6 and 8 has a marked influence on biological activities.

A series of twelve 4(3H)-quinazolinones **CIV** has been synthesized which showed significant antiinflammatory activity [177]. Seth and Khanna [178] synthesized various 2-substituted and 2,3-disubstituted-4(3H)-quinazolinones **CV** and evaluated them for their antiinflammatory activity against carrageen-induced edema in mice; seven compounds **CVa–CVg** at 1/5 LD50 dose i.p. exhibited 20–40% activity, as compared to the control.

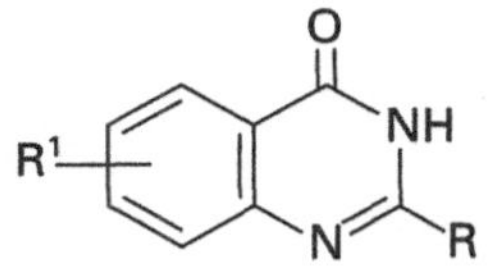

CIV   R = Alkyl, substituted phenyl, R^1 = H, alkyl, Cl, Br
CVa   R = (2-Phenyl)ethylamino, R^1 = H
CVb   R = 1, 2, 4-Triazolyl-3-amino, R^1 = H
CVc   R = 5, 6, 7, 8-Tetrahydronaphthyl-1-amino, R^1 = H,
CVd   R = 3, 4 Dimethoxyphenyl)ethylamino, R^1 = H
CVe   R = 2 (N, N-Diethylamino)ethylamino, R^1 = 6-Cl
CVf   R = 3, 4-Dichlorobenzylamino, R^1 = 6-Cl
CVg   R = N-Phenylpiperazino, R^1 = 7-Cl

T. Oine et al. [179–181, 25–27] synthesized a large number of 2-substituted-1-phenyl-4(1H)-quinazolines **CVI** and found them to be useful ,as antiinflammatory agents. These findings further led to the synthesis of some more derivatives of 1-aryl-4(1H)-quinazolinones as potent antiinflammants [182–184].

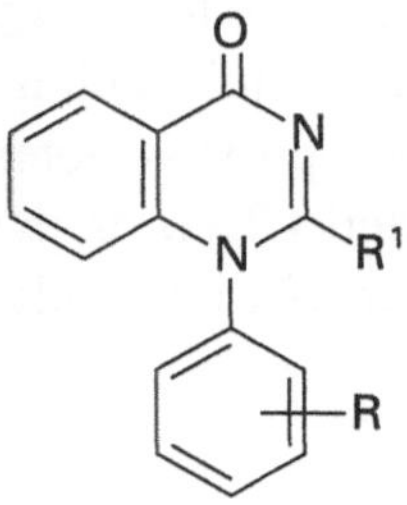

CVI
R = H, 3-CF3, 2-COOH, 4-CONH2, 4-COOH, 2-CONH2, 3, 4(OMe)COOH, R^1 = Me, CH2, Cl, CH2CH2COOMe, CH2CH2COOH, COOEt, CHMe2, cyclo alkyl etc.

A large number of 1-alkyl-4-phenyl-2(1H)-quinazolinone derivatives as antiinflammants have also been synthesized [185–196], among them 1-cy-clopropylmethyl-4-phenyl-6-methoxy-2(1H)-quinazolinone **CVII** ex-hibited activity against carrageenin-induced edema in rat, 1.6 times that of phenylbutazone and ibuprofen, 3.3 times that of mefenamic acid and 6.7 times that of mepirizole. In the yeast-induced edema test in rats, **CVII** showed equal activity to ibuprofen and 4 times that of mepirizole, while in dextran-induced edema in rats, activity of **CVII** was significantly higher than those of ibuprofen and mepirizole. ACOH-induced increase in capillary permeability in mice was observed. In an adjuvant arthritis test in rats, **CVII** showed equipotent activity with phenylbutazone. It strongly inhibited cyclooxygenase activity and leukocyte function but only slightly inhibited lipoxygenase activity [193]. The gastric hemorrhagic effect of **CVII** was significantly less than that of nonsteroidal antiinflammatory drugs. A protective effect of **CVII** against indomethacin-induced intestinal lesions was also observed [191].

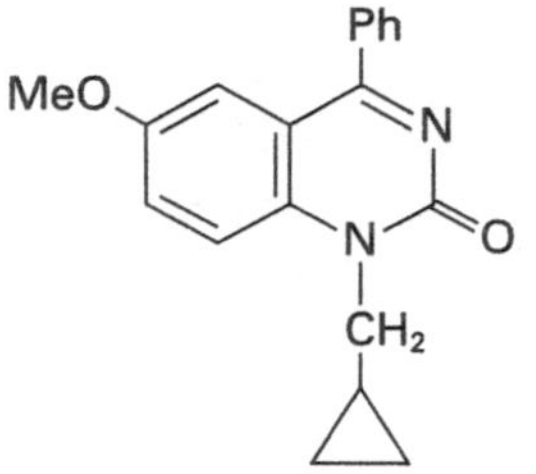

CVII

Yakuri [197] reported that 1-isopropyl-2-phenyl-6-methyl-4(3H)-quina-zolones **CVIII** possess antiinflammatory activity comparable to in-domethacin. A series of 3-arylquinazolones substituted with piperazine or piperidine were synthesized and screened against carrageenin-induced edema at an oral dose of 50 mg/kg [198]. Results indicated that compound **CIXa** was most potent, exhibiting 35.4% inhibition equipotent to phenyl-butazone and devoid of any side effects. It was concluded that quinazolones with a methyl group in aryl moiety linked at position 3 possess potent antiinflammatory activity, and homopiperidino **CIXa** and **CIXb** or pyr-rolidino **CIXc** and **CIXd** groups at position 2 caused an increase in antiin-flammatory activity.

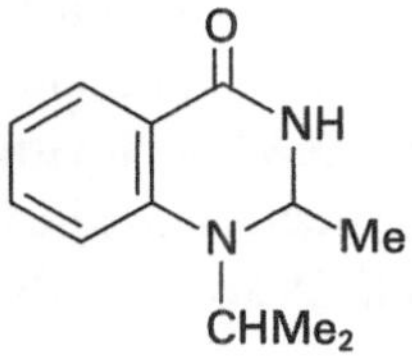

CVIII

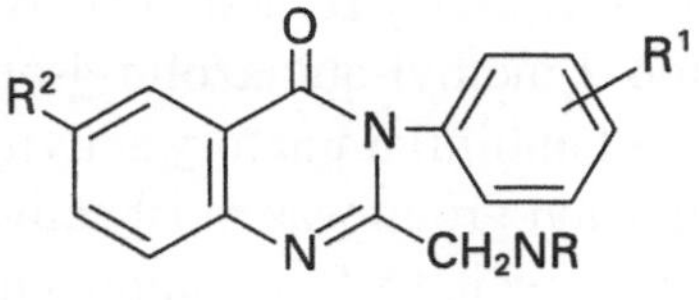

CIX
CIXa R = Homopiperidinyl, R^1 = 2-Me, R^2 = I
CIXb R = Homopiperidinyl, R^1, R^2 = H
CIXc R = Pyrrolidinyl, R^1, R^2 = H
CIXd R = Pyrrolidinyl, R^1 = 2-Me, R^2 = I

Singh et al. [199] synthesized various 3-substituted phenyl4(3H)-quina-
zolinones and evaluated them for activity against edema. All compounds
exhibited inhibition to some extent, 3-(2-chlorophenylmethyl)-3-(2-piper-
azine phenyl)-4(3H)-quinazolinone **CXa** being the most potent showing
54% inhibition, and more active than phenylbutazone. It was apparent from
the results that the chlorophenyl or tolyl group at position 3 and homopiperidino moiety at α- and β-positions **CXb–CXd** enhance the antiinflammatory activity; compound **CXe** bearing morpholino moieties at α- and
β-carbon atom also possessed 53% inhibition.

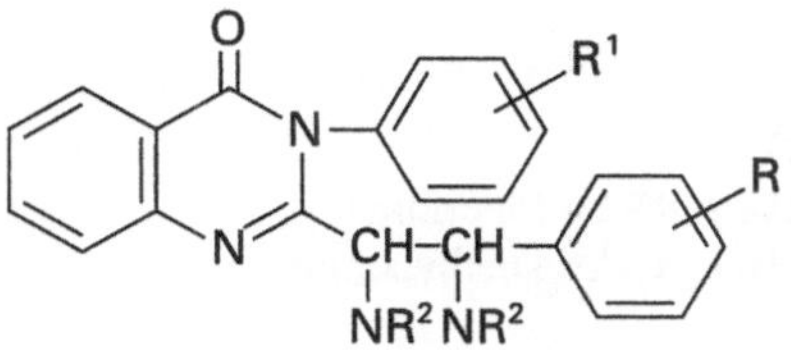

CX
CXa R = 3-Cl, R^1 = 2-Cl, NR^2 = Phenylpiperazino
CXb R = 3-Cl, R^1 = 2-Cl, NR^2 = Homopiperidino
CXc R = 2-OMe, R^1 = 2-Cl, NR^2 = Homopiperidino
CXd R = 2-OH, R^1 = 2-Me, NR^2 = Homopiperidino
CXe R = 2-OMe, R^1 = 2-Cl, NR^2 = Morpholino

Eight quinazoline derivatives with sulfanilamide grouping moiety at N^3
were synthesized by Shanker et al. [103] and tested for antiinflammatory
activity, of which compounds **CXIb** and **CXIe** were quite potent showing
67.5% protection in rat paw edema, which was superior to aspirin, while
activity of **CXIc** followed by **CXIa** was of the order of phenylbutazone.
The rest of these compounds except **CXId** did exhibit a moderate antiinflammatory activity. Further, they synthesized 3-α-(S-substituted mercap-

toacetamido) **LXXXVII** and 3-α-(N,N-disubstituted aminoacetamido)-6,8-dibromo-2-methyl-quinazolin-4-ones **CXII** which exhibited appreciable degrees of antiinflammatory activity [106]. Compound **LXXXVII** with a carboxyphenyl group was most active exhibiting 62% protection against rat paw edema whilst a few compounds, **LXXXVIIe, LXXXVIIc, CXIIa** and **CXIIb**, had activity comparable to phenylbutazone.

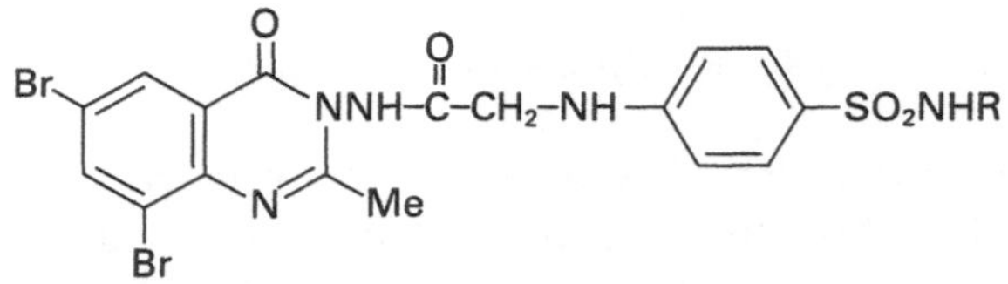

Br—[quinazolinone ring]—NNH–C(=O)–CH$_2$–NH—[phenyl]—SO$_2$NHR, with Br and Me substituents, N

CXI
CXIa   R = H
CXIb   R = Ac
CXIc   R = 5-Methyl-2-(1, 3, 4-thiadiazolyl)
CXId   R = 4, 6-Dimethyl-2-pyrimidyl
CXIe   R = 2, 6-Dimethyl-4-pyrimidyl

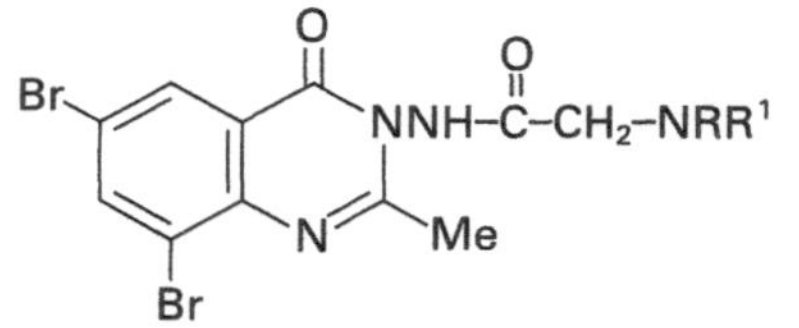

Br—[quinazolinone ring]—NNH–C(=O)–CH$_2$–NRR^1, with Br and Me substituents, N

CXII
CXIIa NRR^1 = Piperidino
CXIIb NRR^1 = Diethylamino

The fact that efficacy of the compounds increased by the presence of a isopropyl group at position 1, viz. proquazone, [200] encouraged Ozaki et al. [201] to synthesize a few derivatives of 4(1H)-quinazolinones **CXIII** and **CXIV**. Structure-activity relationship revealed that 2-iso-propyl-1-phenyl-, 2-cyclopropyl-1-phenyl- and isopropyl-2-phenyl-4(1H)-quinazolinones possess optimal potency, and the presence of a halogen atom is beneficial for activity, 1-isopropyl-(2-fluorophenyl)-4(1H)-quinazolinone **CXIVa** being the most potent.

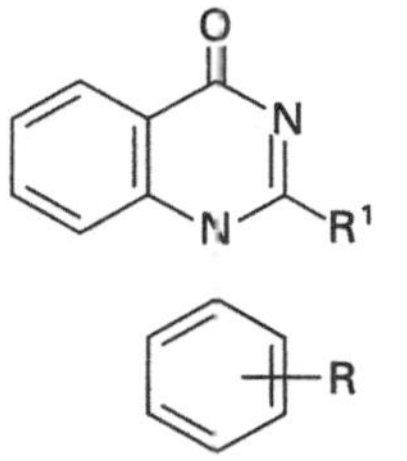

CXIII
CXIIIa R = H, R^1 = Isopropyl
CXIIIb R = H, R^1 = Cyclopropyl
CXIIIc R = 4-Cl, R^1 = Cyclobutyl
CXIIId R = 3-CF$_3$, R^1 = CH$_2$Cl

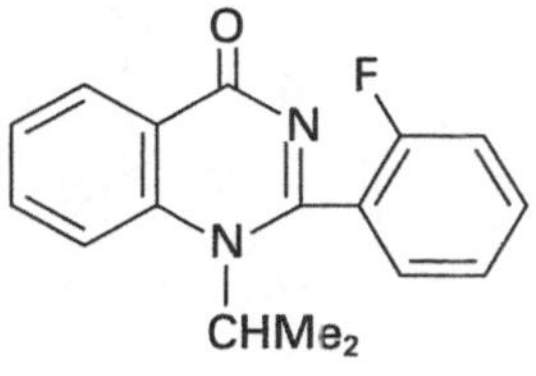

CXIV

Antiinflammatory activity of 1,2,3,4-tetrahydro-4-quinazolinones was studied, and the results suggested that acylation at N' increases the activity [104]. Structure-activity relationship study in a series of 2,3-dihydro-1-(β-phenylethyl)-2-aryl- and 2,3-diaryl-4(1H)-quinazolinones **LXXIVa–LXXXIVb** revealed that 3-N-unsubstituted quinazolinones are more potent than 3-N-phenyl substituted quinazolinones. Introduction of a methyl group at position 4 of the phenyl ring causes reduction in antiinflammatory activity, whereas introduction of an ethoxy substituent at position 2 of the phenyl ring increases the activity of 3-N-phenyl substituted quinazolinones. It was also found that 3,4-dichloro substitution in the phenyl ring of 2-phenyl quinazolinones led to an increase in activity, whereas 2,4-dichlor substitution in the phenyl ring resulted in a decrease of activity [103].

Antiinflammatory activity of 4(3H)-quinazolinones in which a heterocyclic nucleus is attached directly via a methylene group at N^3 was studied. Plescia et al. [202] observed that among 3-(pyrazol-5-yl)quinazolin-4(3H)-ones **CXV**, compounds **CXVa** and **CXVb** exhibited good activity in carrageenin rat paw edema tests. In oxoimidazoline substituted quinazolones **CXVI**, compounds **CXVIa**, **CXVIb**, **CXVIc** and **CXVId** exhibited protection (29.3–56.4%) against carrageenin-induced mice paw edema, whereas compounds **CXVIe**, **CXVIf**, **CXVIg**, **CXVIh** and **CXVIi** showed protection in the range of 11.3–21.6% [203]. SAR studies revealed that compounds with ethyl substitution at position 2 of quinazolinones were more potent than corresponding methyl substituted ones, except **CXVIc**. It is also noteworthy that substitution at position 6 resulted in decreased activity. Quinazolinones, substituted by oxadiazole moiety at N via a methylene group **CXVII** were also found to possess antiinflammatory activity [102]. Highest protection (50–64%) was observed by compounds **CXVIIa**, **CXVIIb** and **CXVIIc**.

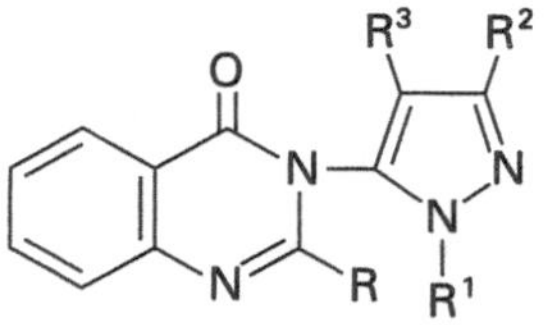

CXV
CXVa R, R^2 = Me, R^1 = Ph, R^3 = H
CXVb R, R^2 = H, R^1 = Me, R^3 = COOEt

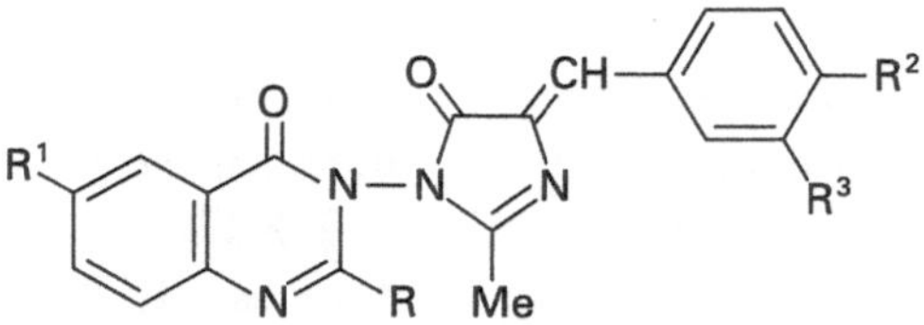

CXVI
CXVIa R = Me, R^1, R^2, R^3 = H
CXVIb R = Me, R^1 = H, R^2, R^3 = OMe
CXVIc R = Et, R^1, R^2, R^3 = H
CXVId R = Et, R^1 = H, R^2, R^3 = OMe
CXVIe R = Me, R^1, R^3 = H, R^2 = OMe
CXVIf R = Me, R^1 = I, R^2, R^3 = OMe
CXVIg R = Et, R^1 = I, R^2, R^3 = H
CXVIh R = Et, R^1 = I, R^2 = OMe, R^3 = H
CXVIi R = Et, R^1 = I, R^2, R^3 = OMe

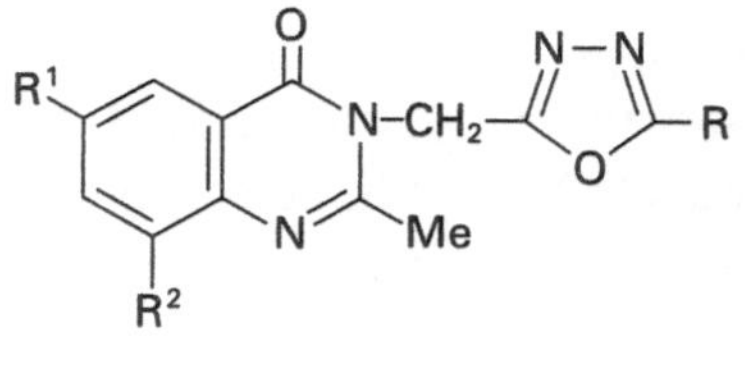

CXVII
CXVIIa R = 4-Hydroxy phenyl, R^1, R^2 = H
CXVIIb R = 2-Chlorophenyl, R^1, R^2 = Br
CXVIIc R = 4-Chloro phenoxy methyl,
          R^1, R^2 = Br

Antiinflammatory activity was also observed in 1-(2-arylindol-3-yl)-2-[3-(p-morpholinophenyl)-6,8-disubstituted-quinazolin-4(3H)-on-2-yl]ethyl enes **CXVIII**. Quinazolinones with a disubstituted carbamoyl phenyl amino grouping at N^3 **XXVI** have also been found to possess antiinflammtory activity ranging from 8–22% in rats [36]. Compound **XXVIa** with a bromo group at position 8 and morpholino with carbamoyl moiety exhibited maximum inhibition of 22%. A series of some new 2-(phenyl/chloromethyl)-3-[4(N,N-disubstitutedaminocarbonyl)phenyl]-8-substituted-4(3H)-quinazolones **XXV** was evaluated for antiinflammatory activity [35]; only two compounds **XXVa** and **XXVb** could exhibit activity of 23 and 31% respectively. Farghaly et al. [204–206] synthesized non-steroidal antiinflammatory agents **CXIX–CXXI**.

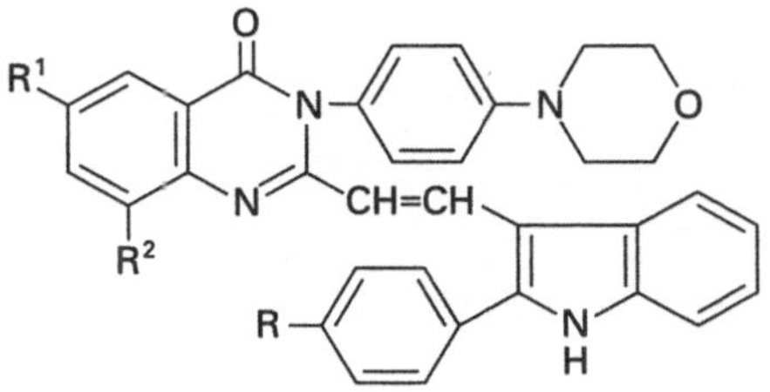

CXVIII
R = H, Me, OMe, Cl, R^1, R^2 = H, Br, I

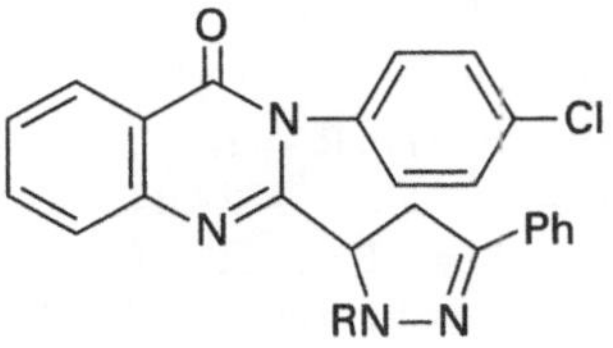

CXIX
CXIXa R = H
CXIXb R = 4-BrPh

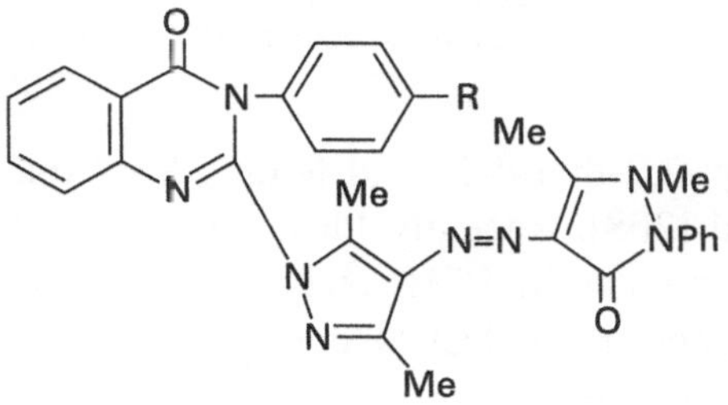

CXX
R = H, Me, Cl, Br

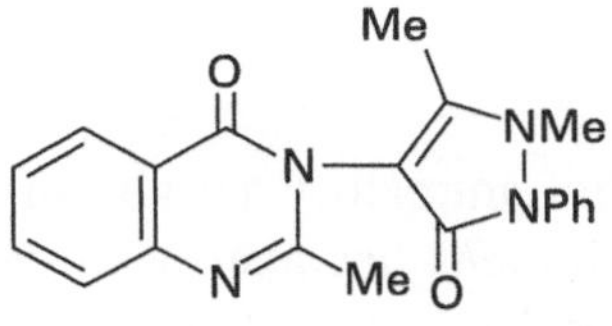

CXXI

In a series of eight quinazolinoformazans [207] almost all compounds exhibited varying degrees (26–57%) of protection against carrageenin-induced edema in rat paw. The results suggest that compounds with methyl at position 2 of the quinazolone nucleus **CXXII** possess higher activity as compared to compounds having arylethenyl moiety (**CXXIII**). Contrary to these observations maximum protection of 56.9% was observed with compound **CXXIIIb**. Four compounds **CXXIIa–CXXIId** exhibited protection of 35, 46, 42 and 57% respectively against carrageenin-induced edema; 10–80% protection against aconitine-induced writhing response in mice. LD50 values ranged from 600–1300 mg/kg, i.p. in mice, indicating low toxicity of the compounds. The most active compounds **CXXIIb** and **CXXIIId** at dose levels of 50, 100 and 150 mg/kg p.o. provided protection against carrageenin-induced edema of 33.6, 46.1 and 55.2% respectively by **CXXIIb** and 37.0, 56.9, 68.1% by **CXXIIId**.

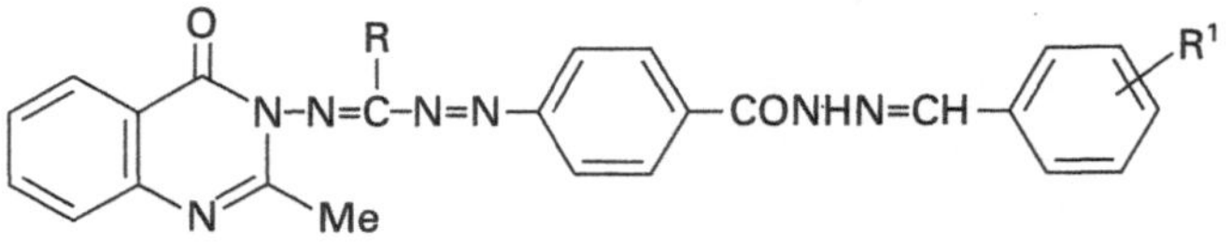

CXXII
CXXIIa   R = Ph, R^1 = H
CXXIIb   R = Ph, R^1 = 2-OH
CXXIIc   R = 2-Furyl, R^1 = H
CXXIId   R = 2-Furyl, R^1 = 2-OH

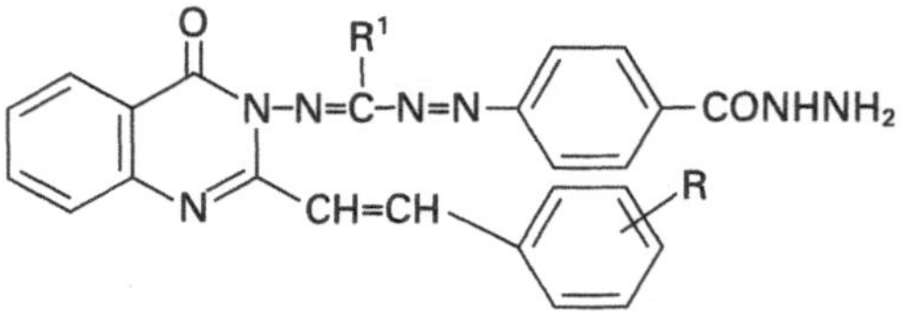

CXXIII
CXXIIIa   R = H, R^1 = Ph
CXXIIIb   R = 2-OH, R^1 = Ph
CXXIIIc   R = H, R^1 = 2-Furyl
CXXIIId   R = 2-OH, R^1 = 2-Furyl

Antiinflammatory activity in 1-acetyl-2,3-diaryl-1,2,3,4-tetrahydro-4-quinazolinones has also been described [208]. Recently Plescia et al. [209] synthesized some 3-(isoxazol-5-yl)-quinazolin-4(3H)-ones, of which one compound showed antiinflammatory activity and LD50 comparable to that of ASA in the carrageenin rat foot edema model.

Various 6,8-disubstituted-3[3/4-(2-hydroxy-3-substituted propoxy)phenyl-2-methyl-4(3H)-quinazolinones **CXXIV** were synthesized and tested for their antiinflammatory activity against carrageenin-induced rat paw edema [210]. A structure-activity relationship study revealed that compounds bearing a substituted propoxy side chain at position 3 of the quinazolinone nucleus via a 1,3-phenyl bridge showed better activity as compared to corresponding compounds with a 1,4-phenyl bridge. Further, phenylpiperazine as R was most beneficial for the activity. Activity was found to decrease when bromine at position 6 was replaced by iodine.

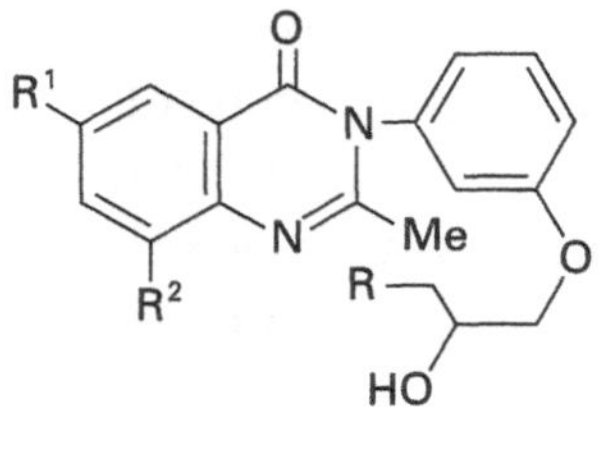

CXXIV
R = Morpholinyl, 4-phenylpiperazino, diethanolamino, R^1, R^2 = H, Br, I

5   Cardiovascular activity

Cardiovasular agents act on the heart or on other parts of the vascular system, thus altering cardiovascular function. The drugs falling into this group include cardiotonic drugs, antihypertensive drugs, antiarrhythmic drugs, vasodilators and lipid-lowering agents.

Quinazolones constitute one of the most important groups of cardiovascular (CVS) drugs. Hess et al. [211] reported antihypertensive activity of 2-di-ethylamino-6,7-dimethoxy-4(3H)-quinazolinone **CXXV** in human models. Further studies on 2-substituted aminoaryl-4(3H)-quinazolinones revealed that compounds containing guanidino moiety **CXXVI** exhibit antihypertensive activity in rats [212,213].

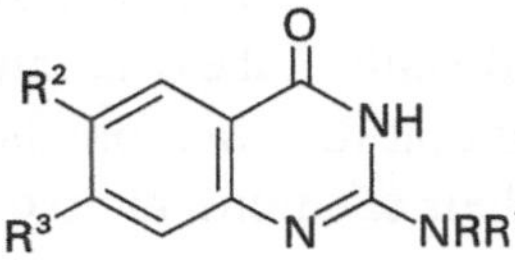

CXXV R, R^1 = Et, R^2, R^3 = OMe
CXXVI R = H, R^1 = 2-OHC$_6$H$_4$

Bandurco et al. [214–217] synthesized various substituted 4-alkyl-2(1H)-quinazolinones **CXXVII** and 5,6-dialkoxy-4-imino-2(1H)-quinozolinone derivatives **CXXVIII** as antihypertensive, bradycardiac and cardiotonic agents. Among these compounds **CXXVIIa** at 13.9 mg/kg dose increased kidney blood flow in dogs by 49%; compound **CXXVIIb** at 40 mg/kg produced 27.5 m.m. lowering of blood pressure in rats whereas 7-ethoxy-6-methoxy-4-methyl-2(1H)-quinazolinone at 100 mg/kg lowered blood pressure in spontaneously hypertensive rats by 27.5 m.m. 5,6-Dimethoxy-4-methyl-2(1H)-quinazolinone **CXXVIIc** is under development as an oral cardiotonic. In 4-imino-quinazolinones, **CXXVIII** at 1.87 mg/kg i.v. dose in anesthetized dogs increased myocardial contractile force by 42%.

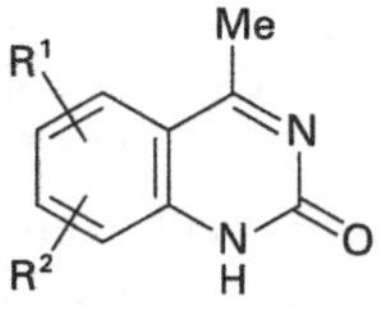

CXXVII
CXXVIIa R^1 = 6-OH, R^2 = 7-OH
CXXVIIb R^1 = 6-OMe, R^2 = 7-OMe
CXXVIIc R^1 = 5-OMe, R^2 = 6-OMe

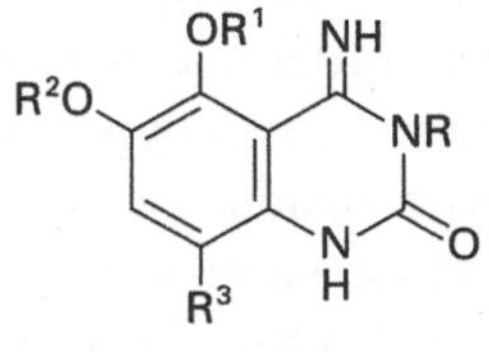

CXXVIII
R = Bu, R^1, R^2 = Me, R^3 = Cl

Synthesis and evaluation of 1- and 3-(1-substituted 4-piperidinyl)-1,2,3,4-tetrahydro-2-oxoquinazolines **CXXIX** as antihypertensive agents [218, 219] revealed that compounds containing Z as H, OH were effective in lowering blood pressure in spontaneous hypertensive rats; compound **CXXIXa** at 1 mg/100 kg orally in rats decreased the blood pressure by 29 mm. In 3-[1-(ω-aryl-ω-hydroxyalkyl)-4-piperidinyl]-1,2,3,4-tetra-hydro-2-oxoquinazolines, the presence of two methoxy substituents at R and R^1 led to weakly active compounds. However, a single methoxy substitution (at 4- position) provided the most potent antihypertensive activity in this series. As regards the chloro substituent, substitution at position 3 led to weakly active compounds whereas substitution at position 4 or 3,4-disubstitution, provided about the same antihypertensive activity as that of the compound with an unsubstituted phenyl group. It was also observed that chlorine at position 6 resulted in a compound with the same activity as the corresponding compound without this substituent. Results of the α-adrenergic blocking activities of the compounds revealed that the compounds of this series exert their hypotensive effect through their α-adrenergic blocking activities.

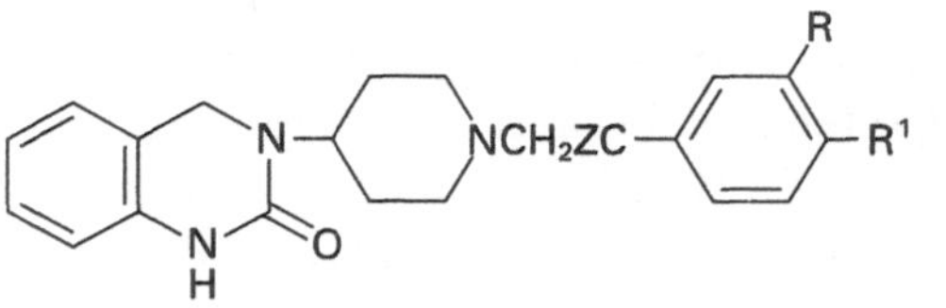

CXXIX
CXXIXa R, R^1 = OMe, Z = O

Amschler et al. [220] found antihypertensive activity in some piperazine alkyl quinazolones; under the assumption that substituted arylpiperazines possess potent α-adrenoceptor blocking property along with their ability to lower systemic blood pressure in renal hypertensive rats, Dubey et al. [221] synthesized substituted 2-methyl-3-(γ-piperazinopropiophenyl)-4-quinazolones **CXXX** and evaluated their cardiovascular activity in anesthetized dogs. It was observed that seven compounds **CXXXa–CXXXg** exhibit marked and sustained hypotensive activity. Compounds **CXXXa–CXXXc** induced hypotension and bradycardia and inhibited carotid occlusion response without significantly affecting noradrenaline response whereas compounds **CXXXd, CXXXf, CXXXg** exhibited hypotensive activity due to α-adrenoceptor blockade. It was concluded from the results that monobromo substituted quinazolones with a 4-methoxyphenyl substituent in the

Table 1
Effect of 2-methyl-3-(γ-piperazinopropiophenyl)-4-quinazolone hydrochloride (CXXX) on blood pressure (B.P.), heart rate (H.R.) and pressor responses in anesthetized dogs.

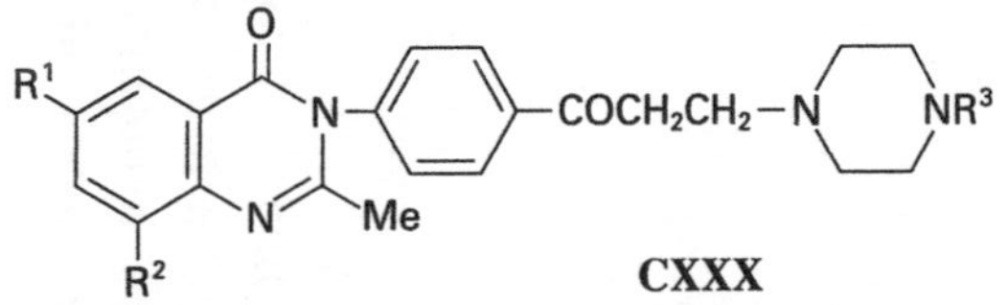

CXXX

Compound No.	R^1	R^2	R^3	Dose i.v. (mg/kg)	Control B.P. (mm/Hg)	B.P. after the drug (mm/Hg)	Control (L.H.R.) (beat/min)	H.R. after the drug (beat/min)	Effect on C.O. response	Effect on N.E.R.
a.	H	H	CH_3	2	140	60	208	150	blocked	–
b.	H	H	C_6H_5	3	160	40	210	170	blocked	partially inhibited
c.	H	H	$2\text{-}OCH_3\text{-}C_6H_4$	2	144	84	206	180	partially inhibited	–
d.	Br	H	C_6H_5	3	200	60	130	200	blocked	blocked
e.	I	H	CH_3	3	150	50	190	170	blocked	–
f.	I	H	C_6H_5	3	120	60	210	210	blocked	partially inhibited
g.	I	H	$2\text{-}OCH_3\text{-}C_6H_4$	3	180	70	220	220	partially inhibited	partially inhibited
h.	Cl	H	CH_3	2	170	130	170	170		markedly potentiated
i.	Cl	H	$3\text{-}Cl\text{-}C_6H_4$	2	170	170	170	250	–	slightly potentiated
j.	Cl	Cl	C_6H_5	3	170	150	250	250	–	–
k.	Br	Br	C_6H_5	2	140	80	190	170	blocked	partially inhibited
l.	Br	Br	$4\text{-}OCH_3\text{-}C_6\text{-}H_4$	2	110	110	260	260	–	–

piperazine moiety lead to a vasopressor compound (Table 1). Sato et al. [222] described sympatholytic 2-thio-quinazolinones **CXXXI** which at 15 µg/kg i.v. inhibited 50% phenyl-ephrine-induced hypertension in rats. Antihypertensive activity was also detected in 3-(1-piperazinylalkyl)-2-thioxoquinazolin-4-ones [223].

A series of 3-[4-{3-(4-aryl-1-piperazinyl)-isopropanoloxy}phenyl]-4(3H)-quinazolinones **CXXXII** was synthesized by Botras and Saad [224], in which **CXXXIIa** was found to possess pronounced and sustained hypotensive effects in anesthetized normotensive rabbits and also showed adrenoceptor antagonist properties with respect to the α- and β-receptors.

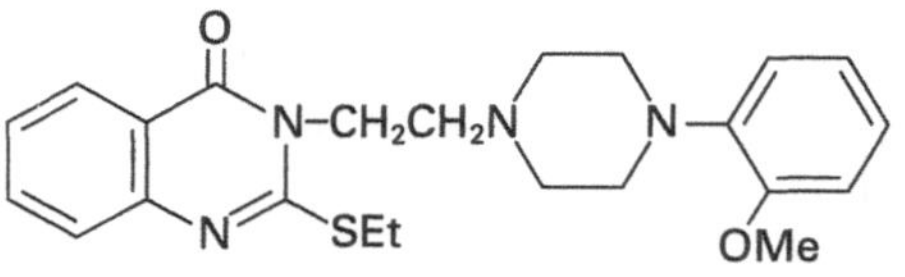

CXXXI

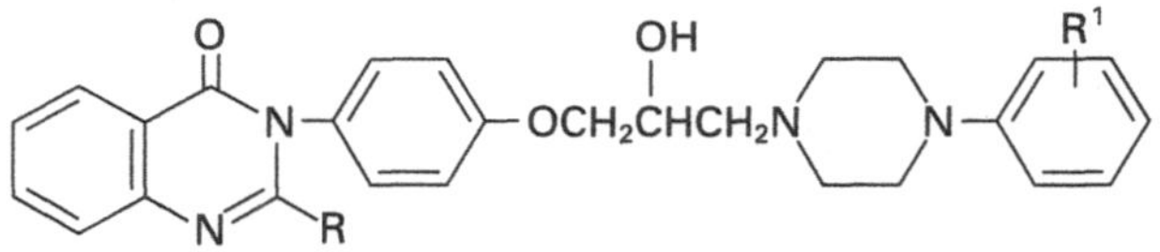

CXXXII   R = H, Me, R^1 = H, Me
CXXXIIa   R, R^1 = H

Agarwal et al. [225] synthesized various quinazolinone derivatives **CXXXIII** and **CXXXIV** and tested their cardiovascular activity in dogs; out of them, **CXXXIII** exhibited potent dose-dependent hypotensive and bradycardiac effects. Structure-activity relationship in these compounds revealed that conversion of 2-substituted-3[(3-alkylamino)ethyl]6,8-disubstituted-4-quinazolones **CXXXIII** to the corresponding 2-substituted-3[3-{(N-alkyl-N-arylthioureido)   ethyl}]6,8-disubstituted-4-quinazolinones **CXXXIV** yielded compounds with higher hypotensive activity.

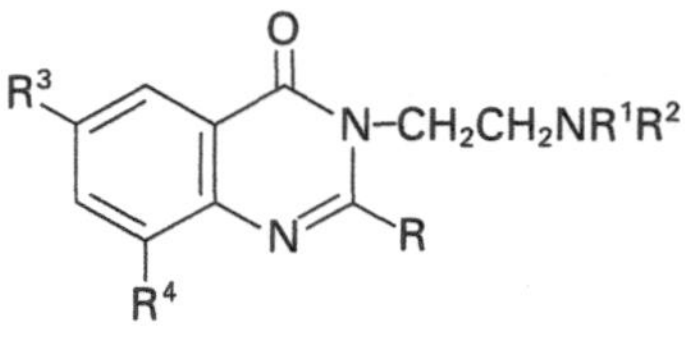

CXXXIII
CXXXIIIa R = Me, R^1, R^4 = H, R^2 = Et, R^3 = I

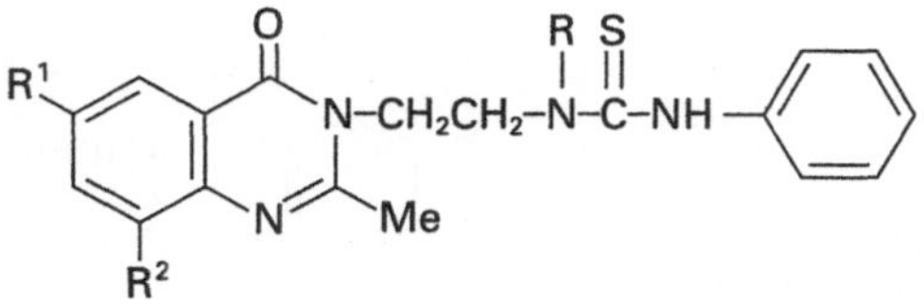

CXXXIV
R = Et, Pr, R^1, R^2 = H, Br, I

A novel quinazolinone calcium antagonist, MCl-176 (2-(2,5-dimethoxy-phenylmethyl)-3-(2-dimethyl-aminoethyl)-6-isopropoxy]-4(3H)-quinazo linone hydrochloride **CXXXV** dose-dependently increased blood flow in blood-perfused sinoatrial (SA) node, atrioventricular (AV) node and papillary muscle preparation of dogs when given intraarterially [226, 227]. Sekiya et al. reported a similar type of quinazolinone **CXXXVI** as cardiovascular agent; compound **CXXXVIa** at 0.3 μM inhibited $CaCl_2$-induced contraction of rat aorta *in vitro* [228].

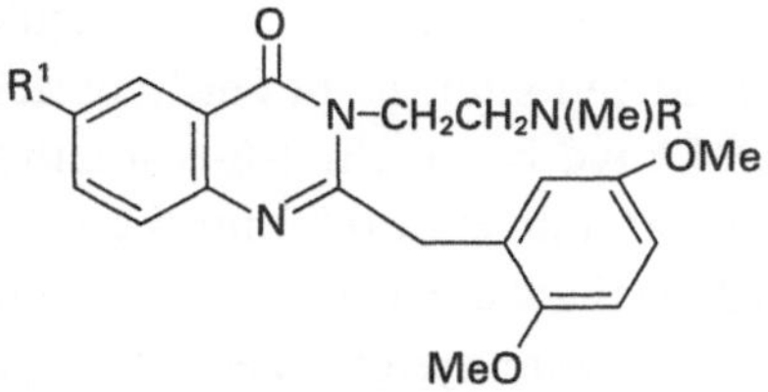

CXXXV R = Me, R^1 = $OCH(Me)_2$
CXXXVI R = $CH_2CH_2C_6H_3(OMe)_2$-3, 4, R^1 = H

Antihypertensive activity [229] was also observed with quinazolin-4(3H)-ones **CXXXVII** and **CXXXVIII**. Liu et al. [230] synthesized new quinazolinones with a phenylamino grouping at position 3 **CXXXIX** and found them to be potent antihypertensives.

Nigam et al. [36] observed that CVS activity was retained in quinazolinones with N,N-disubstituted carbamoyl-phenylamino at position 3 **XXVI**. They also observed that substitution at position 8 causes a decrease in activity. Synthesis of new 2-(phenyl/chloromethyl)-3-[4(N,N-disubstituted amino-carbonyl)phenyl]-8-substituted-4-(3H)-quinazolones **XXV** had been carried out [35], but only compounds **XXVa** and **XXVb** could exhibit mild hypotensive effect, and it was concluded that the N-phenylpiperazino group was responsible for the activity and also that -NH- between N^3 of quinazolone and the substituted amino carbonyl group **XXVI** causes a decrease in activity as compared to compounds **XXV** where the substituted amino carbonyl group is directly attached to N^3 of quinazolone.

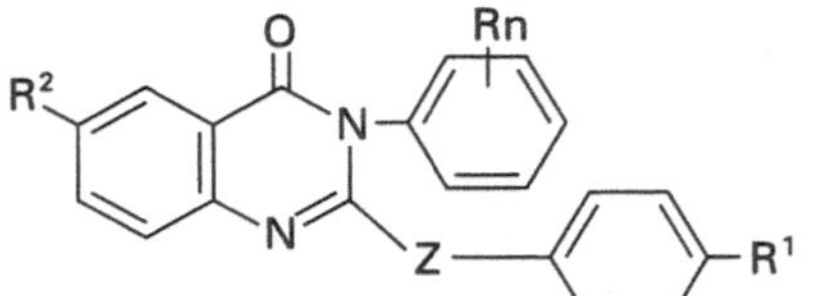

CXXXVII   Z = CH=CH, CHBr–CHBr, Rn = 2, 6-Cl$_2$,
2,4-Cl$_2$, 4-Cl, R^1 = OMe, NMe$_2$, R^2 = H, Br, I
CXXXVIII   Z = CH————CH, Rn = 2, 6-Cl$_2$, 2, 4-Cl$_2$, 4-Cl

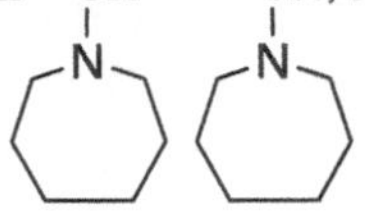

R^1 = OMe, NMe$_2$, R^2 = H, Br, I

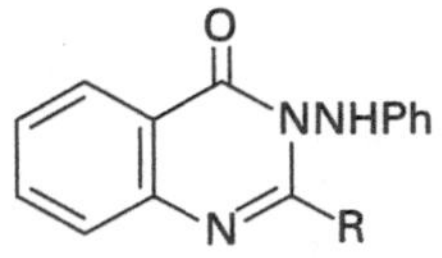

CXXXIX
R = H, Me

Wright et al. [231, 232] synthesized some new quinazolinones **CXL** in order to study the effect of a heteroaryl alkyl group at position 3 on cardiovascular activity. Five compounds **CXLa–CXLe**)showed significant antihypertensive effects in rats at 100 mg/kg. p.o. 4,5-Dihydro-5-methyl-6-(4-methyl-aminoquinazolin-7-yl)-3(2H)-pyridazinone at a dose of 0.03 mg/kg i.v. in dogs increased myocardiac contractility [233]. Few derivatives of 3[-(tetra-zolylbiphenylyl]methyl]-4(3H)-quinazolones were synthesized, in which **CXLI** at 30 mg/kg, oral dose showed ≥ 70% inhibition of pressor action of i.v. angiotensin II in rats [234].

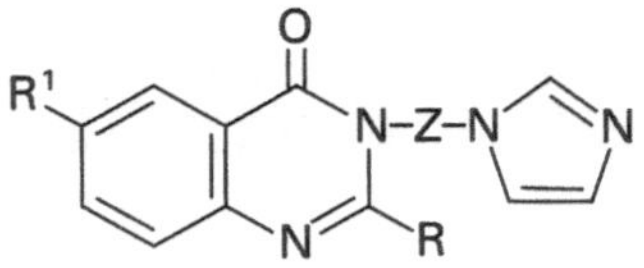

CXL
CXLa R = H, Z = (CH$_2$)$_6$, R^1 = H
CXLb R = H, Z = (CH$_2$)$_4$, R^1 = Cl
CXLc R = H, Z = CH$_2$CH$_2$CH(Me), R^1 = Cl
CXLd R = Me, Z = (CH$_2$)$_4$, R^1 = Cl
CXLe R = Et, Z = (CH$_2$)$_4$, R^1 = Cl

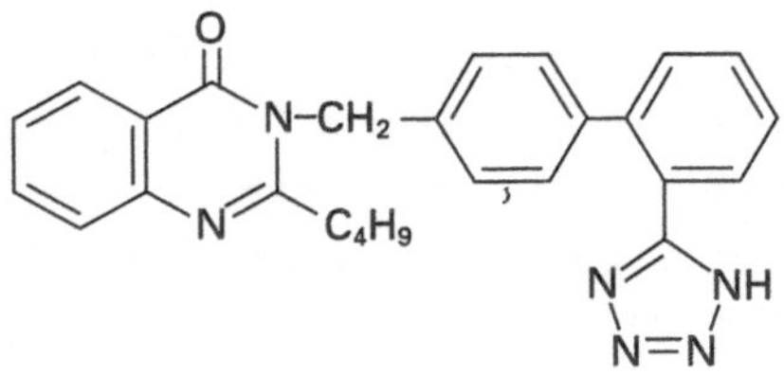

CXLI

Recently, Vishnoi et al. [235] synthesized some propanolamino quinazolinones **CXLII** and **CXLIII** and screened them for hypotensive and β-adrenoceptor blocking activities. A few compounds were also evaluated for their antiarrhythmic activity. Most of the compounds exhibited marked hypotensive activity in normotensive anesthetized cats, maximum activity of 88% fall in blood pressure at 5 mg/kg dose level was obtained by compounds **CXLIIa** and **CXLIIb** suggesting that the 3-diethylamino-2-hydroxypropyl side chain attached either directly to position 3 of the quinazolinone nucleus or through an oxygen bridge is essential for hypotensive activity. Almost all the compounds produced a lowering of heart rate per sc. Compound **CXLIIIa** showed maximum bradycardia (41%) at a 5 mg/kg dose. Most of the compounds had an inconsistent blocking effect on the depressor and positive inotropic effect of isoprenaline. Compounds **CXLIIc** and **CXLIIIb** possessed potent antiarrhythmic activity, **CXLIIc** was equipotent to quinidine at 3 μg/ml.

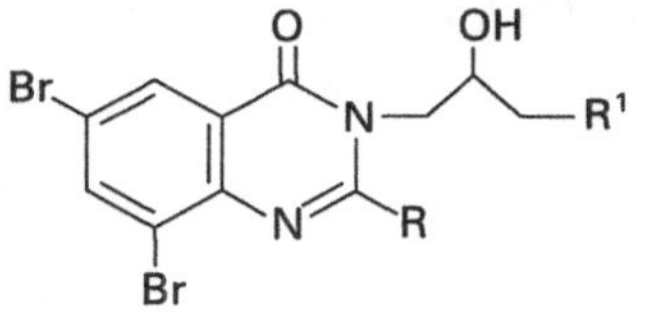

CXLII
CXLIIa R = Me, R^1 = –NH–CMe$_3$
CXLIIb R = Me, R^1 = morpholinyl
CXLIIc R = H, R^1 = morpholinyl

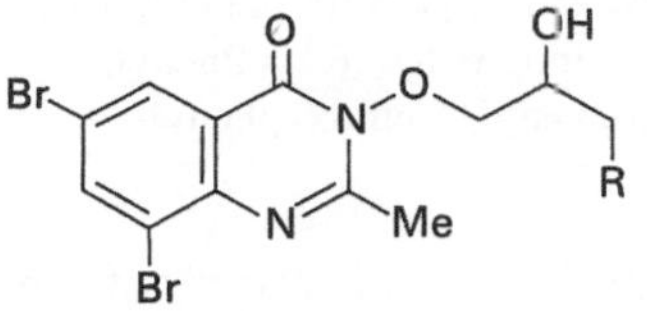

CXLIII
CXLIIIa R = –NEt$_2$
CXLIIIb R = –NHCMe$_3$

6   Antimicrobial activity

There has been a vast development in the chemotherapy of various microbial ailments affecting mankind as well as plants during the last several decades. The causative organisms of these ailments include bacteria, fungi, viruses, protozoa and mycobacteria. The search for curative drugs for microbial ailments is very old; use of quinine in malaria; ipecae and emetine in amoebic dysentry; arsenical drugs in experimental trypanosome infection in mice is well known. Recent development in chemotherapy begins with the use of sulphonamides, antibiotics and various other synthetic molecules. Quinazolinone molecules are known to display a wide range of antimicrobial activity.

6.1   Antibacterial

Bhargava et al. [236] synthesized a series of 5-nitro-3-aryl-2-substituted thio-4(3H)-quinazolinones **CXLIV** aiming at antibacterial agents. They observed that substitution of chloro, ethoxy at 4-position in the aryl enhanced the activity of these compounds. Bhargava and Prakash [29] further synthesized new quinazolinones **CXLV** and screened them against *Staphylococcus aureus, Staphylococcus typhi* and *Escherichia coli* but none of them showed a remarkable antibacterial activity.

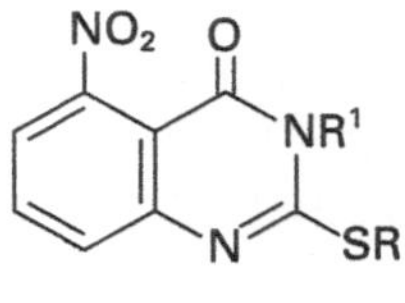

CXLIV
R = 2-Nitrobenzyl, N, N-methylphenyl, carboxamido methyl, R^1 = Phenyl, 4-chlorophenyl, 4-ethoxyphenyl

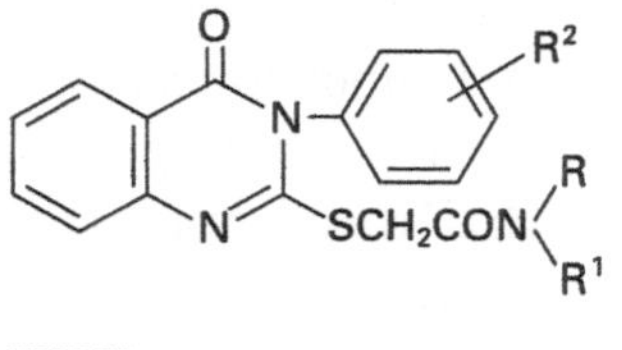

CXLV
R, R^1 = Isobutyl or benzyl, R^2 = Me, Cl, OMe

High antibacterial activity of urea derivatives prompted Bahadur et al. [130] to synthesize new quinazolinones **CIII** in which 4-aryloxy-phenylureido moiety was substituted at position 3 of quinazolinone via mercaptoacetyl bridge. The compounds were evaluated for their antibacterial activity against *Staphylococcus aureus, Escherichia coli, Bacillus subtilis* and *S. typhi*. It was observed that all the quinazolinones with 6- and 8-bromo substituents displayed significant antibacterial activity against gram positive strains and also that the quinazolinones were more active against gram positive bacteria than gram negative bacteria.

Antibacterial activity was also shown in quinazolinones with a 5-mercapto-1,2,4-triazolyl group at position 3 **CXLVI**. Compound **CXLVIa** had a bactericidal effect at 0.2×10^{-4} mg/l [237].

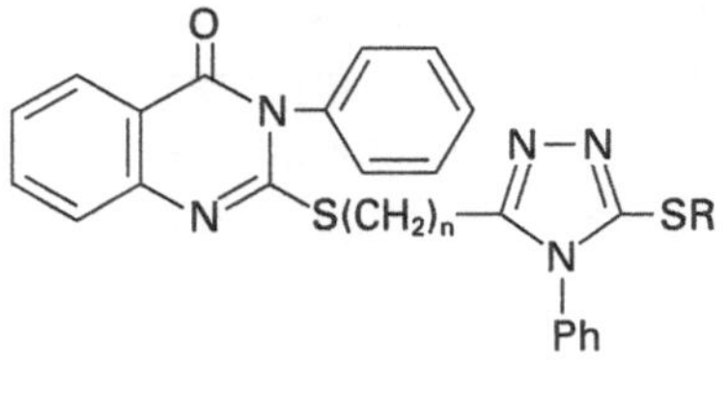

CXLVI
CXLVIa R = 4-MeC$_6$H$_4$NHCOCH$_2$, n = 3

Lakhan and Rai [238] synthesized 2-[ω-(dialkylamino)-alkylthio]-3-aryl, or alkyl-6,8-disubstituted-4(3H)-quinazolinones **CXLVII**; among them compounds with a diisopropylamino ethyl substituent at position 2 were found to be more active at higher concentrations (100 µg/ml) against *S. aureus* than *E. coli*, showing that compounds were more active against gram positive bacteria than gram negative strains. In a series of N-[S-(3-arylquinazolinon-2-yl) mercaptoacetyl] hydrazines **CXLVIII** and their corresponding thiosemicarbazides and triazoles **CXLIX**, antibacterial activity was exhibited against gram positive and gram negative bacteria by few compounds [239].

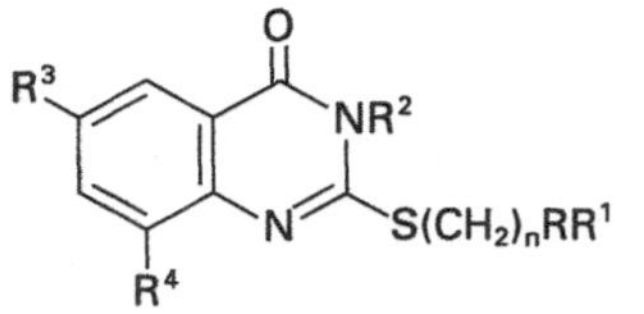

CXLVII
R, R^1 = H, Et, isopropyl, R^2 = Et, substituted phenyl, R^3, R^4 = H, Br, n = 2, 3

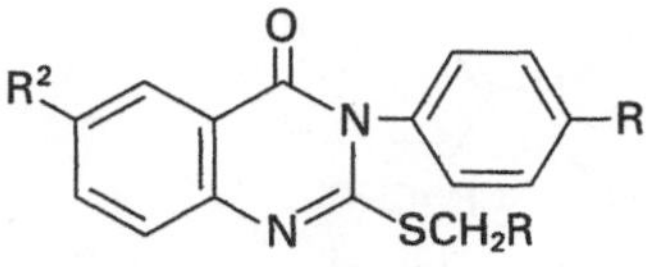

CXLVIII R = CONHNR^{3}R^4, R^1 = H, Me, R^2 = H, Br, R^3, R^4 = H

CXLIX R = [triazole structure] R^3, R^1 = H, Me, R^2 = H, Br, X = NPh, S, R^3 = OH, SH

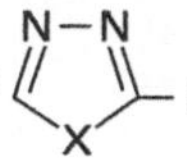

Varma [240] synthesized a series of 2-methyl/styryl-3-aryl- 4(3H)-quinazolinones {CL} and screened them against *Bacillus megaterium, E. coli, S. aureus* and *Salmonella typhosa*. Only moderate inhibition was observed with compounds **CLa** and **CLb** against *B. megaterium*. Varma and his co-workers [241, 242] further synthesized similar types of compounds **CLI**, in which morpholino/piperidino moiety was incorporated at N^3-aryl, but antibacterial activity was shown only by compound **CLIa** against *B. subtilis*.

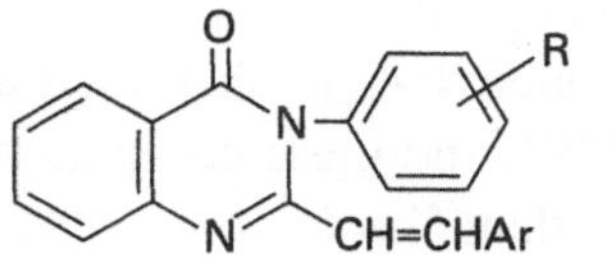

CL
CLa R = 4-COOMe, Ar = 2-furyl
CLb R = 3-COOMe, Ar = 4-OMePh

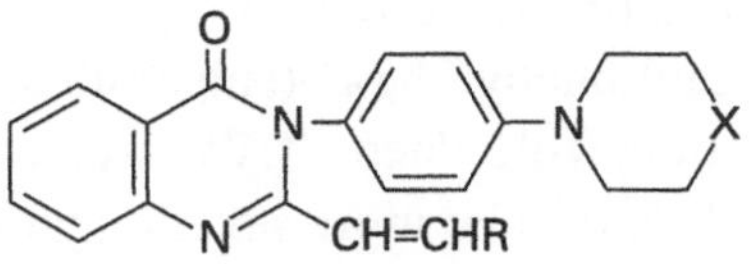

CLI
CLIa R = 4-OMePh, X = CH$_2$

Takashi and Yamane [243, 244] synthesized 2-(3',4'-dimethoxy styryl)-3-phenylquinazolinones **CLII** in which **CLIIa** at 1 µg/ml *in vitro* inhibited

Escherichia coli. Antimicrobial 2-[aryl-4(3H)-quinazolinon-2-yl]pyr-rolino[5,4-b]2,3-dihydro-4H-benzopyran-4-ones **CLIII** have also been reported recently [245].

Antibacterial activity was also exhibited by 3-(4'-bromophenyl)-1,2,3,4-tetrahydroquinazolinon-4-ones **CLIV** and **CLV** against *S. aureus.* Compound **CLV** had a minimum bactericidal concentration of 250 µg/ml against *E. coli* [246, 247].

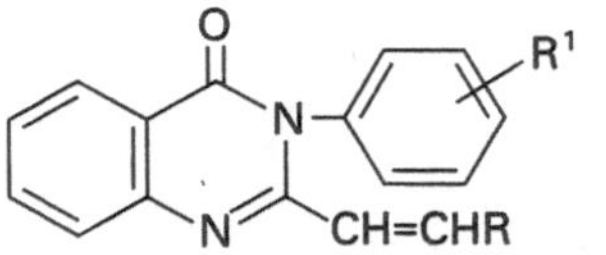

CLII R = 3, 4(OMe)$_2$Ph, R^1 = H, Cl, Br

CLIII R = , R^1 = H, Me, Br, R^2, R^3 = H, Me, Cl

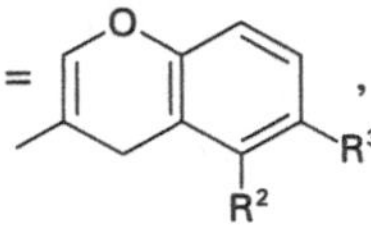

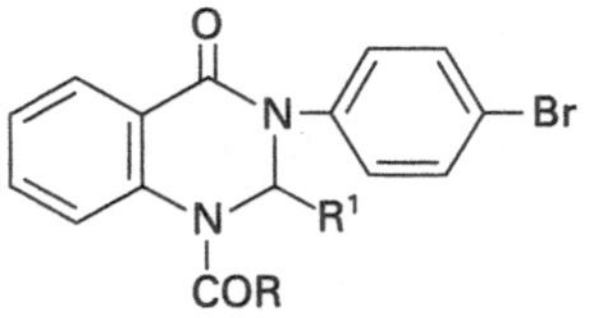

CLIV R = CH$_2$CH$_2$Cl, morpholino ethyl,
piperidino ethyl, R^1 = H

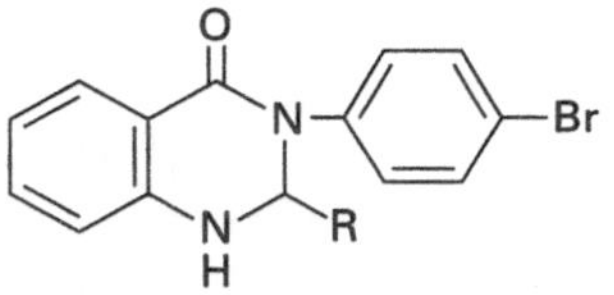

CLV
R = 3-OMe, 4-OHPh

Sen Gupta et al. [248] synthesized some substituted 2-phenyl-3-arylquina-zol-4-ones **CLVI** and found them to be potent antibacterials. With a view to evaluating the effect of diphenyl-ether-group at position 3, synthesis of 2-methyl/phenyl-3-[4'-(substituted   phenoxy)phenyl]-6,8-substituted-4-(3H)-quinazolinones **CLVII** was carried out [249], and these compounds were found to be more potent against *B. subtilis* than *Sarcina lutea.* Their efficacy reaches a maximum when there is bromine substituted at position 6, a phenyl group at position 2 and fluorine or chlorine in the phenoxy phenyl part of the molecule. Further substitution of bromine at position 8 results in loss or decrease of activity with the exception of 2-methyl-3[4'-(fluorophenoxy)phenyl]-6,8-dibromo-4(3H)-quinazolinone which offers a greater protection against *B. subtilis.*

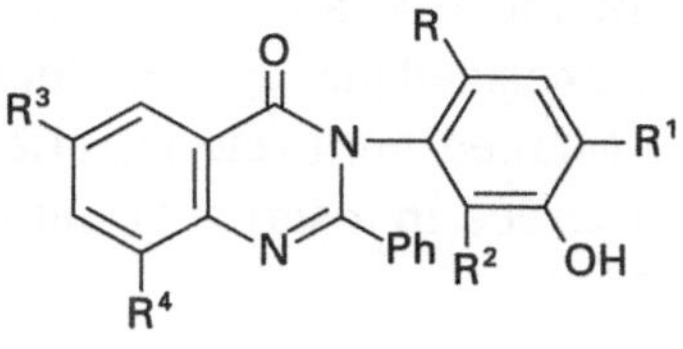

CLVI
CLVIa R, R^2, R^3 = H, R^1 = COOH,
          R^4 = Br
CLVIb R, R^2, R^4 = Br, R^1 = COOH,
          R^3 = H

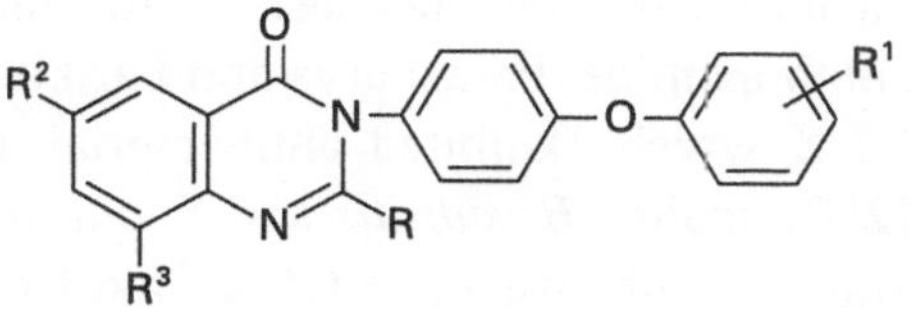

CLVII
R = Ph, Me, R^1 = 4-Cl, Me, F, 2-Me, H, R^2,
R^3 = H, Br

Shanker et al. [250] observed that substitution of sulfonamido moiety at methyl of position 2 **CLVIII** resulted in active compounds and among them **CLVIIIa** was active against all the tested microorganisms, viz. *S. lutea*, *E. coli*, *B. megaterium*, *P. flourescence* and *P. vulgaris*. It was also concluded that compounds with a N'-acetylsulfonamido grouping at position 2 were more active than those with N,N-dimethylamino or morpholino/piperidino at position 2. A series of 2,3,6-trisubstituted-4-quinazolylsulfonyl-thioureas **CLIX** was synthesized [251] and evaluated for antibacterial activity. Most of them were found to be effective against *B. subtilis*, *S. aureus*, *B. megaterium* and *E. coli*. The activity of the compounds was attributed to the presence of a thiourea group.

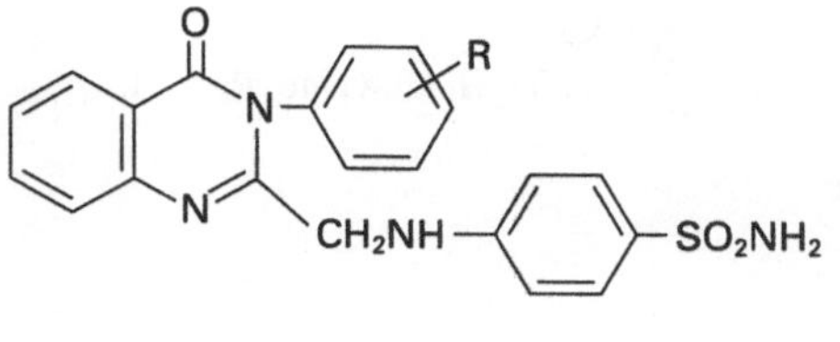

CLVIII
CLVIIIa R = 4-Me

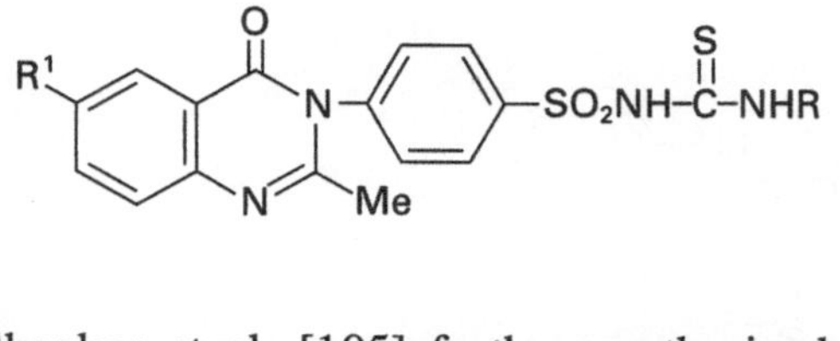

CLIX
R = Me, Et, Br, n-Bu, Phenyl,
R^1 = H, I

Shanker et al. [105] further synthesized N^4-[N-(6,8-dibromo-2-methyl-quinazolin-4(3H)-onyl)acetamido]-N^1-substituted sulfanilamides **LXXXVI** and screened them for antibacterial activity against *B. megaterium*, *B. pumilus*, *E. coli* and *Pseudomonas ovalis*, but none showed bactericidal effect because of the blocking of the free amino group of sulphonamide. Parasharya and Parikh [252] synthesized new quinazolones **CLX** which exhibited antibacterial activity. Marked antibacterial effect [253] against *B. subtilis* and *S. aureus* was observed in a series of quinazolones with structures **CLXI** and **CLXII**.

Substitution at position 3 by a heterocyclic moiety resulted in active compounds. Rida and co-workers [254] synthesized a series of 3-[1-(1H-benzimidazol-2-yl)alkyl]-2-substituted-4(3H)-quinazolinones in which five compounds exhibited marked antibacterial activity. Hussain et al. [40] incorporated aryl substituted oxothiazolidine moiety at position 3 of quinazolinones **XXX** and screened them against *B. cereus, S. aureus, Micococcus flavus, S. lutea* and *B. subtilis*. Some compounds were found to be inactive against *B. subtilis* whereas maximum inhibition was observed against *B. cereus*. It was concluded that the presence of an electron-attracting group and methoxy group at the phenyl ring of thiazolidone increases the antibacterial activity. They further synthesized 3-(N,N-disubstituted amino methyl)-5-[6,8-disubstituted-4-oxoquinazolin-3-yl)imino]-4-oxo-1,3-thia zolidine-2-thiones **CLXIII** as antibacterial agents [255].

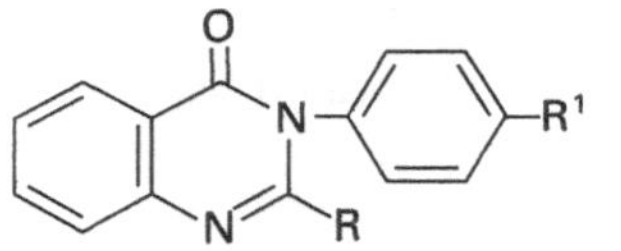

CLX
CLXa R = CH=CHR^2, R^1 = OH, OMe,
         R^2 = Ph, substituted Ph
CLXb R = CHBrCHBrR^2, R^1 = OH, OMe,
         R^2 = Ph, substituted Ph

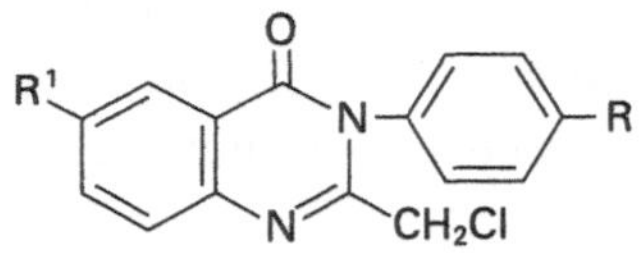

CLXI
R = NO$_2$, H, Cl, OMe, R^1 = H, I

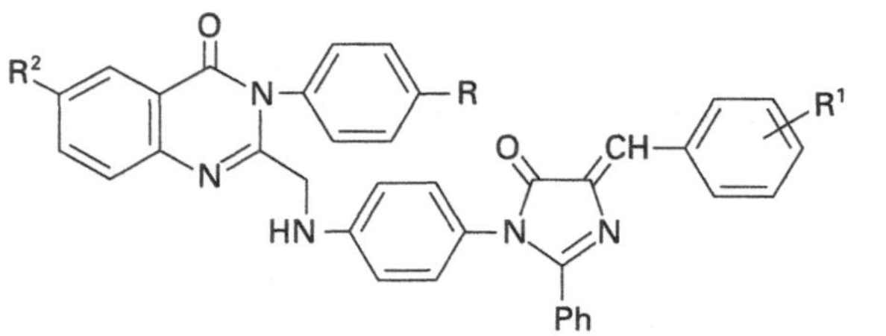

CLXII
R = NO$_2$, H, Cl, OMe, R^1 = H, 4-OH, 2-OH, 4-OMe, 4-Cl, 3-NO$_2$, R^2 = H, I

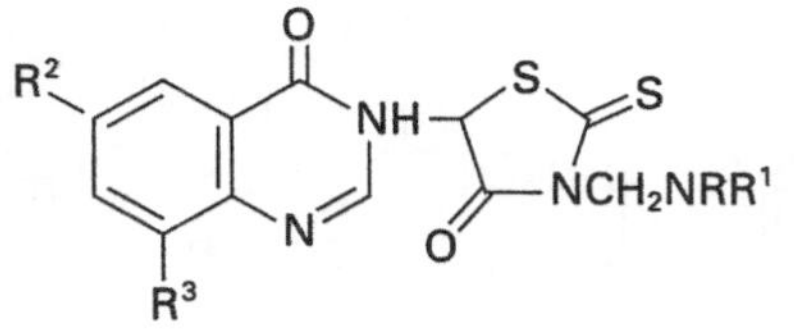

CLXIII
NNR^1 = NMe$_2$, NEt$_2$, NEtPh, piperidino, morpholino

Rao et al. [102] synthesized 3-(5-aryl-1,3,4-oxadiazol-2-ylmethyl)-2-methyl-4(3H)-quinazolinones **LXXXIII** and tested them against *B. megaterium* and *E. coli* but none of the compounds were found to be active. Bactericidal activity in thiadiazoloquinazolinones **CLXIV** was reported by Khalil and Habib [256].

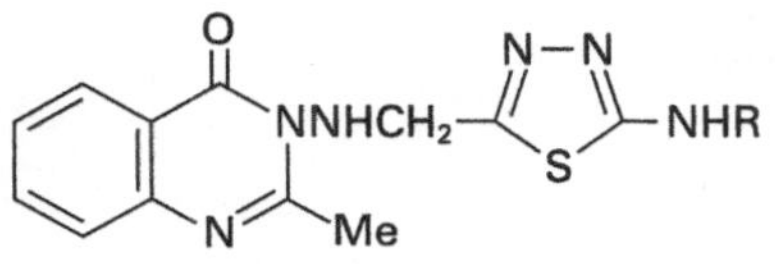

CLXIV
R = Bu, Ph, CH$_2$C$_6$H$_4$, ClC$_6$H$_4$

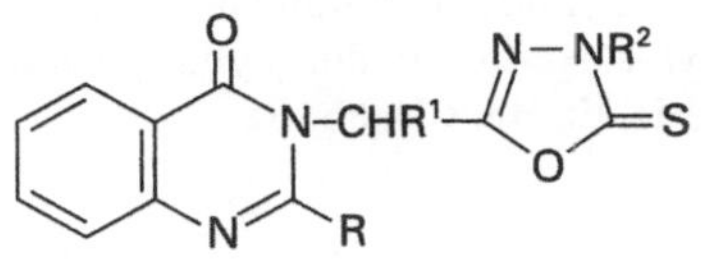

CLXV
R = Ph, 2-ClC$_6$H$_4$, R^1 = H, Me
R^2 = H, Et$_2$NCH$_2$, morpholinomethyl

Ahmed et al. [257] synthesized some quinazolin-containing oxadiazolin-5-thiones **CLXV** in which he found promising antibacterial activity in compounds with a morpholino group. Quinazolinones with indolinones at position 3 **CLXVI** also exhibited a bactericidal effect [258].
Zohry and co-workers [259] synthesized new quinazolinones in which the imidazolyl, benzimidazolyl or naphthyl group is attached to position 3 via an alkyl sulphide or sulphone group **CLXVII**; few compounds exhibited antimicrobial activity. Recently Achaiah and Reddy [260] synthesized new quinazolinones, with chromone moiety **CLXVIII**, as antibacterial agents. Antimicrobial activity [261] has also been reported for quinazolinones **CLXIX**.

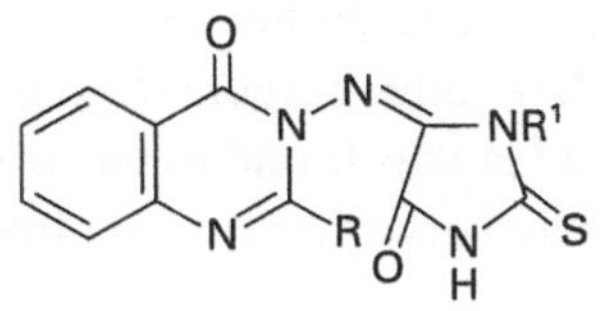

CLXVI
R = Me, Ph, R^1 = H, Br

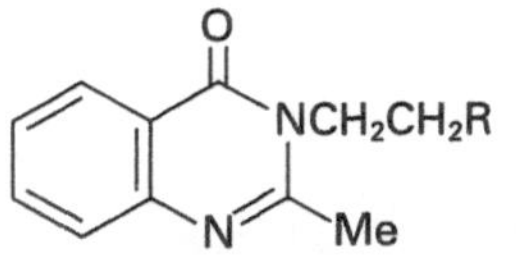

CLXVII
R = SAr, Ar = Ph, 4-ClC₆H₄,
2-imidazolyl, 2-benzimidazolyl,

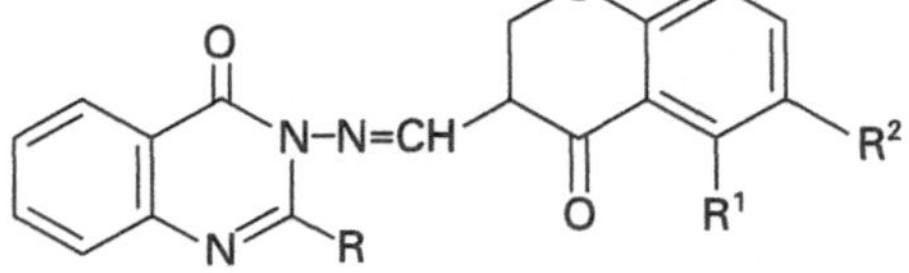

CLXVIII
R = Me, Ph, R1 = H, Me, R2 = H, Cl, Me

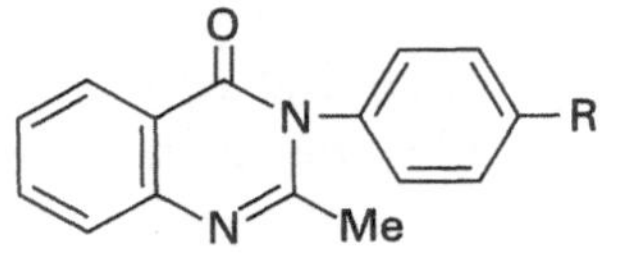

CLXIX
R = 3-Alkyl-4-aryl-2, 3-dihydrothiazol-2-ylideneamino,
3-alkyl-4-oxo-thiazolidin-2-ylideneamino, NHCSNHR^1
R^1 = Me, Et, Bu, CH₂Ph, Bz

Substitution at positions 6 and 8 by chlorine also resulted in active compounds. Ammar et al. [262] reported bactericidal 2-methyl-3-(p-tolyl)-6,8-dichloroquinazolinone **CLXX** as well as a number of related compounds [263, 264]. They further synthesized new quinazolinones **CLXXI** and tested them against *E. coli, S. aureus* and *Streptococcus*. Only two compounds **CLXXIa** and **CLXXIb** exhibited activity against all the three tested organisms, and it was concluded that incorporation of sulfonamido moiety in the quinazolinone nucleus confers high activity against the tested organisms.

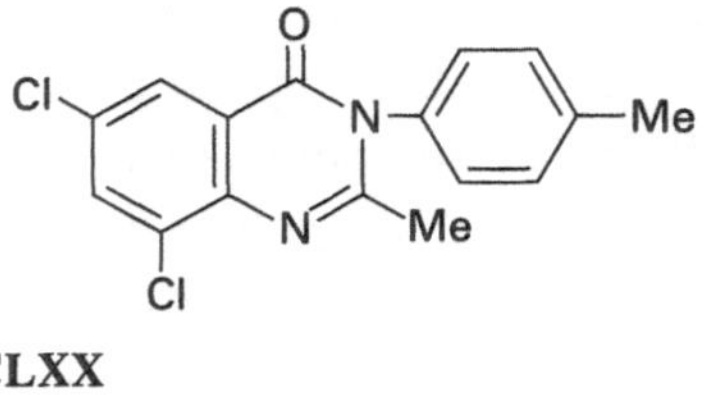

CLXX

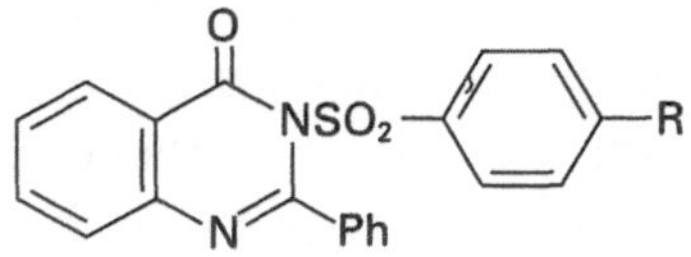

CLXXI
CLXXIa R = Cl
CLXXIb R = Me

Kulkarni et al. [266, 267] synthesized 2-methyl-6,8-substituted-3[substituted-aminoacetyl]-4(3H)-quinazolinones **CLXXII** and screened them against *B. subtilis* and *S. aureus*. Compound **CLXXIIa** was found to be very effective against *B. subtilis* whereas **CLXXIIb** was very effective against *S. aureus*.

Few derivatives of 2-aryloxymethyl-3-substituted-quinazolin-4(3H)-ones and 2-aryloxymethyl-3-(2-substituted ethyl)-quinazolin-4(3H)-ones have been reported as bactericides [268]. Chernobrovin and co-workers [269, 270] reported 2-benzyloxymethyl-3-(3'-tolyl)-4(3H)-quinazolinone and 2-benzyloxymethyl-3-(4-methoxyphenyl)-4(3H)-quinazolinone as potent antibacterial agents.

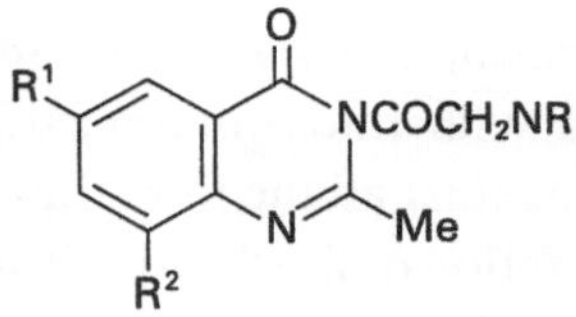

CLXXII
CLXXIIa   NR = Phenyl piperazino, R^1 = H, R^2 = I
CLXXIIb   NR = Phenyl piperazino, R^1, R^2 = Br

Synthesis   of   2-alkyl/aryl-3(arylhydrazino)quinazolin-4(3H)-ones **CLXXIII** and **CLXXIV** has been carried out and a few compounds exhibited *in vitro* antibacterial activity [41]. Gupta et al. [271] synthesized some schiff bases of 3-amino-2-methylquinazolin-4(3H)-ones **CLXXV**, out of which five compounds showed bactericidal activity with MIC of 60–100 µg/ml.

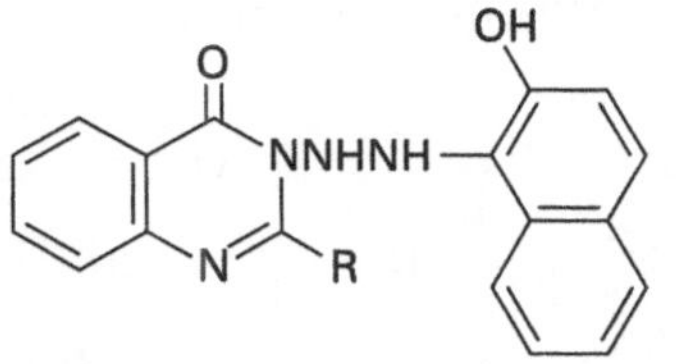

CLXXIII
R = Alkyl

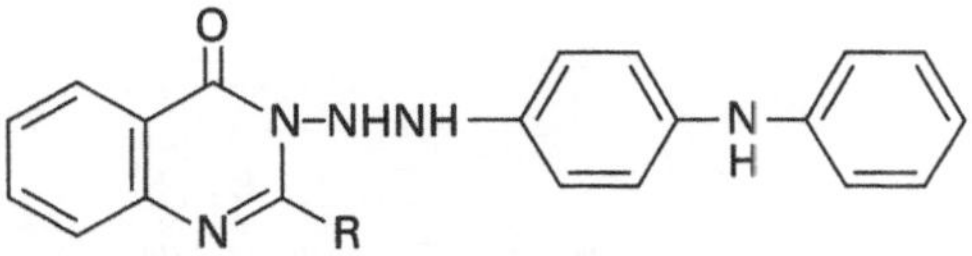

CLXXIV
R = Aryl

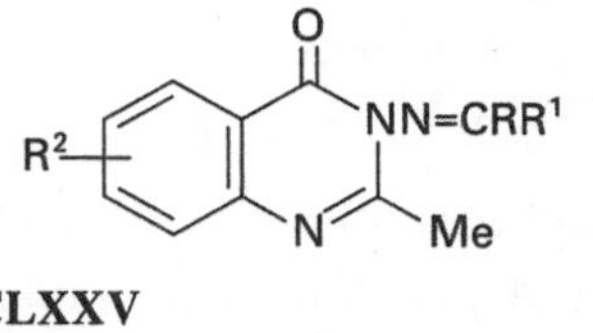

CLXXV
R = H, Me, Ph, R^1 = Me, styryl, Ph, substituted Ph , R^2 = H, Br

6.2   Antifungal activity

Fungicidal action of 2-amino-4(3H)-quinazolinones **CLXXVI** has been reported by Bullock et al. [272]; among them **CLXXVIa** exhibited 100% inhibition at 3 ppm against powdery mildew. 2-Thienylvinyl-4(3H)-quina-zolinones **CLXXVII** also exhibited fungicidal activity [273].

Joshi and Joshi [274] synthesized new quinazolinones with thiosemicar-bazide, triazole and triazolo thiazine moieties at position 3 **CLXXVIII** and screened them against *Alternaria alternata, Drechslera papendorfii* and *Helminthosporium oryzae*. Only quinazolinones with thiosemicarbazide moiety possessed measurable antifungal activity against all the three fungi at a concentration of 2%. It was inferred that cyclization of the thiosemicarbazides into corresponding triazole or triazolo thiazines resulted in a loss of activity.

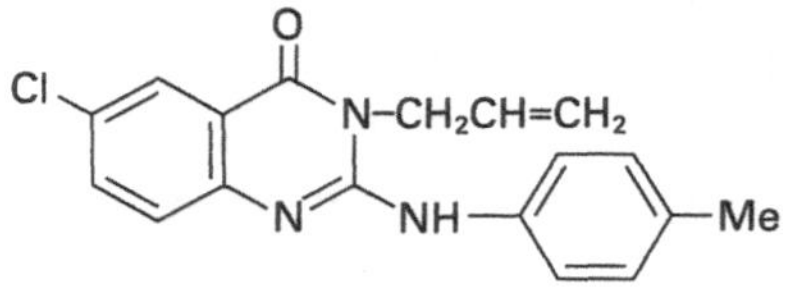

CLXXVI

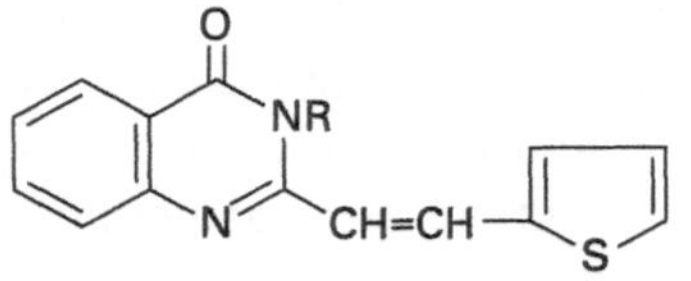

CLXXVII
R = H, NH2NHPh, NHCONH2

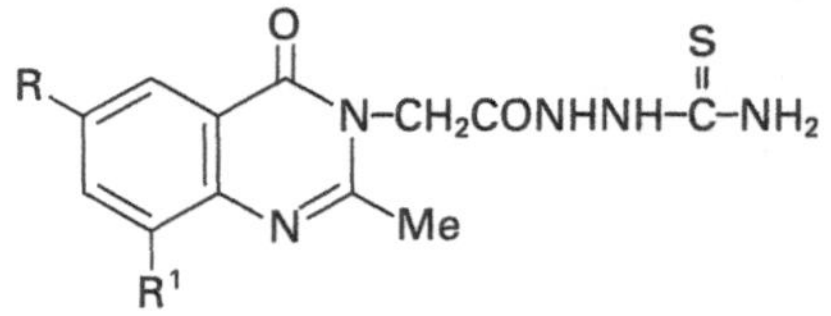

CLXXVIII
R = H, Br, Cl, R^1 = H, Br, I, Cl

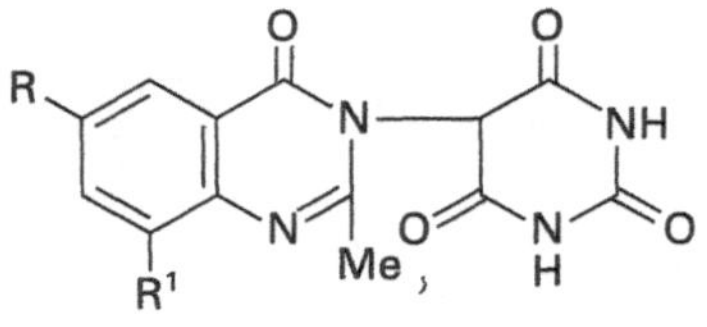

CLXXIX
CLXXIXa R = H, R^1 = Br
CLXXIXb R = H, R^1 = I
CLXXIXc R, R^1 = Cl
CLXXIXd R, R^1 = I

Fungicidal action was observed with quinazolinyl barbiturates **CLXXIX**, compounds **CLXXIXa** and **CLXXIXb** inhibited *Aspergillus niger* and *A. terreus*; **CLXXIXc** inhibited *A. niger* only and **CLXXIXd** *A. terreus* only [275]. The presence of a thiol group at position 2 produced compounds with high fungicidal activity; in view of this finding, Shakhidoyatov et al. [276] synthesized 2-mercaptoalkyl-quinazolin-4-one **CLXXX** and found that lengthening of the alkyl chain, beyond ethyl, resulted in a decrease of fungicidal effect.

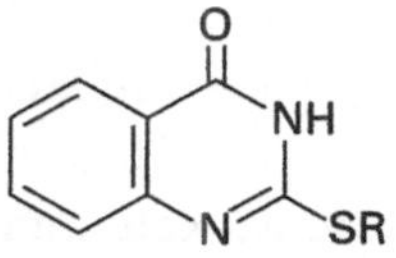

CLXXX
R = Me, Et, Pr, Bu, C$_6$H$_{11}$, n-C$_6$H$_{13}$

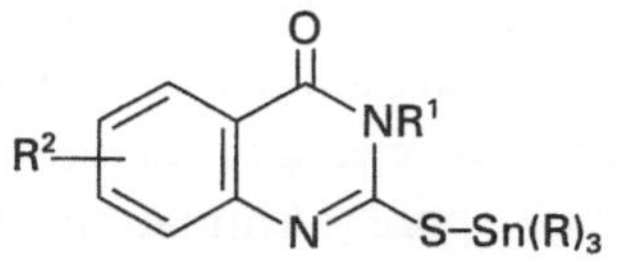

CLXXXI
CLXXXIa R = Bu, R^1 = Ph, R^2 = Cl, Br, I

Bahadur et al. [128] reported fungicidal activity of 2-mercaptoacetyl-N-(4-aryloxy)phenylureido-3-aryl-4(3H)-quinazolinones **CIII** against *A. niger* and *Helminthosporium* spp. 5-Mercapto-1,2,4-triazolylquinazolinone **CXLVIa** also exhibited fungicidal activity at 0.2×10 mg/l [237]. Edwards [277] synthesized 2-thio-organotin-4(3H)-quinazolinones **CLXXXI**, among them **CLXXXIa** exhibited an effectiveness comparable to Difolatan in mycelial inhibition tests against a variety of fungi. Fungicidal activity of 3-substituted-2-aminothio-4-oxo-3,4-dihydroquinazolines **CLXXXII** has recently been reported by Chaurasia et al. [278].

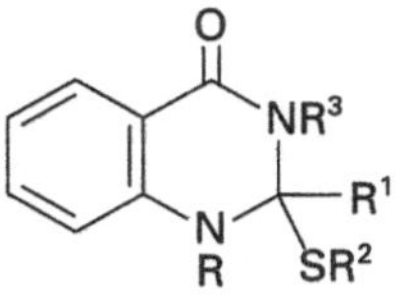

CLXXXII
CLXXXIIa RR^1 = bond, R^2 = NH$_2$, R^3 = (Un)substituted alkyl, alkenyl, (hetero)aryl

Substituted 2-phenyl-3-arylquinazol-4-ones **CLVI** tested as antibacterials, also exhibited antifungal activity [248]. In 2-methyl/phenyl-3-[4'-(substituted phenoxy)phenyl]-6,8-substituted-4(3H)-quinazolinones **CLVII** [249], two compounds **CLVIIa** and **CLVIIb** were evaluated as fungicides against *Fusarium moniliforme* and *Calytrotrichum C. falcatum Went*.

Chaurasia and Sharma [279] synthesized benzothiazolyl quinazolinones **CLXXXIII** and found them active against *Aspergillus niger* and *Drechslera australiensis*. They further observed [280] that substitution by chlorine at position 6 and 8 produced more potent compounds; **CLXXXIIIa** and **CLXXXIIIb** inhibited *Alternaria alternata* growth, while **CLXXXIIIc** was active against *A. fumigatus*. They [281, 282] also synthesized benzothiazolyl quinazolinones with a phenyl group at position 2 **CLXXXIV** and these compounds were found to be active against *A. fumigatus* and *A.*

alternata. It was observed that replacement of hydrogen by a methyl, chloro, methoxy or ethoxy group in benzothiazolyl moiety increases the activity except methoxy at position 6 which causes decrease in activity against *A. fumigatus*. The introduction of 6,8-dibromo groups in the 4(3H)-quinazolinone ring appeared to enhance the antifungal action as compared to unsubstituted ones and the 6,8-dibromo substituted quinazolinones inhibited 100% spore germination of both fungi at low dilutions. Retention of antifungal activity against *A. niger* and *A. alternata* was observed [283] in compounds with chlorine at position 6 and 8 **CLXXXIV** and it was concluded that replacement of hydrogen by methyl or chlorine in the benzothiazolyl nucleus increases the activity, and a decrease in activity was observed with methoxy or ethoxy groups.

Lakhan and Rai [284] reported antifungal activity in 3-(2'-benzothiazolyl)-4(3H)-quinazolinones **CLXXXV** which was comparable to Dithan M-45. Some new thiazolyl quinazolones **CLXXXVI** were synthesized by Dash et al. [285] which at 500 ppm inhibited *Helminthosporium sativum* by 50–70% *in vitro*.

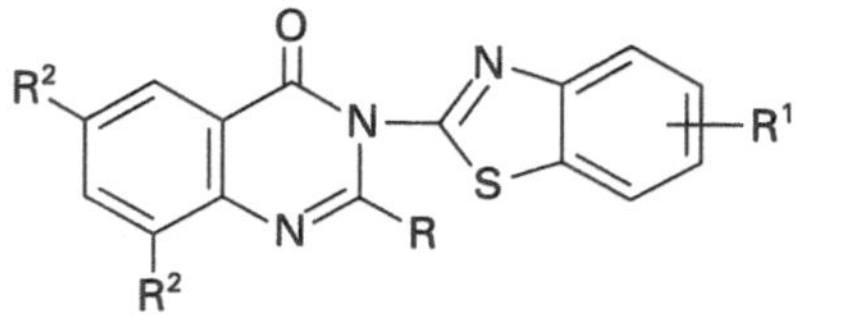

CLXXXIII
CLXXXIIIa   R = CH$_2$CH$_2$NEt$_2$, R^1 = 4-Cl, R^2 = Cl
CLXXXIIIb   R = CH$_2$CH$_2$NEt$_2$, R^1 = 6-OMe, R^2 = Cl
CLXXXIIIc   R = CH$_2$CH$_2$NEt$_2$, R^1 = 5-Cl, R^2 = Cl
CLXXXIV   R = Ph, R^1 = 6-Me, 5-Cl, 6-Cl, R^2 = H, Cl

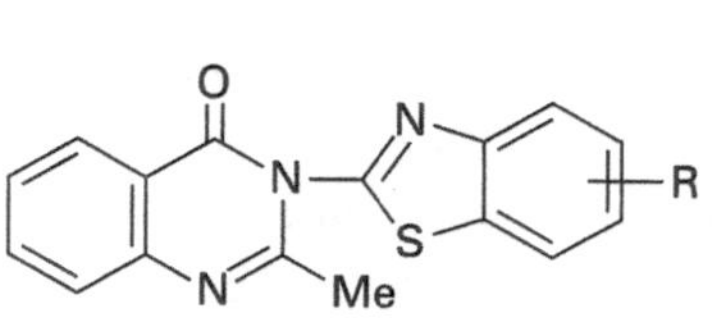

CLXXXV
R = NO$_2$, Cl

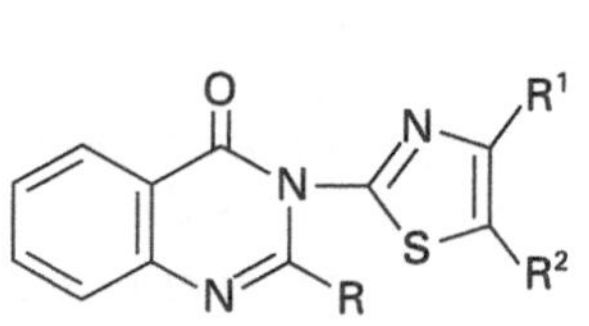

CLXXXVI
R = Me, Ph, R^1 = thienyl, Ph, R^2 = H, Ph, 4-ClPh

Reddy et al. [286] synthesized 2-(2-methyl-4-oxoquinazolin-3-yl)methyl-5-arylamino-1,3,4-thiadiazoles **CLXXXVII** which inhibited (90–100%) *F. solani* at a concentration of 600–840 µg/ml. Khalil and Habib [256] also reported fungicidal thiadiazoloquinazolinones **CLXIV**. Mitra et al. [287] evaluated some rhodanines of type **CLXXXVII** as potential fungicides. Fungicidal imidazolyl and triazolylquinazolines had been reported in literature [288]. Gauss et al. [289] reported fungicidal activity in 2-(3-methyl-1H-pyrazol-1-yl)-4(3H)-quinazolinone **CLXXXIX** which had a minimum inhibitory concentration of <0.1 mg/l, *in vitro* against *Coniophora puteana in vitro*. Synthesis of 2-(4-aryl-2-pyrazolin-3-yl)-3-aryl-4(3H)-quinazolinones **CXC** was carried out by Reddy et al. [290], among them **CXCa** inhibited spore germination in *Drechslera rostrata* (ED50 24.80) and *Fusarium oxysporum* (ED50 22.20).

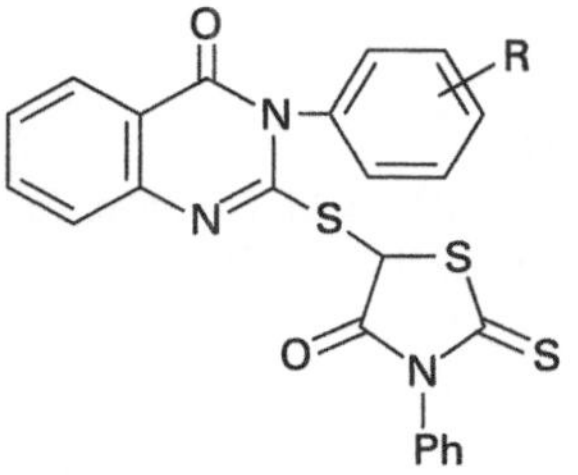

CLXXXVII
R = Cl, COOMe, Me, OMe

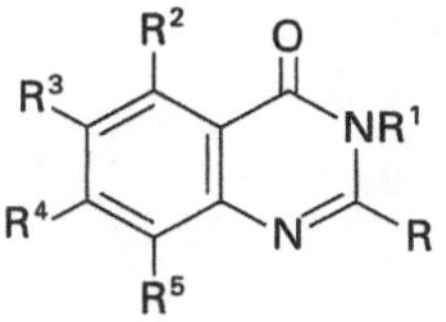

CLXXXVIII
R = 1-imidazolyl, 1, 2, 4-triazol-1-yl, R^1 = aryl,
R^2, R^3, R^4, R^5 = H, Cl, Br, I, Me, OMe

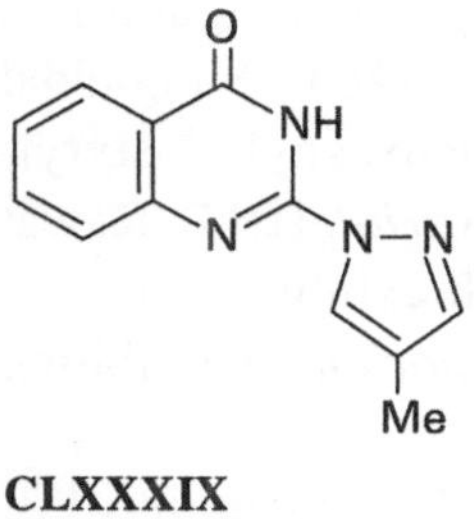

CLXXXIX

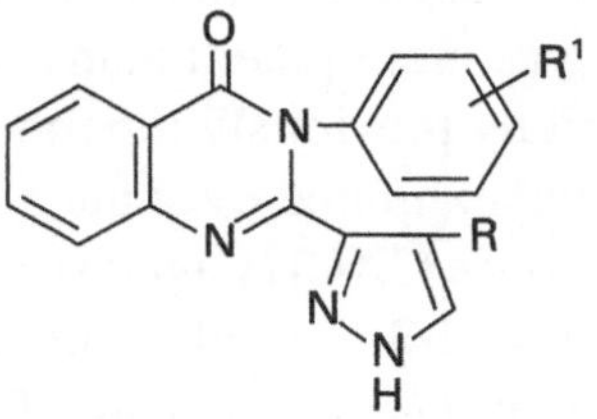

CXC
R = Ph, substituted Ph, R^1 = H, 2-Me, 2-Cl,
4-Me, 4-Br

Shanker et al. [250] synthesized new quinazolinones in which they incorporated sulphonamide moiety at position 3 **CLVIII**. The compounds exhibited antifungal activity in addition to antibacterial effect. Rao and Shanker [291] further synthesized 3-aryl-quinazolinones **CXCI** and **CXCII**, out of them **CXCIIa** at 800 µg/ml totally controlled *Corvularia lunata* and *Fusarium oxysporum*. Findings suggested that among **CXCII**, 4-nitro phenyl at position 3 was effective in checking fungal growth, 2-tolyl and 2-nitrophenyl groups were moderate in their fungicidal effect. Amongst substituents in sulphonamide moiety at position 2 in compounds **CXCI**, the nitro-substituent was more effective than the methyl and methoxy substituents, and compound **CXCII** is more active than **CXCI**.

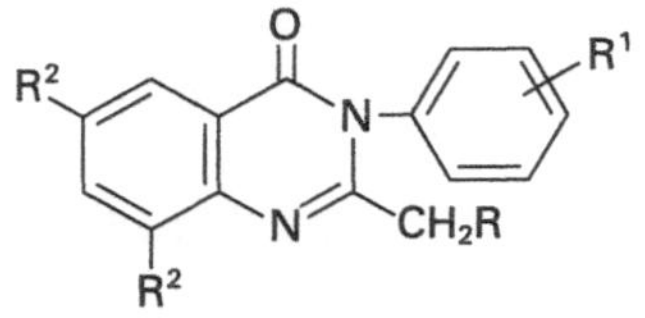

CXCI
R = NMe2, NEt2, piperidino, morpholino,
R^1 = 4-Me, 2-Me, 4-N02, R^2 = H, Br

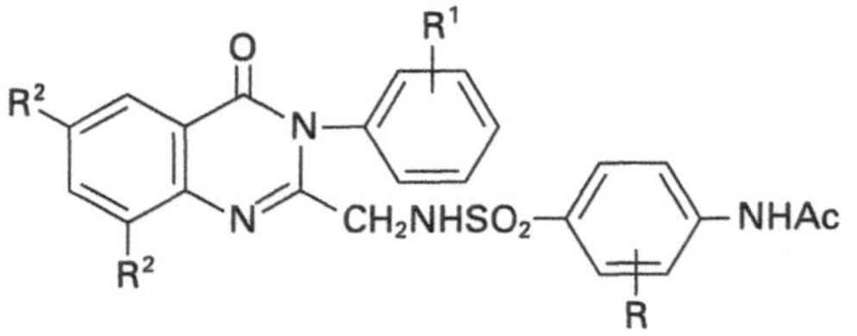

CXCII
R = H, 2-NO2, 3-Me, 3-OMe,
R^1 = NO2, Me, R^2 = H, Br

Reddy et al. [292] evaluated 2-methyl/phenyl-3-anilino quinazolinones for antifungal activity. Both of the compounds totally inhibited spore germination of *Fusarium oxysporum* and *Corvularia lunata* at 360 μg/ml, and 2-phenyl analog was more potent than 2-methyl analog. Antifungal effect was also exhibited by previously reported antibacterials [263]. Fungicidal action has also been exhibited by some 3-(5-methyl-3-isoxazoyl)-2-styryl-quinazolin-4(3H)-ones **CXCIII** against *Paecilomyces varioti* [293]. Rawat [294] reported 2-styryl-3-O-tolyl-4-quinazolone which exhibited fungicidal effect against *Corvularia lunata* and *Fusarium oxysporum* by inhibiting 22.5–40.3% growth.

In vitro antifungal activity was also observed by 3-[1H-benzimidazol-2-yl)alkyl]-2-substituted-4(3H)-quinazolinones [254]. Achaiah [260] reported the antifungal activity of 3-[N-(4-oxo-2-substituted-3-quinazolinyl)formimidoyl]chromones **CLXVIII**.

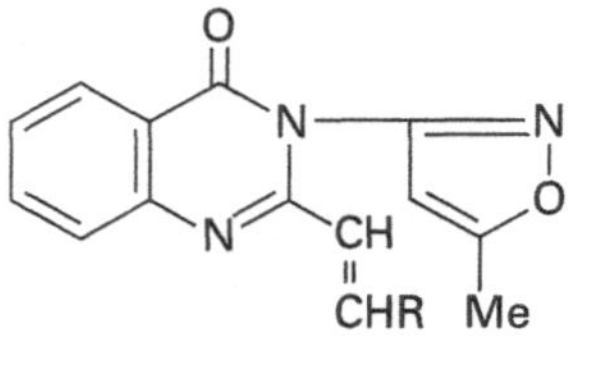

CXCIII
R = Ph, OMeC6H4, NMe2C6H4, NO2C6H4, ClC6H4, thienyl

6.3 Antiviral activity

Virucidal 6-nitro substituted-2(1H)-quinazolinones **CXCIV** were synthesized by Yamamoto et al. [295, 296]. The minimum inhibitory concentration of 1-tetrahydrofurfuryl-4-phenyl-6-nitro-2(1H)-quinazolinone on vaccinia virus multiplication in chick embryo fibroblast cell culture was observed to be 1.0 erg/ml.

A series of 4(3H)-quinazolone derivatives was evaluated for their activity against Ranikhet disease virus (RDV) *in vitro* (chorioallantoic membrane) and *in vivo* (Chick embryo) [297]. 3-[Benzoxazolin-2'-thion-3'-yl-5'-vinyl]-2-[4-chlorophenyl]-4(3H)-quinazolone **CXCV** was the most active, exhibiting inhibition of RDV *in vitro* (62.5%) and *in vivo* (72.5%), whereas 7-chloro-2(2'-benzimidazolyl)-methylthio]-3-phenyl-4(3H)-quinazolone showed inhibition of RDV *in vitro* (50%) and *in vivo* (55%). A structure-activity relationship study indicated that presence of chlorophenyl group at position 3 enhanced the virucidal activity.

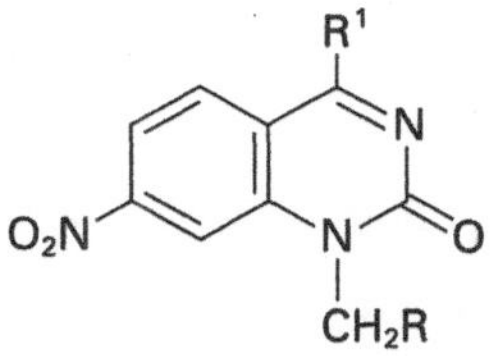

CXCIV
R = 2-Furyl, 2-thienyl, 2-pyridyl,
R^1 = Ph, thienyl

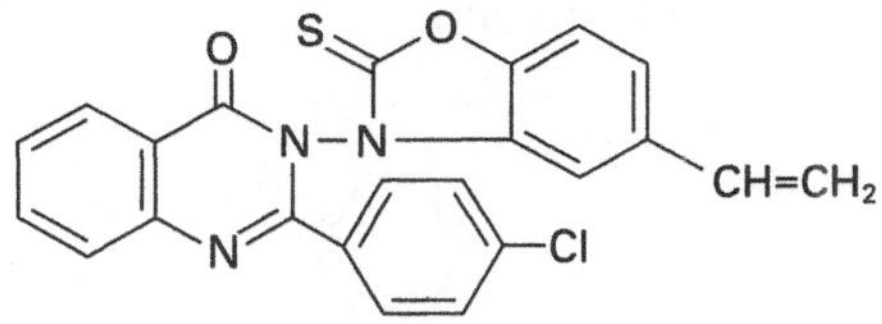

Nautiyal et al. [298] synthesized new 3(4-aryl)-substituted carbamidoacetyl-aminomethyl-4(3H)-quinazolinones **CXCVI** and screened them for antiviral activity in Tobacco Mosaic virus *in vivo* and *in vitro*. Maximum inhibition was observed with 6-nitro-3(O-tolyl carbamidoacetyl)amino methyl-4(3H)-quinazolone which exhibited inhibition *in vivo* (86%) and *in vitro* (81%). Similarly 6-nitro-3-(O-anisylcarbamidoacetyl)amino methyl-4(3H)-quinazolone and 6-bromo-(3-(carbamidoacetyl)aminomethyl-4(3H)-quinazolone also exhibited *in vivo* (81 and 73%) and *in vitro* (57 and 46%) respectively. It was noticed that all the compounds described decreased virus multiplication in the case *in vivo* study, and substitution at positions 6 and 8 of the quinazolone ring increases antiviral activity, the nitro group at position 6 producing a more potent compound than its 6-bromo analog.

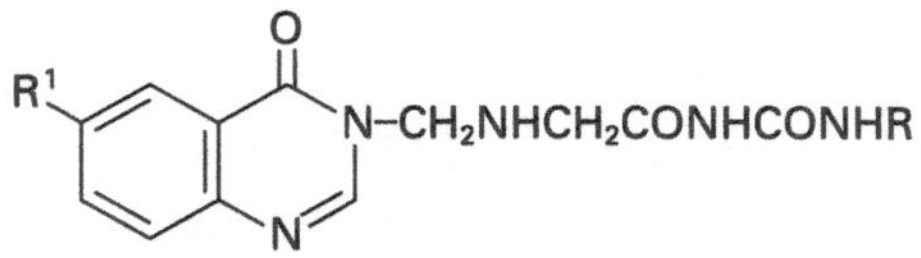

CXCVI
R = Ph, 2-MeC$_6$H$_4$, 4-ClC$_6$H$_4$, 4-MeC$_6$H$_4$, R^1 = H, Br, NO$_2$

Pandey et al. [299] synthesized 1-(2'-phenyl-3'-ethyl-4-oxoquinazo-lyl)benzophenothiazines **CXCVII** and tested them for antiviral activity. Compounds **CXCVIIa** and **CXCVIIb** inhibited multiplication of en-cephalomyocarditis, Ranikhet disease and Newcastle disease viruses in tissue culture. Further they [300] observed that the presence of a cinnamoyl-phenyl group at position 3 also resulted in active compounds, thus **CXCVIIIa** and **CXCVIIIb** showed 80% inhibition of Ranikhet disease virus at 1 mg/ml/ culture. It was also observed that a methoxy substituent at position 4 was largely responsible for the antiviral activity and that the 2-hydroxy-5-methoxy substituent was more active than 4-hydroxy-3-methoxy substituent.

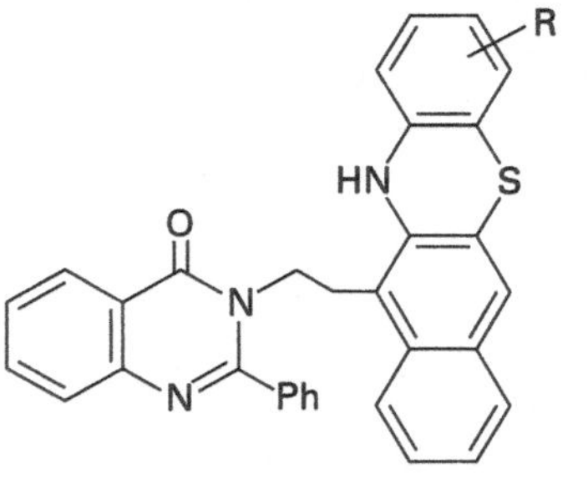

CXCVII
CXCVIIa R = 6-Me
CXCVIIb R = 7-OMe

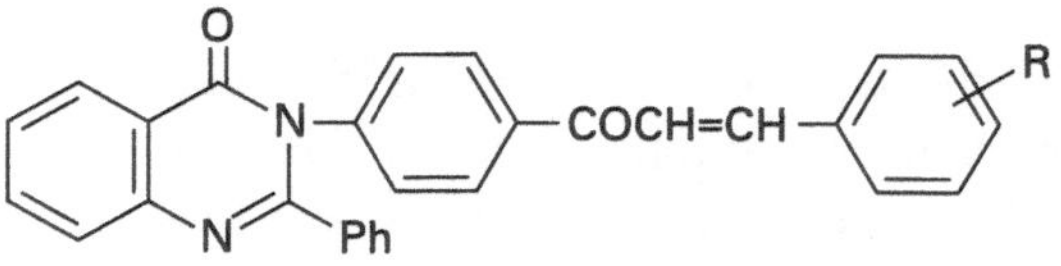

CXCVIII
CXCVIIIa R = 4-OMe
CXCVIIIb R = 2-OH, 5-OMe

6.4   Antimyocobacterial activity

Bhargava and Singh [301] observed antitubercular activity in 5-nitro-3-aryl-2-substituted thio-4(3H)-quinazolinones **CXCIX** against *M. tuber-*

culosis var *hominis* (Strain H$_{37}$ RV) *in vitro*. Four compounds **CXCIXa–CXCIXd** exhibited maximum inhibition and also the compounds prepared from the halides with tertiary nitrogen were highly potent **CXCIXc** and **CXCIXd**. It was also evident that substitution by chloro or ethoxy group in phenyl at position 3 enhanced the activity of the compounds.

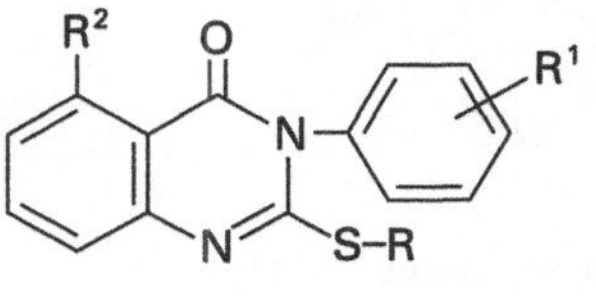

CXCIX
CXCIXa R = Et, R^1 = 4-OEt, R^2 = NO2
CXCIXb R = C$_5$H$_{10}$N–CO–CH$_2$, R^1 = 4-Cl, R^2 = NO$_2$
CXCIXc R = CH$_2$CON(Me)Ph, R^1 = 4-Cl, R^2 = NO$_2$
CXCIXd R = CH$_2$CON(Ph)CH$_2$Ph, R^1 = 4-OEt, R^2 = NO$_2$
CXCIXe R = 2-CH$_2$COOMeC$_6$H$_4$, R^1 = 4-Cl, R^2 = H
CXCIXf R = 2-C$_2$H$_2$COOMeC$_6$H$_4$, R^1 = 4-Cl, R^2 = H

The same type of compounds were further synthesized by Srivastava [302] and screened against *M. tuberculosis* var. *hominis* (Strain H$_{37}$ RV); only two compounds **CXCIXe** and **CXCIXb** were found to be weakly active. Rao and Sharma [303, 304] reported antitubercular activity in compound **CC**; only two compounds **CCa** and **CCb** had minimum inhibitory concentration below 100 µg/ml.

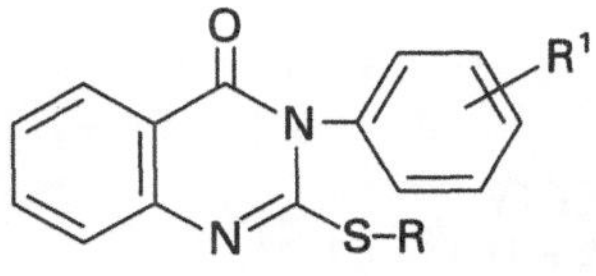

CC
CCa R = Me, R^1 = 4-Me
CCb R = Me, R^1 = 4-Br
CCc R = Alkyl, R^1 = cyclohexyl

Habib and Hazzaa [305] reported antitubercular 2-methyl-3-arylamino-4(3H)-6,8-disubstituted quinazolones. In a series of 2-phenyl-3-(5-substituted mercapto-1,3,4-thiadiazol-2-yl)-quinazolin-4(3H)-ones, few compounds were found to be active against *M. smegmatis* and *M. tuberculosis* (H$_{37}$ RV) *in vitro* [306].

7   Antimalarial activity

Bhargava and Shyam [307] reported antimalarial 4(3H)-quinazolinones **CCI**. A series of twenty-five 3-substituted amino-4-quinazolinones **CCII** was synthesized by Chen and Zhang [308] and evaluated for their antimalarial activity against *Plasmodium berghei*, but none would exhibit activity.

Singhal et al. [309] synthesized new quinazolinone derivatives **CCIII** and screened two compounds against *P. berghei* and *P. gallinaceum* in mice; only compound **CCIIIa** exhibited promising results in arresting the growth of the parasite.

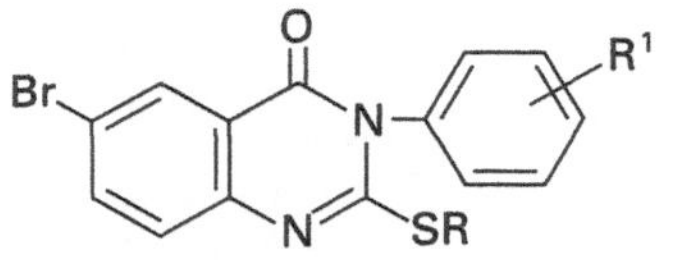

CCI
R = CH2CONPhCH2CH2CHMe2,
R^1 = H, 3-Me, 4-Me, 4-Cl, 4-Br, 4-OMe, 4-OEt

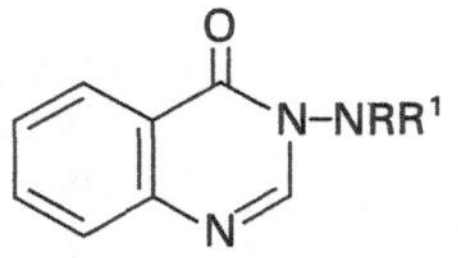

CCII
R = H, nitroso, substituted benzyl,
R^1 = substituted benzyl, RR^1 = substituted benzylidene

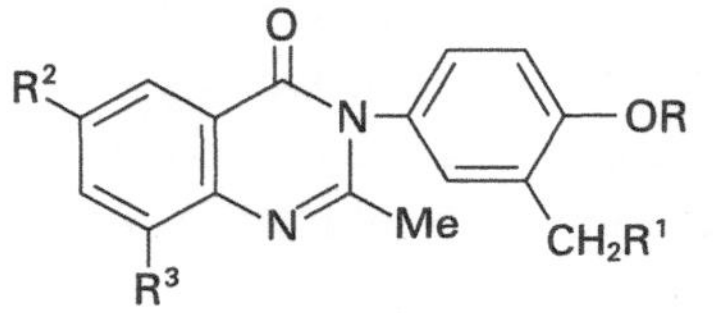

CCIII
CCIIIa R = Et, R^1 = NEt2, R^2 = Cl, R^3 = H

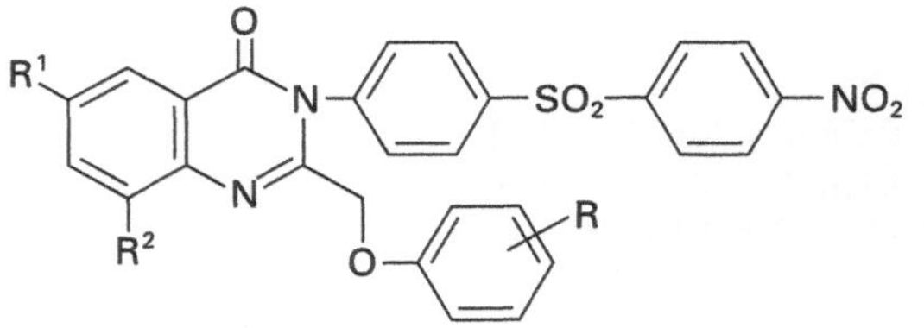

CCIV
R = H, Me, Cl, R^1,
R^2 = H, Br, I

High antimalarial activity was observed in a series of 2-aryloxymethyl-3-[4-nitrophenyl-sulfonyl)phenyl]-quinazolin-4(3H)-one **CCIV** against *P. berghei* [310]. All the compounds had shown very high antimalarial activity at a dose of 1 mg/kg. It was observed that the 4-chloro and 3-methyl group as well as the bromo group at position 6 and 8 enhanced the activity. The dibromo compounds were more potent than unsubstituted or mono iodo derivatives. The compounds also exhibited activity against *P. yoelli nigeriensis* in mice at doses of 1 mg/kg to 4 mg/kg.

Lakhan et al. [311] synthesized new derivatives of quinazolinones **CCV** with a view that compounds might be potent antimalarials. The compounds were screened against *P. berghei* but found to be inactive at 1 quinine equivalent of the dosage.

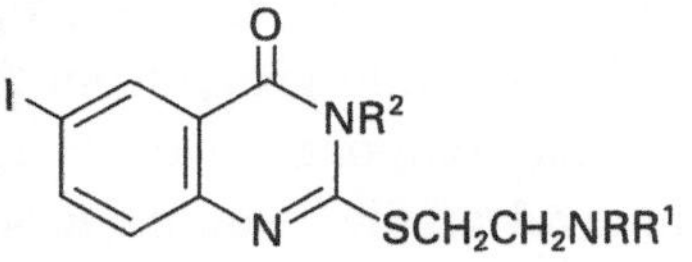

CCV
R, R^1 = H, Et, CHMe$_2$, RR^1 = (CH$_2$)$_5$
R^2 = Me, Et, PhCH$_2$

8   Antitumor activity

The recent discovery of potent and selective inhibitors of thymidylate synthetase (TS) and glycinamide ribonucleotide (GAR) transformylase [312] provided the impetus for renewed interest in the unexplored potential of antifolates in cancer chemotherapy.

In 1981, Jones and co-workers reported [314] that 10-propargyl-5,8-dideaz-afolic acid **CCVI** CB3717 was a selective tight-binding inhibitor of thymidylate synthetase (TS); it inhibited TS from L1210 cells competitively with respect to the substrate methylene-tetrahydrofolate. Treatment of animals bearing the L1210 tumor with CB3717 **CCVI** at 125 or 200 mg/kg/day for 5 days resulted in cures, >120 days survival in 90% of animals. The high therapeutic efficacy of CB3717 may be due to preservation of *de novo* purine synthesis which is inhibited by other antifolates. *In vitro* results further suggest that CB3717 could be active against methotrexate-resistant tumors.

CB3717 showed activity against ovarian, liver and breast cancer, however, with troublesome hepatic toxicity and dose-limiting renal toxicity [315–321]. This drug is poorly soluble at neutral or acidic pH, which posed problems for its clinical use and is probably responsible for the renal toxicity. It is known that the drug precipitates in the renal tubule, in mice [322] and in renal tubule and bile duct in mice [323].

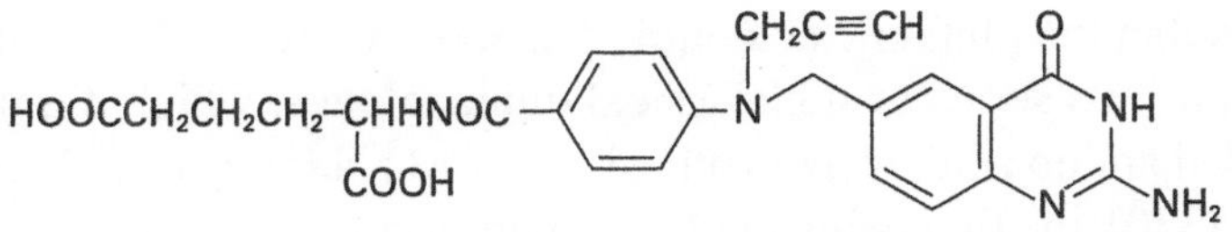

CCVI

An analog program designed to increase aqueous solubility may have found early success. Although extensive modifications at N^{10} position [324, 325], the benzoyl ring [326], and the amino acid terminus, provided no advantage; modification of the substituent on the 2-carbon has shown promise [327].

Further, Jones et al. [328] synthesized five new 2-desamino analogs **CCVIIa–CCVIIe** with a view that the removal of amino group from the position 2 might increase its water solubility. These compounds were tested against L1210 TS and it was found that removal of the 2-amino group caused a slight (3–9 fold) loss of TS inhibition; **CCVIIe** was only 8-fold a lesser TS inhibitor than the parent drug. All five compounds **CCVIIa– CCVIIe** were more cytotoxic to L1210 cells in culture than their 2-amino counter parts, **CCVIIe** was 8.5-fold more active with an ID50 of O.4 μM. This remarkable result is probably related to increased cellular penetration. **CCVIIe** was 5-fold more soluble than CB3717 **CCVI** at pH 5.0 and >340-fold more soluble at pH 7.4.

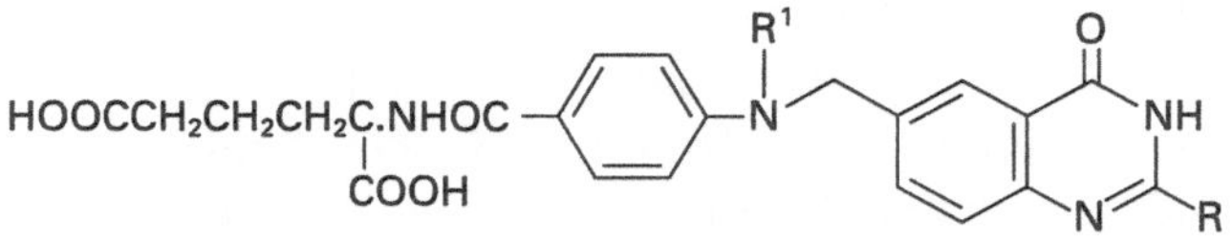

CCVII
CCVIIa   R, R^1 = H
CCVIIb   R = H, R^1 = Me
CCVIIc   R = H, R^1 = Et
CCVIId   R = H, R^1 = allyl
CCVIIe   R = H, R^1 = propargyl

While considering the structure-activity relationship regarding the role of the glutamate moiety in TS inhibition and cytotoxicity, Jones et al. made two observations. Firstly the role of glutamate in the transport of CB3717 is unclear, and secondly and more importantly, the polyglutamates of CB3717 are more potent inhibitors of TS than the parent drug; specifically the compound with three additional glutamates attached to CB3717. It clearly indicates that the glutamic acid moiety is required for high activity. With this in mind, two series of nonclassical quinazolones, which did not bear the appended amino acid, were synthesized by Mc Namara et al. [329] and Bisset et al. [330], the first being the 10-propargyl-5,8-dideazafolic acid derivatives **CCVIII** and the second comprised analogous 2-desamino derivatives **CCVIII**, both bearing a more lipophilic substituent on the phenyl ring than the co-glutamate of classical antifolates. Compounds **CCVIII** with 2-amino group were generally potent inhibitors of L1210 TS with IC50s within the range of 0.51–11.5 μM compared to 0.05 μM for

CB3717. The order of potency for phenyl substitution at the 4-position in this series was as: $COCF_3 \geq NO_2 \geq CONH_2 \geq COCH_3 \geq SO_2NMe_2 > CN >> OCF > F$. The 2-desamino target compounds also exhibited significant TS inhibition. Both series were growth inhibitory to cells in tissue culture and this inhibition could be reversed by thymidine alone, indicating that the primary target was TS. None of the compounds was a potent inhibitor of dihydrofolate reductase. These studies indicate that the presence of the glutamate moiety in folate analogs is not an absolute requirement for potent inhibition of TS. Jones et al. [331] also reported for the compound **CCVIIIa** thymidylate synthase inhibition constant Ki in *Escherichia coli* and humans as 0.015 and 0.075 µM, respectively.

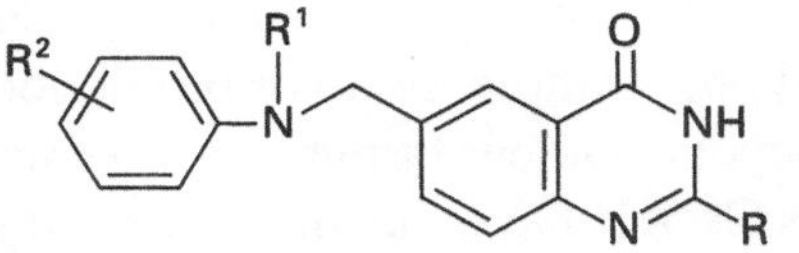

CCVIII
R = H, Me, NH_2, R^1 = Me, Et, allyl, R^2 = 3, 4-Cl_2, 4-COMe, 3, 4, 5(OMe)3, 4-F, 4-CN, 4-$CONH_2$, 4-SO_2NMe_2, 4-NO_2, 4-$COCF_3$, 4-OCF_3
CCVIIIa R = H, R^1 = allyl, R^2 = 4-F_3CSO_2

Hughes [332, 333] reported the synthesis of N-[[(quinazolinyl methyl) amino]aroyl] amino acids **CCIX** and observed that they inhibited thymidylate synthetase and the growth of leukemia L1210 cells with IC50 of 0.03 µM and 0.18 µM, respectively. Compound **CCX** showed an IC50 of 3.9 µM against L1210 cell line [334].

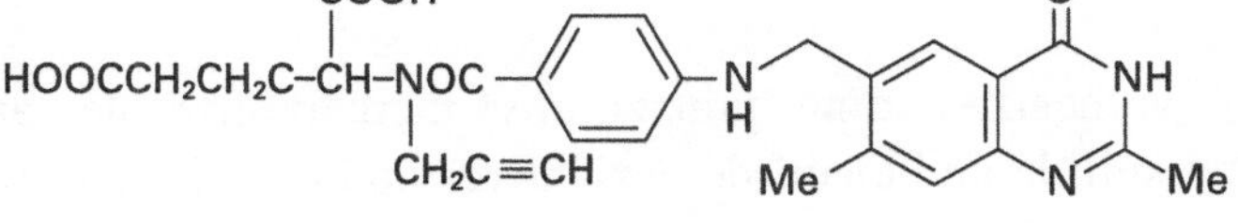

CCIX

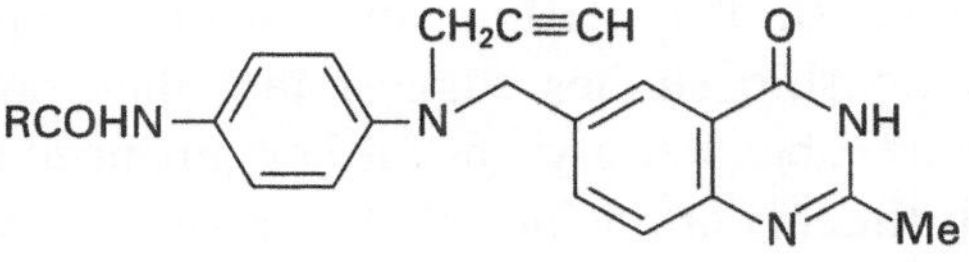

CCX
R = 2-Pyridylmethyl

Mc Namara et al. [335] reported that 6-{[(hetero)arylamino]-methyl}quinazolinones *in vitro* inhibited L1210 murine leukemia cell line with IC50 of 2.4 to 26.1 μM. Kunzel et al. [336] synthesized 2-phenyl-4(3H)-quinazolone derivatives **CCXI** and observed that compound **CCXIa** at 100 mg/kg dose (4 × i.p.) showed in mice the best cytostatic activity.

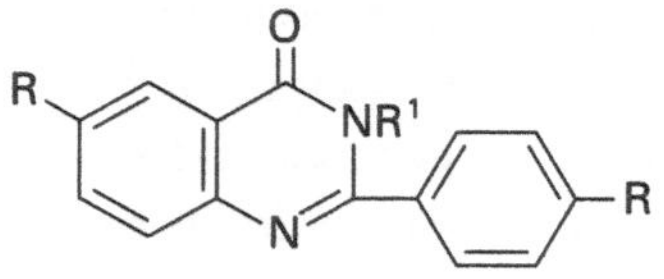

CCXI
R = $NHCOOR^2$, R^1 = Me, Ph, OMe, Cl, ClCH$_2$, substituted phenyl, R^2 = Me, Et, 4-tert-butyl-cyclohexyl
CCXIa R = NHCOOMe, R^1 = Ph

A number of 2-alkyl-3-aryl-derivatives of 4(3H)-quinazolinone **CCXII** have been synthesized which contained one or more mono or bifunctional mustard grouping attached to the heterocyclic nucleus through an enzymatically hydrolyzable linkage. Compounds **CCXII** have shown reduced activity in various biological test systems *in vitro* and on subcutaneous administration; the monofunctional compounds were more toxic than the bifunctional analogs. None of the monofunctional compounds produced leucopenia at the LD50 dose level which was in contrast with marked leucopenia produced by the bifunctional compounds against L1210 system [337].

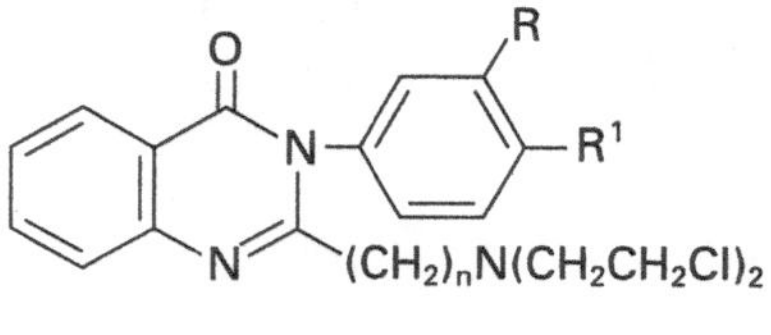

CCXII
n = 0, 1, 2, R = CH$_2$N(CH$_2$CH$_2$OH)$_2$, CH$_2$NHCH$_2$CH$_2$Br, R^1 = OH, OEt, N(CH$_2$CH$_2$Cl)$_2$

Joshi et al. [338] synthesized some quinazolonyl mercaptotriazoles and their corresponding sulfide and disulfide derivatives and tested their antitumor activity. None of the compounds showed activity. 2-Styrylquinazolin-4(3H)-ones **CCXIII**, synthesized by Jiang et al. [339], inhibited tubulin polymerization and the growth of L1210 murine leukemia cells. Extensive structure-activity relationship studies suggest that the entire quinazolinone structure was required, but activity was further enhanced by halide or small hydrophobic substituents at position 6. These analogs did not substantially interfere with the binding of radio-labeled colchicine, vinblastine or GTP to tubulin. Several analogs have shown *in vivo* tumor growth inhibitory activity in the L1210 leukemia model, with the lead compound **CCXIII** exhibiting good antitumor activity against murine solid tumors as well as human tumor xenografts. Ebeid et al. [340] synthesized N-(p-substituted sulfamoyl phenyl)-11-oxo-11H-pyrido(2,1-b)-quinazolin-6-carboxamides as antitumor agents.

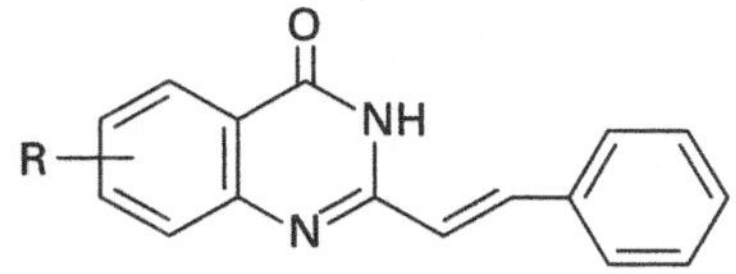

CCXIII
R = 5-, 6-, 7-, 8-Cl, 6-Br, 6-F, 6-NH2, 6-OMe, 5-, 6-Me, 6-OH, 6-OEt
CCXIIIa R = 6-OMe

9 Antihistaminic and antiulcer activities

Peet et al. [341] reported that 3-(1H-tetrazol-5-yl)-4(3H)-quinazolinone sodium salt monohydrate (MDL-427) **CCXIV** inhibited passive cutaneous anaphylaxis (PCA) in the rat when administered by parenteral and oral routes. MDL-427 **CCXIV** has an oral ED50 of 1.5 mg/kg. Peak activity was observed within 5 min. of oral administration and appreciable activity persisted for several hours. In contrast, the activity of **CCXVa** diminished to a negligible level within 1 hour. A possible explanation for this discrepancy is that when **CCXIV** is converted to **CCXVa** in the acidic medium of the stomach, it is deposited as a microprecipitate, and thus more bioavailable than the crystalline quinazolinone **CCXVa**. The observed inhibition of the PCA was due to the inhibition of a mediator release. The compounds were also tested for their ability to inhibit histamine release from the mixed population of cells in the peritoneal cavity of rats passively sensitized with IgE antibodies to ovalbumin. In this system, compound **CCXIV** has an IC50 of 0.3 µg/ml. Substitution at the position 2 also affects the activity, all the 2-substituted compounds **CCXVb–CCXVd** are decidedly less active than **CCXVa** which suggests the need for an accessible electrophilic center for interaction at the site of activity. Vinogradoff [342] also synthesized 3-tetrazol-5-yl-4(3H)-quinazolinones as a mediator release inhibiting agent.

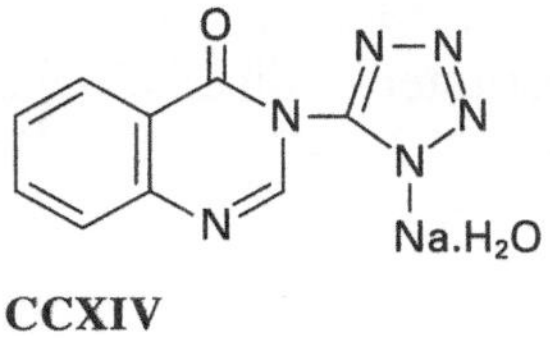

CCXIV

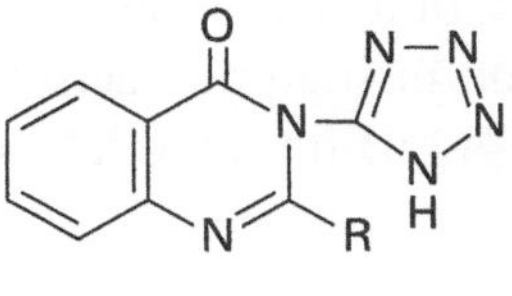

CCXV
CCXVa R = H
CCXVb R = Me
CCXVc R = Et
CCXVd R = Ph

Agelastine hydrochloride **CCXVI** is an orally effective antihistamine, useful in the treatment of asthma and nasal allergy. This drug is known as Azeptin®. It appears to inhibit the release of histamine, in addition to antagonizing its action [343–345].

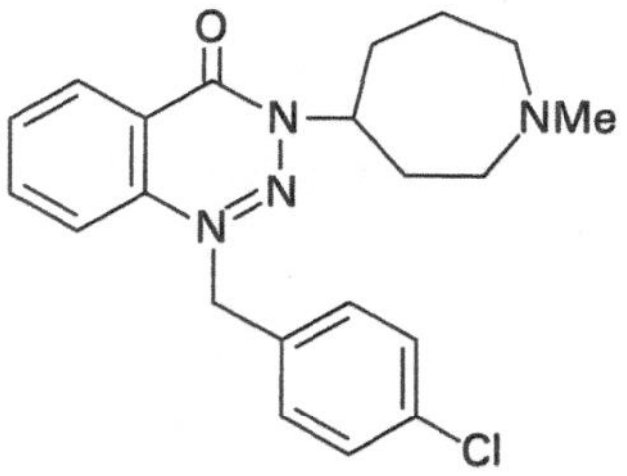

CCXVI

Coates et al. [346] synthesized a series of 2-(2-alkoxyphenyl)-4(3H)-qui-nazolinones **CCXVII** and their analogs and observed that compound **CCXVII** showed 34% reduction of 9,11-methanoepoxy PGH-induced bronchoconstriction in guinea pig at 10 μmol/kg i.v. 1-Aryl-4(1H)quina-zolones possessed antitussive activity at a dose of 5–30 mg/kg [182], and 3,4-dihydro-2(1H)quinazoline derivatives showed histamine H_2-receptor inhibiting activity [190], while quinazolinones **CCXVIII** showed antiallergic activity [347].

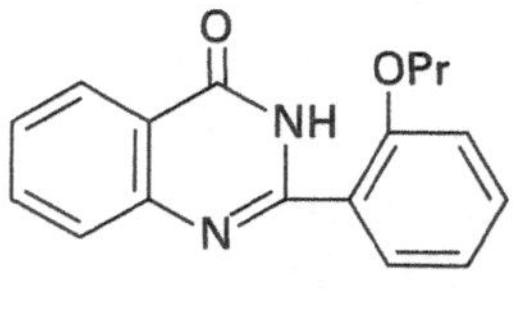

CCXVII

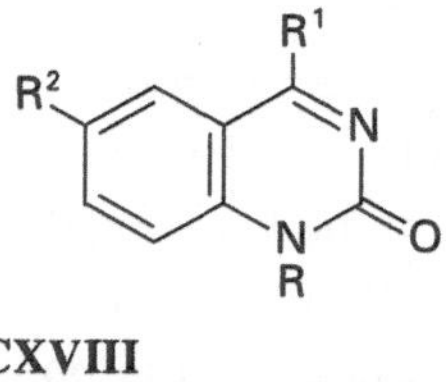

CCXVIII
R = Alkyl, piperazino alkyl,
R^1 = NH2, alkylamino, piperazino, alkyl amino,
R^2 = H, Br, I

Amschler et al. [348] reported the synthesis and antihistaminic activity of piperazinyl alkyl-4-quinazolinone analogs **CCXIX**. Hardtman [349] also investigated the antihistaminic activity of 1-substituted-2-disubstituted amino quinazolin-4(1H)-ones **CCXX** in guinea pigs.

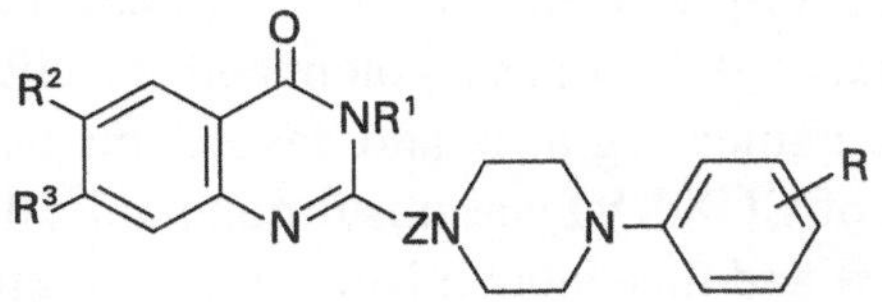

CCXIX
R = H, 2-, 3-, 4-Me, OMe, Cl, F, CF$_3$, OEt,
R^1 = H, Me, PhCH$_2$CH$_2$, Me$_2$CHCH$_2$CH$_2$, cyclohexyl,
R^2, R^3 = H, OMe, Me, Z = CH$_2$, (CH$_2$)$_2$, (CH$_2$)$_3$, CHEt, CH=CH–CH$_2$

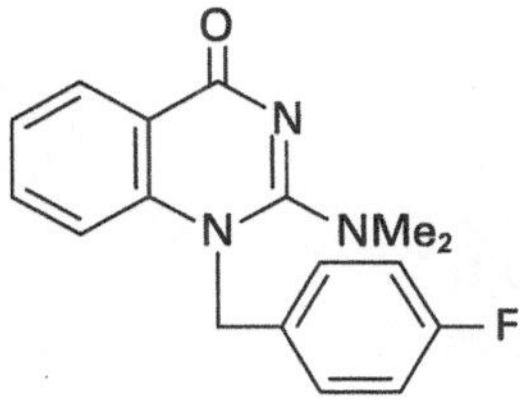

CCXX

ω2-Aryl-2,3-dihydro-4(1H)-quinazolinonyl)-alkyl substituted ureas and cyanoguanides were synthesized by Buyuktimkin et al. [350] as H$_1$/H$_2$ antihistaminics. Antihistaminic activity of piperidinyl benzimidazolyl quinazolone **CCXXI** has been reported by Janssens et al. [351].

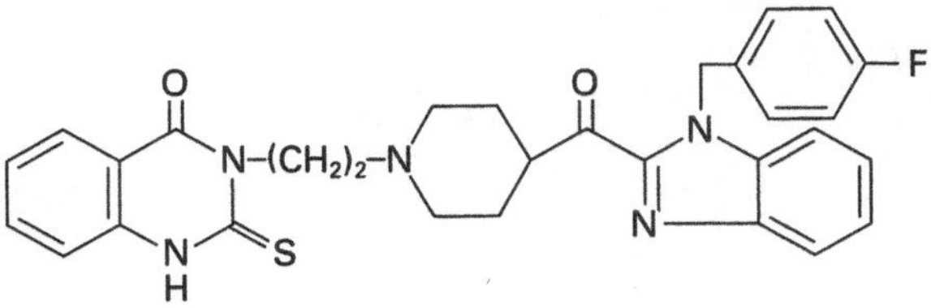

CCXXI

Takahashi et al. [243] synthesized 2-(3',4'-dimethoxy-styryl)-3-phenylquinazolinones and observed that these are intermediates for allergy inhibitors. 2-Aryl-4(3H)-quinazolinon-2yl]pyrrolino[5,4-b]2,3-dihydro-4-H [I] benzopyran-4-ones **CLIII** were reported to posses antihistaminic activity [245]. 11-Oxo-11-H-pyrido-(2,1-b)-quinazolin-2-carboxylic acid was developed as a new antiallergic drug [353–355].

Cimetidine [356], the first antiulcer agent to exhibit histamine H$_2$-antagonist activity, has been widely used clinically, and subsequently, many other H$_2$-antagonists such as ranitidine **CCXXIII**, famotidine **CCXXIV** and roxatidine acetate **CCXXV** have been developed [357].

2-[3-(3-1-piperidinyl   methyl)phenoxy)-propylamino)-4(3H)-quinazolin-one **CCXXVI** was reported by Oshita et al. [358] as a potent and selective histamine H_2-receptor antagonist in guinea pig atria and gastric mucosal cells. In guinea pig atria antagonism of **CCXXVI** was unsurmountable, the onset of action of **CCXXVI** was slow and this antagonism was apparently irreversible not only on the guinea pig atria but also on the gastric mucosal cells. It also inhibited gastric acid secretion in pylorus ligated rats on intraduodenal administration. Thus **CCXXVI** is a powerful and unique histamine H_2-receptor antagonist and may be useful in the treatment of peptic ulcer.

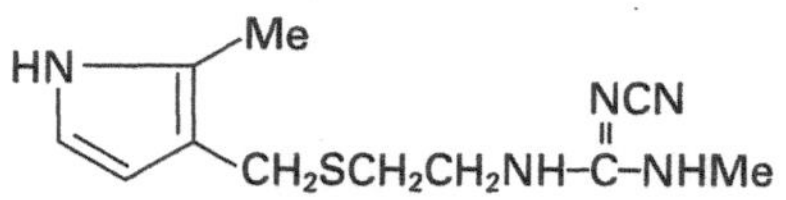

CCXXII

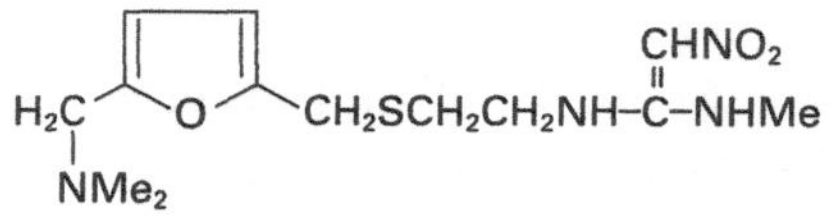

CCXXIII

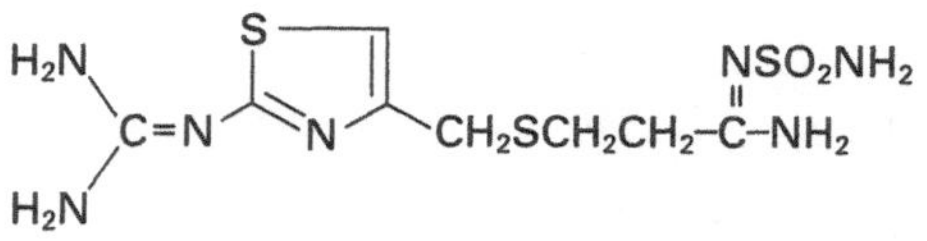

CCXXIV

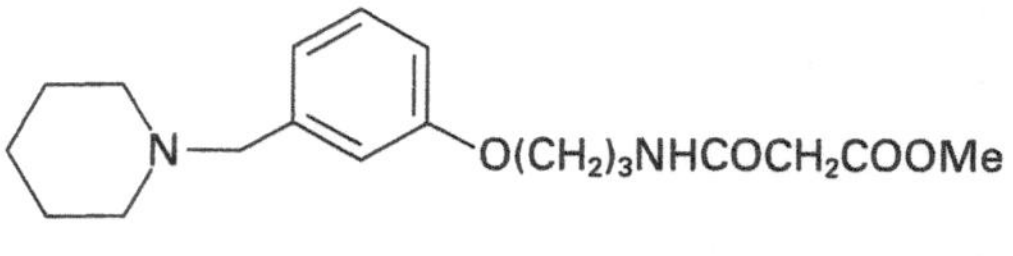

CCXXV

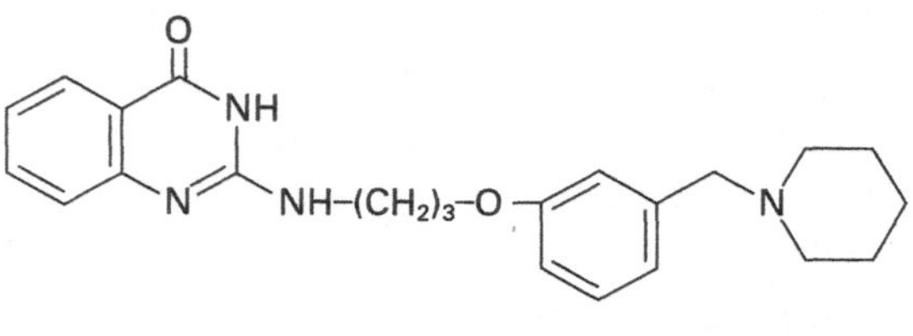

CCXXVI

Further histamine H_2-antagonist activity of 4-quinazolone derivatives **CCXXVII** was examined using excised atria from guinea pig [359]. Results showed that **CCXXVIIa**, with a benzene ring, possessed the highest log

KB value 7.39 which was higher than that of ranitidine (7.06). Whilst the compounds with furan ring **CCXXVIIIa** and **CCXXVIIIb** showed low activity. Compound **CCXXIX** in which the alkyl amino group of **CCXXVIIa** is replaced by alkylthio group showed a fairly low log-KB value (Table 2). The activity of **CCXXVIIb** and **CXXVIId** with pyrrolidinyl and 3-methylpiperidino groups respectively was almost equal to that of **CCXXVIIa**.

Table 2

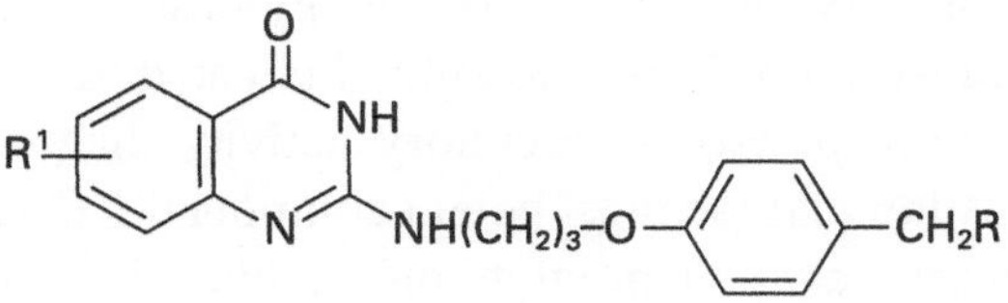

CCXXVII

Compd. No.	R	R'	-log KB	Antisecretory activity	
				Dose mg/kg	Inhibition %
CCXXVIIa	piperidinyl	H	7.39	5.0	82.5
				2.5	72.0
CCXXVIIb	pyrrolidinyl	H	7.55	1.25	51.1
				5.0	71.5
				2.5	30.1
CCXXVIIc	4-methyl-piperidinyl	H	6.91	5.0	37.0
				2.5	29.8
CCXXVIId	3-methyl-piperidinyl	H	7.31	5.0	74.7
				2.5	39.2
CCXXVIIe	piperidinyl	6-Me	7.15	5.0	68.2
				2.5	17.0
CCXXVIIf	piperidinyl	7-Cl	6.96	5.0	14.4
				2.5	−7.9

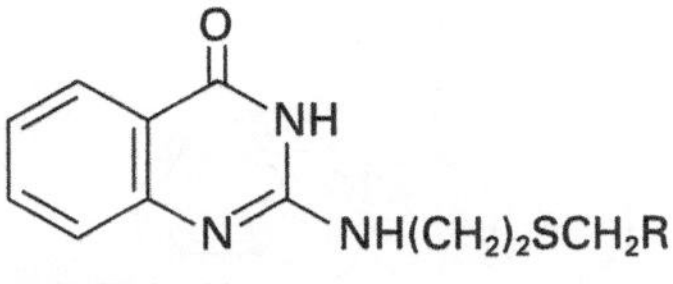

CCXXVIII

CCXXVIIIa R =

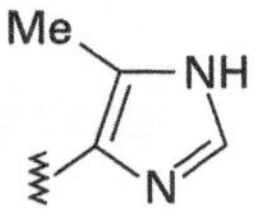

CCXXVIIIb R =

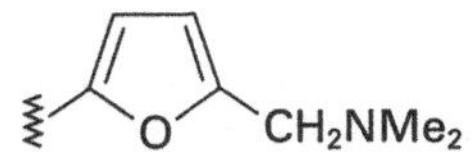

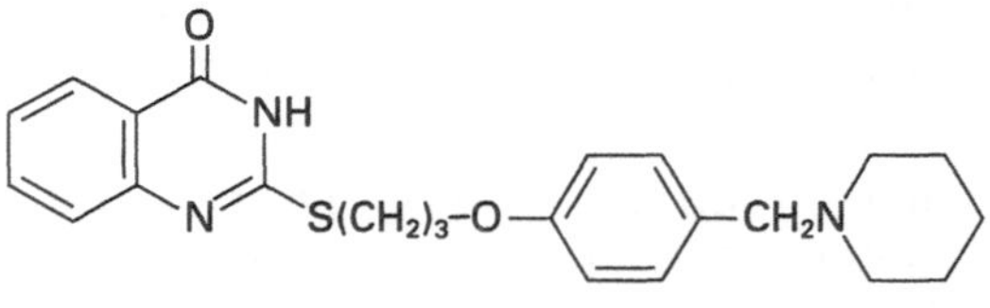

CCXXIX

Ganellin has suggested that the conformation of the guanidine moiety and an increase in its lipophilicity may possibly enhance H_2-antagonist activity [360]. Antisecretory activity was tested in pylorus-ligated rats by intraduodenal administration [359]. Results indicated that **CCXXVIIa–CCXXVIIe** had more potent antisecretory activity than ranitidine. It is particularly interesting that the most potent compound **CCXXVIIa** has the same benzene ring moiety as lamtidine; on the other hand **CCXXXa** and **CCXXXb** lacking a NH group failed to show potent antisecretory activity in spite of their high H_2-antagonist activity. **CCXXVIIa** (ED50 0.4 mg/kg) was the most potent antisecretory compound being 10 times more potent than ranitidine **CCXXIII** (ED50 12.3 mg/kg).

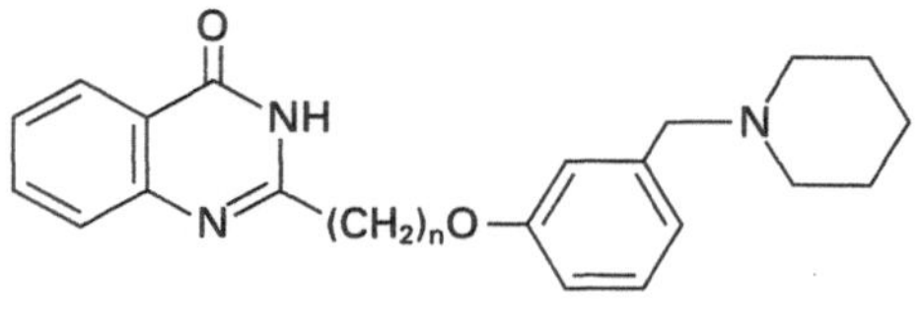

CCXXX
CCXXXa   n = 3
CCXXXb   n = 4

Takahashi et al. [361] synthesized 2-(heterocyclylalkyl)-quinazolin-4-ones **CCXXXI**, which showed 40–96% inhibition of indomethacin-induced ulcers in mice at a 100 mg/kg oral dose. Further they observed that 2-(aralkylsulfinyl)-4(3H)-quinazolinones **CCXXXII** at a 100 mg/kg oral dose in mice suppressed 83% of indomethacin-induced ulcers [362].

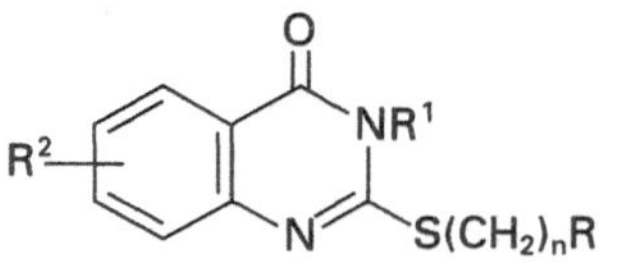

CCXXXI

R = C_{1-6} alkyl amino, substituted phenyl, heterocyclyl, geranyl, dipyridyl methylalkyl,
R^1 = H, C_{1-6} alkyl, substituted aryl, aralkyl,
R^2 = H, Cl, Br, I, C_{1-6} alkyl

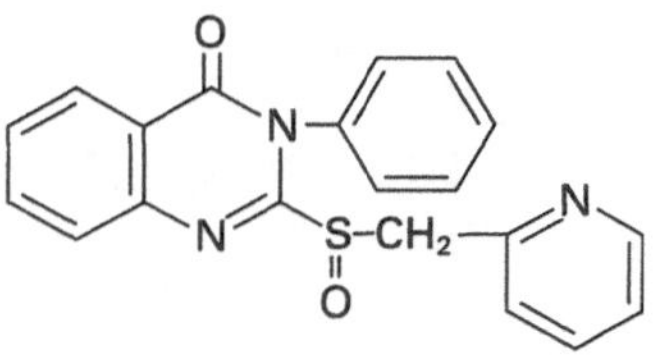

CCXXXII

2-Indolyl-3-phenyl-4-quinazolinones **CCXXXIII** were reported as useful agents in treating gastrointestinal disorders [363]. Doria et al. [364] reported the antiulcer activity of pyrrolo and pyrido [2,1-b] quinazolines. 1-(Substituted phenyl)-2-substituted-4(1H)-quinazolinones **CVI** also exhibited antiulcer activity [25, 179, 180]. Ito et al. [365, 366] synthesized some 2-(substituted-phenoxy alkyl)-3-substituted)-4-(3H)-quinazolinones **CCXXXIV** and **CCXXXV** and reported that they are inhibitors of stomach acid secretion.

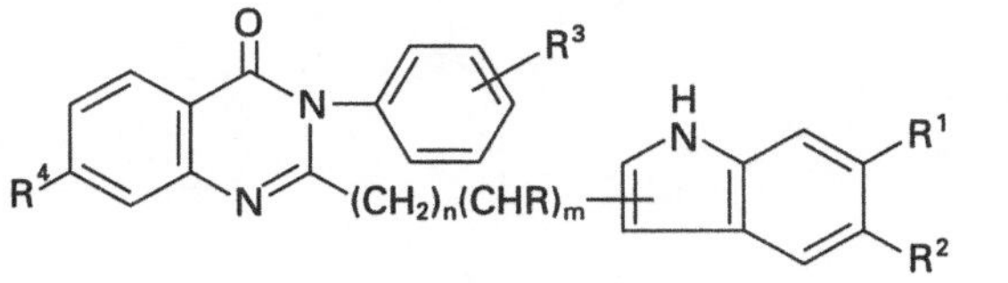

CCXXXIII
R = H, alkyl, CH$_2$Ph, Ph, R^1, R^2 = H, alkyl, alkoxy, halo, CF$_3$,
R^3 = Cl, Br, I, CF$_3$, alkoxy, alkyl, alkylthioamino, R^4 = H, Cl, Br, n = 1, 2, m = 0, 1

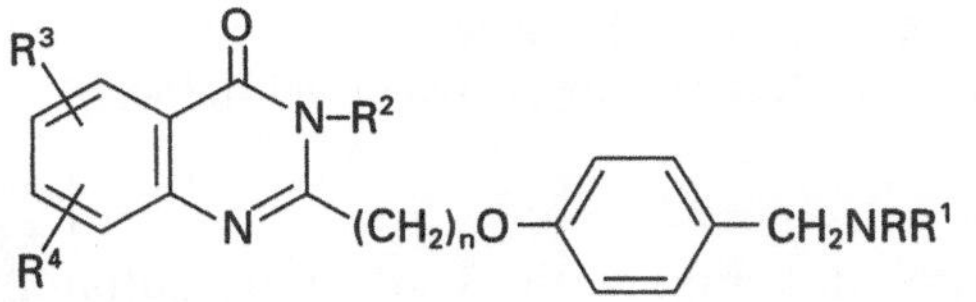

CCXXXIV
R, R^1 = Alkyl, alkylene, R^2 = H,

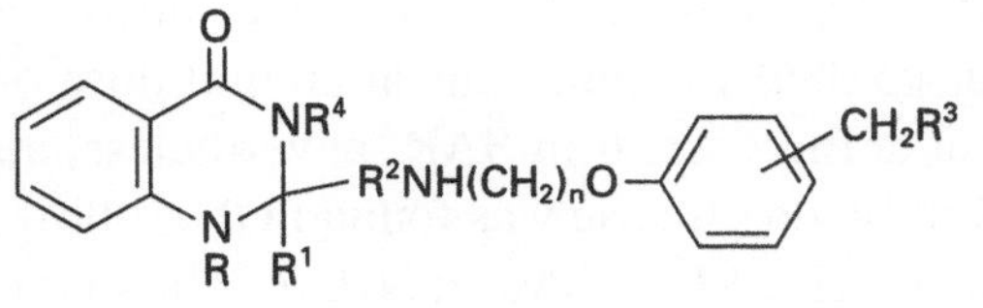

CCXXXV
R, R^4 = H, alkyl, R R^1 or
R^1, R^4 = bond, R^2 = H, alkyl,
R^3 = Phenyl, piperidino,
1-piperidinomethyl

10   Hypoglycemic activity

Gupta et al. [376] synthesized 2-piperazino-3H-4-quinazolone monoacetate **CCXXXVI** and reported that it was an effective blood sugar lowering agent, exhibiting activity in male and female albino rats at doses ranging between 10–100 mg/kg of body weight. **CCXXXVI** was found to be equipotent to tolbutamide in lowering the blood sugar of rabbits. The LD50 of **CCXXXVI** i.p. in albino mice is greater than 50 mg/kg, which is higher than the LD50 of tolbutamide. 2-Substituted and 2,3-disubstituted 4(3H)-quinazolones **CVa–CVg** showed weak hypoglycemic and diuretic activity compared to tolbutamide and chlorthiazide, respectively [178]. 2,3-Diphenyl-2,3-dihydro-4-(1H)-quinazolinone **CCXXXVII** and 3,4-dihydro-2(1H)-quinazolone derivatives **CCXXXVIII** possess choleretic and antidiabetic activities [368, 369].

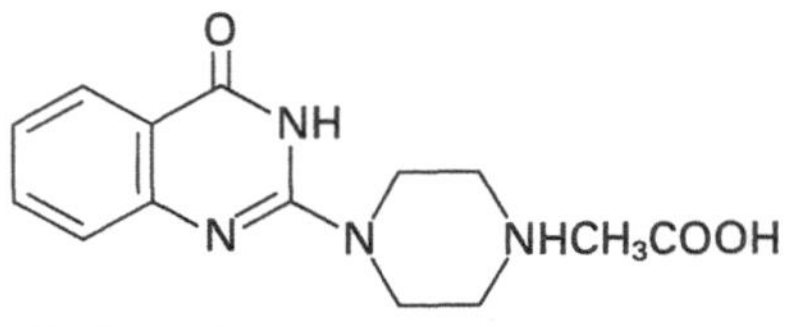

CCXXXVI

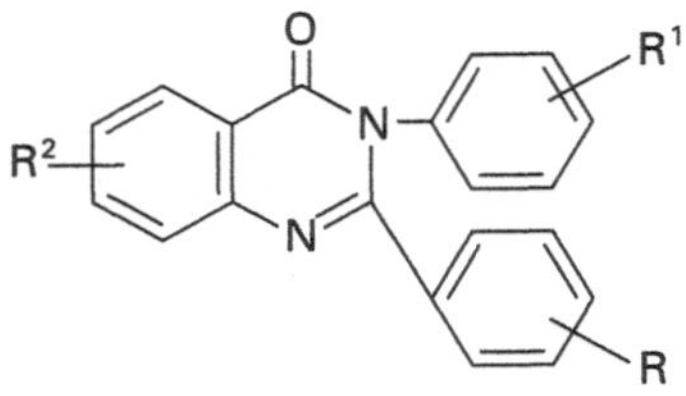

CCXXXVII
R, R^1 = 4-Cl, 4-OMe, 3, 4(OMe)$_2$,
R^2 = H, 5, 8-Cl$_2$

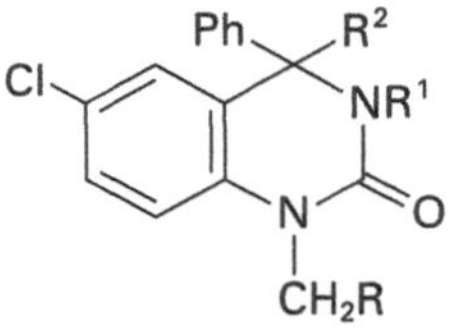

CCXXXVIII
R, R^1, R^2 = Cyclopropyl, Me, H; cyclopropyl, Et, H;
cyclopropyl, Et, Me; cyclopropyl, Me, Et and H, Me, Et

A series of N -(2-aryl-6,8-substituted-4-quinazolin-3-yl)-N-arylsulphonyl ureas **CCXXXIX** have been synthesized by Husain et al. [370] and evaluated for their hypoglycemic activity. Compound **CCXXXIX** showed a reduction in blood sugar level up to 38% in albino rats at an oral dose of 250 mg/kg. It is difficult to see a definite trend in SAR, nevertheless, an increasing trend in the reduction of blood glucose was found in the following order of the phenyl substituents: H < Me < OMe < NHAc. The maximum reduction of 38.0% in blood glucose was shown by compound **CCXXXIXa**. Replacement of a phenyl group at position 2 by a styryl group results in the decrease of hypoglycemic activity as shown by compounds **CCXXXIXb–CCXXXIXd** 0, 11.0 and 8.0%, respectively. The effect of substituents in the phenyl ring of quinazolone nucleus showed an increasing trend of hypoglycemic activity in the order: Unsubstituted phenyl < 8-bromophenyl < 6,8-dibromophenyl.

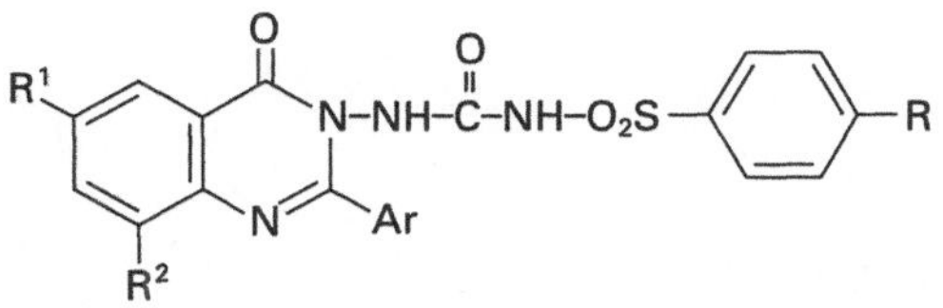

CCXXXIX
CCXXXIXa R = NHCOMe, R^1 = H, R^2 = Br, Ar = Ph
CCXXXIXb R, R^1, R^2 = H, Ar = CH=CHPh
CCXXXIXc R = NHCOMe, R^1 = H, R^2 = Br, Ar = CH=CHPh
CCXXXIXd R = OMe, R^1, R^2 = H, Ar = CH=CHPh

Further Husain et al. reported the hypoglycemic activity of 2-(substituted phenoxymethyl)-3-(thiadizol-2-yl)-4-quinazolones (**CCXL**). Compounds **CCXLa** and **CCXLb** caused 15 and 17% decrease in blood sugar level at 250 mg/kg orally in rats. Introduction of a nucleophile decreased the activity [311].

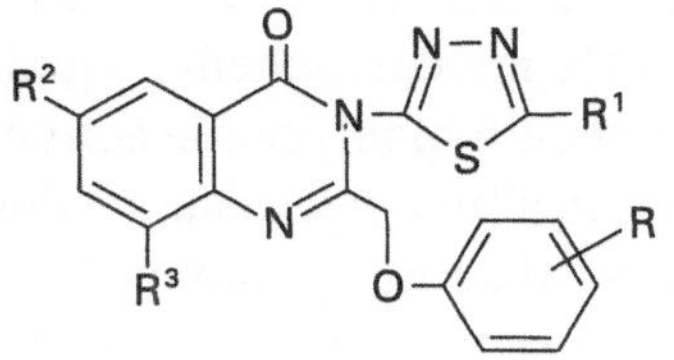

CCXL
CCXLa R = 4-Me, R^1 = Me, R^2, R^3 = H
CCXLb R = 3-Me, R^1 = Me, R^2, R^3 = H

Some new 1-(arylideneamino)-3-(substituted phenylamino/4-quinazolon-3-yl methyl)guanidines were synthesized by Husain et al. [372] as hypoglycemic agents. Husain et al. [373] also synthesized N^1-{p-[[(3-aryl-4-oxo-quinazolin-2-yl)-methyl]amino]benzoyl}-N^4-arylthiosemicarbazides **CCXLI** and 2-(arylamino)-5-{p-[[(3-aryl-4-oxoquinazolin-2-yl)-methyl]amino]phenyl-1,3,4-thiadiazoles and oxadiazoles **CCXLII**, expecting that the incorporation of thiadiazole or oxadiazole moiety in quinazolone nucleus might enhance their hypoglycemic activity. In the case of thiosemicarbazides **CCXLI**, a maximum reduction of 7% was shown by the compound with R as 4-OMe and R^1 as Me. It was also observed that incorporation of a thiadiazole moiety in substituted quinazolones results in a greater hypoglycemic activity than oxadiazole moiety. However the presence of 4-OMe(R^1) and Me(R) in compounds **CCXLI** and **CCXLII** caused maximum reduction in blood glucose.

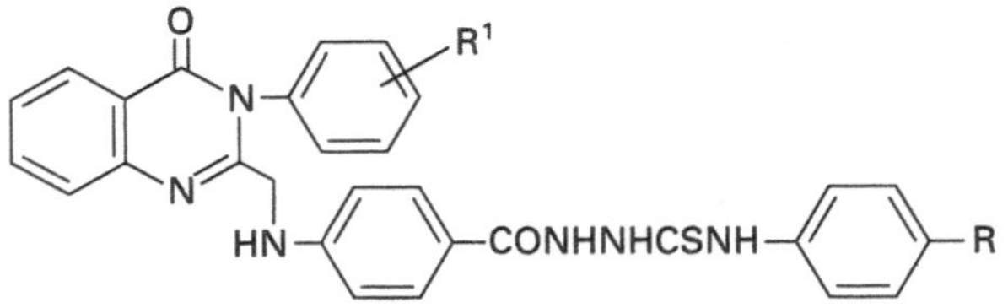

CCXLI

R = 2-Me, 4-OMe, 4-NO$_2$, R^1 = H, Me, OMe, Cl, Br

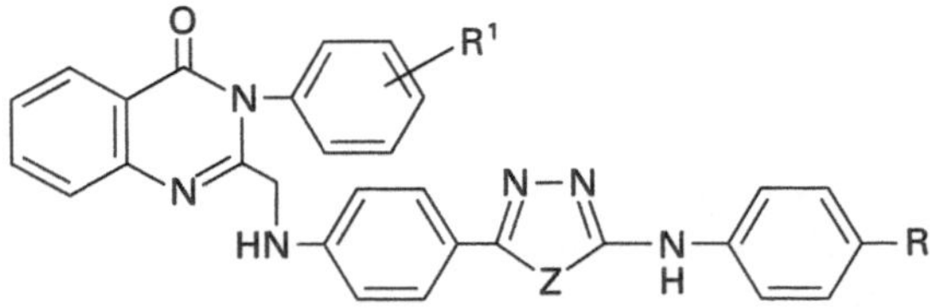

CCXLII

R = 2-Me, 4-OMe, 4-NO2, R^1 = H, Me, OMe, Cl, Br, Z = O, S

Agarwal et al. [374] synthesized some hitherto unknown substituted-2-phenyl-3-[2-substituted anilinothiadiazolyl-5-(N-mercaptophenyl)]quinazolin-4-one **CCXLIII** with a view to studying their hypoglycemic activity, which was found to be in the range of 227.56% in albino rats at single dose of 250 mg/kg. Compounds **CCXLIIIa–CCXLIIId** have shown 27.56, 22.39, 25.13 and 20.0% inhibition in blood glucose level in comparison to 40.0% of tolbutamide. Compounds **CCXLIIIe** and **CCXLIIIf** showed 14.12 and 15.5% inhibition respectively, while the rest of the compounds either showed very low or almost nil inhibition in blood glucose. From these results it was concluded that a minimum substitution on the quinazolone nucleus increased its hypoglycemic activity.

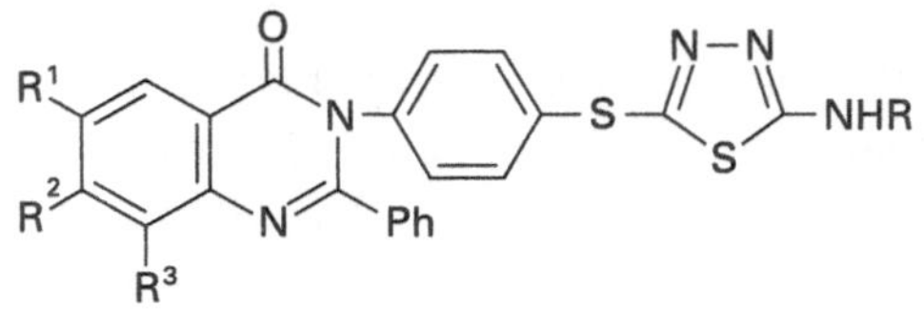

CCXLIII

CCXLIIIa	R = Ph, R^1, R^2, R^3 = H
CCXLIIIb	R = 2-MeC$_6$H$_4$, R^1, R^2, R^3 = H
CCXLIIIc	R = 4-BrC$_6$H$_4$, R^1, R^3 = Br, R^2 = H
CCXLIIId	R = 4-ClC$_6$H$_4$, R^1, R^3 = H, R^2 = NO$_2$
CCXLIIIe	R = Ph, R^1 = Br, R^2, R^3 = H
CCXLIIIf	R = 4-ClC$_6$H$_4$, R^1, R^3 = Br, R^2 = H

References

A   A. H. Amin, D. R. Mehta and S. S. Samarth: Prog. Drug Res. *14*, 218 (1970).

B   C. M. Gupta, A. P. Bhaduri and N. M. Khanna: J. Sci. Ind. Res. *30*, 101 (1971).

C   L. N. Yakhontov, S. S. Libermann, G. P. Zhikhareva and K. K. Kuzmina: Khim. Farm. Zh. 11, *14* (1977).

D   S. Johne: Pharmazie *36*, 583 (1981).

E   S. Johne: Prog. Drug Res *26*, 259 (1982).

1   R. J. Alaimo, C. J. Hatton and M. K. Eckman: J. Med. Chem. *13*, 554 (1970).

2   R. J. Alaimo and C. J. Hatton: J. Med. Chem. *15*, 108 (1972).

3   M. I. Husain and S. K. Agarwal: J. Indian Chem. Soc. *51*, 1015 (1974).

4   S. S. Tewari and S. B. Misra: J. Indian Chem. Soc. *52*, 1073 (1975).

5   Z. Budesinsky, P. Lederer and J. Danek: Collect. Czech. Chem. Commun. *42*, 3473 (1977).

6   Z. Budesinsky, P. Lederer and J. Danek: Czech. 190854 (1981) Dec. 15: Chem. Abstr. *98*, 89378 y (1983).

7   S. Kumar, V. K. Kansal and A. P. Bhaduri: Indian J. Chem. *20*B, 1068 (1981).

8   J. S. Shukla, M. Singh and R. Rastogi: Indian J. Chem. *22*B, 306 (1983).

9   J. S. Shukla and M. Fadayan: Asian J. Chem. *1*, 208 (1989).

10   J. S. Shukla and B. Srivastava: Indian J. Pharm. Sci. *7*, 168 (1985).

11   J. S. Shukla and B. Srivastava: Curr. Sci. *54*, 1162 (1985).

12   B. Srivastava, J. S. Shukla, V. S. Prabhakar and A. K. Saxena: Indian J. Chem. *30*B, 332 (1991).

13   J. S. Shukla, K. Agarwal and R. Rastogi: Arch. Pharm. *316*, 525 (1983).

14   R. R. Mohan, R. Agarwal and V. S. Misra: Indian J. Chem. *24*B, 78 (1985).

15   J. S. Shukla and R. Rastogi: Indian J. Chem. *25*B, 774 (l986).

16   V. K. Pandey and P. Garg: Indian J. Pharm. Sci. *49*, 172 (1987).

17   D. P. Gupta, S. Ahmad, A. Kumar and K. Shanker: Indian J. Chem. *27*B, 1060 (1988).

18   J. S. Shukla and Roli Shukla: Indian J. Pharm. Sci. *51*, 175 (1989).

19   K. Noda, A. Nakagawa, S. Yamazaki, H. Noguchi and I. Terumi: Jpn 7778, 888 (1977) July 2.

20   T. Oine, T. Yamada, K. Ozaki and W. S. Wakamoto: Jpn 77, 153, 984 (1977) Dec. 21.

21   T. Oine, Y. Yamada and B. Ozaki: Jpn 153, 982 (1977) Dec. 21.

22   J. P. Osselarese and L. A. Charles: Ger. 2, 075, 454 (1977) Aug. 25.

23   B. V. Shelly: US *4060*, 526 (1977) Nov. 29.

24   T. Oine, K. Ozaki and S. Wakamoto: Jpn.. 7805, 179 (1978) Jan. 18: Chem Abstr *88*, 190884 d (1978).

25   T. Oine, K. Ozaki and Y. Yamada: Jpn. 7909, 290 (1979) Jan. 24: Chem. Abstr. *91*, 39517 c (1979).

26   T. Oine, K. Ozaki and Y. Yamada: Jpn. 7909, 290 (1979) Jan. 24: Chem. Abstr. *91*, 157758 e (1979).

27   A. K. Sen Gupta, K. C. Agarwal and P. K. Seth: Indian J. Chem. *14*B, 1000 (1976).

28   A. G. Glasser, L. Diamond and G. Combs: J. Pharm. Sci. *60*, 127 (1971).

29   P. N. Bhargava and S. Prakash: Indian J. Pharm. *39*, 18 (1977).

30   P. N. Bhargava and H. D. Singh: Indian J. Chem. *15*B, 659 (1977).

31   S. S. Tewari, R. K. Satsangi and S. Misra: Indian J. Pharm. *40*, 40 (1978)

32   S. S. Tewari, S. Misra and R. K. Satsangi: Indian J. Chem. *18*B, 283 (1979).

33   S. Singh, M. Sharma, C. Nath, P. Bhargava and K. Shanker: Curr. Sci. *52*, 585 (1983).

34   R. Agarwal, C. Agarwal, C. Singh and V. S. Misra: J. Chem. Soc. Pak. *6*, 89 (1984).

35   R. Agarwal, C. Singh and V. S. Misra: Indian Drugs *25*, 185 (1988).

36   R. Nigam, V. K. Saxena and S. R. Chowdhury: Indian Drugs *27*, 169 (1990).

37   R. Nigam, S. Swarup, V. K. Saxena, P. R. Dua and R. C. Srimal: Indian Drugs *27*, 238 (1990).

38   R. K. Saxena and M. A. Khan: Indian J. Chem. *27*B, 295 (1988).

39   Y. D. Kulkarni, A. Bishnoi and P. R. Dua: Indian J. Pharm. Sci. *51*, 201 (1989).

40   M. I. Hussain and S. Shukla: Indian J. Chem. *25*B, 545 (1986).

41   R. K. Saxena and M. A. Khan: Indian J. Chem. *28*B, 443 (1989).

42   R. Lakhan and R. L. Singh: Indian J. Pharm. Sci. *52*, 1 (1990).

43   R. Lakhan and R. L. Singh: Farmaco. Ed. Sci. *43*, 745 (1988).

44   D. D. Mukerjee, S. R. Nautiyal and C. R. Prasad: Indian J. Pharm. Sci. *40*, 44 (1978).

45   D. D. Mukerjee and S. R. Nautiyal: J. Indian Chem. Soc. *56*, 1226 (1979).

46   D. D. Mukerjee, S. R. Nautiyal and B. N. Dhawan: Indian J. Pharm. Sci. *41*, 33 (1979).

47   D. D. Mukerjee, S. R. Nautiyal and C. R. Prasad: J. Prakt. Chemie *382*, 855 (1980).

48   S. R. Nautiyal, V. R. Agarwal and D. D. Mukerjee: Indian J. Pharm. Sci. *50*, 26 (1988).

49   D. D. Mukerjee, S. R. Nautiyal, C. R. Prasad and B. N. Dhawan: Indian J. Med. Res. *71*, 480 (1980).

50   D. D. Mukerjee and S. R. Nautiyal: J. Indian Chem. Soc. *55*, 709 (1978).

51   T. Junichi, J. R. Agar, D. R. Harenson and J. B. Taylor: J. Med. Chem. *20*, 3379 (1977).

52   T. Junichi, Y. Yoshihisa, O. Toyonari, O. Tokashi, I. Ryuichi and I. Ichizo: J. Med. Chem. *22*, 95 (1979).

53   T. Ochiai, R. Ishida, S. Nurimoto, I. Inove and Y. Kowa: Japan J. Pharmacol. *22*, 431 (1972).

54   K. C. Joshi and V. K. Singh: Indian J. Chem. *11*, 430 (1973).

53   K. C. Joshi, V. K. Singh, D. S. Mehta, R. C. Sharma and L. Gupta: J. Pharm. Sci. *64*, 1428 (1975).

56   S. Sato and G. T. Tsukamoto: Jpn. 76, 133, 287 (1986) Nov. 18; Chem. Abstr. *87*, 68405 n (1977).

57   Tanabe Seiyaku Co. Ltd.: Jpn. 59, 128, 376 (1984) Jul. 24; Chem. Abstr. *102*, 6537 b (1985).

58   J. D. Bianchi, M. T. Rikimanu, R. J. Gujman and C. R. Thompson: Anesthesia and Analgesia *50*, 231 (1971).

59   C. Bianchi and A. David: J. Pharm. and Pharmacol. *12*, 501 (1960).

60   S. C. H. Boeehringer: Fr. 1,412615 (1965) Oct. 7; Chem. Abstr. *64*, 5113 (1966).

61   S. C. H. Boeehringer: Fr. 1,446523 (1966) July 22; Chem. Abstr. *66*, 76030 t (1967).

62   S. C. H. Boeehringer: Fr. 1,446078 (1966) July 15; Chem. Abstr. *66*, 76032 v (1967).

63   F. K. Kirchner and A. W. Zalay: US 3,217,005 (1965) Nov 9; Chem. Abstr. *64*, 3570 (1966).

64   N. V. Gloeilampen-fabrieken Philips: Neth 6,403,115 (1965) Sept. 27; Chem. Abstr. *64*, 5114 c, (1966).

65   A. G. Glasser, L. Diamond and G. Combs: J. Pharm. Sci. *60*, 127 (1971).

66   J. S. Shukla and Shradha Saxena: Indian Drugs *17*, 96 (1980).

67   J. S. Shukla, Shradha Saxena and Ranjana Misra: J. Indian Chem. Soc. *59*, 1196 (1982).

68   M. I. Husain and E. Singh: Pharmazie *37*, 6 (1982).

69   M. I. Husain, G. C. Srivastava and P. R. Dua: Indian J. Chem. *21*B, 381 (1982).

70   J. P. Barthwal, S. K. Tandon, V. K. Agarwal, K. S. Dixit and S. S. Parmar: J. Pharm. Sci. *62*, 613 (1973).

71   O. El-Nasser, R. Abdel and S. El-Sayed Barakat: Arch. Pharm. Chem. Sci. Ed. *14*, 37 (1986).

72   V. S. Misra, P. N. Gupta, R. N. Pandey, C. B. Nath and G. P. Gupta: Pharmazie *35*, 400 (1980).

73   V. S. Misra, R. N. Pandey and K. N. Dhawan: Pol. J. Pharmacol. Pharm. *29*, 543 (1978).

74   V. K. Rastogi, S. S. Parmar, S. P. Singh and T. K. Arora: J. Heterocycl. Chem. *15*, 497 (1978).

75   R. S. Misra, A. Chaudhari, A. Chaturvedi, S. S. Parmar and B. V. R. Sastry: Pharmacol. Res. Commun. *9*, 437 (1977).

76   O. L. Vizyunova, Yu. V. Kozhevnikov, L. M. Obvintseva and V. S. Zalesov: Khim. Farm. Zh. *20*, 1047 (1986).

77   S. Buyuktimkin: Arch. Pharm. *319*, 933 (1986).

78   M. J. Kornet: Eur. J. Med. Chem. Chim. Ther. *21*, 529 (1986).

79   C. Dwivedi, G. W. Omodt: PCT Int. 9213,535 (1992) Aug. 20; Chem. Abstr. *117*, 234037 d (1992).

80   M. Shrimali, R. Kalsi, K. S. Dixit and J. P. Barthwal: Arzneim. Forsch. *41*, 514 (1991).

81   A. Lata, R. K. Satsangi, V. K. Srivastava and K. Kishor: Arzneim. Forsch. *32*, 24 (1982).

82   J. F. Wolfe, T. L. Rathman, M. C. Sleevi, J. A. Campbell and T. D. Greenwood: J. Med. Chem. *33*, 161 (1990).

83   M. A. Khalil and M. M. M. El-Din: Alexandria J. Pharm. Sci. *3*, 190 (1989).

84   S. Buyuktimkin: Istanbul Univ. Eczacilik Fak. Mecm. *21*, 26 (1985).

85   N. Despande, Y. V. Rao, R. P. Kandlikar, A. D. Rao and V. M. Reddy: Indian J. Pharmacol. 18, 127 (1987).

86   S. Buyuktimkin: Istanbul Univ. Eczacilik Fak. Mecm. *21*, 37 (1985).

87   S. Buyuktimkin: Arch. Pharm. *319*, 933 (1986).

88   M. J. Kornet, T. Varia and W. Beaven: J. Heterocycl. Chem. *21*, 1709 (1984).

89   M. J. Kornet: J. Heterocycl. Chem. *29*, 103 (1992).

90   M. L. Gujral and R. P. Kohli: J. Ass. Physns. India 2, 29 (1955).

91   J. G. Swift, E. A. Dickens and B. A. Becker: Arch. Int. Pharmacodyn. Ther. *128*, 112 (1960).

92   S. K. Rastogi, J. N. Sinha and K. P. Bhargava: Indian J. Med. Res. *69*, 1008 (1979).

93   G. N. Gordiichuk, S. A. Andronati, T. A. Voronina, I. Kh. Rakhmankulova, P. B. Terent'ev, P. A. Sharbatyan and A. S. Yavorshii: Fiziol. Akt. Veshchestva *74*, 36 (1982).

94   K. Kottke, H. Kuehmstedt, I. Graefe, H. Wehlan and D. Knoke: Ger. 253,622 (1988) Jan. 27; Chem. Abstr. *109*, 170452k (1988).

95   Sumitomo Chem. Co. Ltd.: Brit. 1,054,718 (1967) Jan. 11; Chem Abstr. *66*, 76031 u (1987).

96   Drugs of Future: *3*, 728 (1978).

97   Drugs of To-day: *14*, 210 (1978).

98   K. P. Bhargava, S. K. Rastogi and J. N. Sinha: Brit. J. pharmacol. *44*, 805 (1972).

99   L. Fisnerova, B. Brunova, E. Maturova, J. Grimova, J. Tibalova and Z. Kocfeldova: Czech. 269,461 (1991) Jan. 21; Chem. Abstr. *115*, 29377 g (1991).

100   L. Fisnerova, B. Brunova, Z. Kocfeldova, J. Tikalova, E. Maturova and J. Grimova: Collect. Czech. Chem. Commun. *56*, 2378 (1991).

101	A. Gursoy, S. Buyuktimkin, S. Demirayak and A. C. Ekinci: Arch. Pharm. *323*, 623 (1990).

102	A. D. Rao, C. R. Shanker, A. B. Rao and V. M. Reddy: Indian J Chem. *25*B, 665 (1986).

103	Y. S. Sadanandam, K. R. M. Reddy and A. B. Rao: Eur. J. Med. Chem. *22*, 169 (1987).

104	O. E. Sattarova and L. G. Mardanova: Deposited Doc. 1984, 4703; Chem. Abstr. *104*, 68806 p (1986).

105	C. R. Shanker, A. D. Rao, A. B. Rao, V. M. Raddy and P. B. Sattur: Curr. Sci. *53*, 1069 (1984).

106	C. R. Shanker, A. D. Rao, V. M. Reddy and P. B. Sattur: Indian Drugs *22*, 465 (1985).

107	S. S. Parmar and S. P. Singh: J. Heterocycl. Chem. *16*, 448 (1979).

108	P. Kumar, C. Nath, K. P. Bhargava and K. Shanker: Pharmazie *37*, 11 (1982).

109	P. Kumar, J. C. Agarwal, C. Nath, K. P. Bhargava and K. Shanker: Pharmazie *36*, 780 (1981).

110	V. K. Srivastava, S. Singh, A. Gulati and K. Shanker: Indian J. Chem. *26*B, 652 (1987).

111	S. S. Tewari and V. K. Pandey: J. Indian Chem. Soc. *52*, 736 (1975).

112	R. Khanna, A. K. Saxena, V. K. Srivastava and K. Shanker: Indian J. Chem. *29*B, 1056 (1990).

113	V. K. Srivastava, G. Palit and K. Shanker: Indian Drugs *24*, 335 (1987).

114	V. K. Srivastava, G. Palit, A. K. Agarwal and K. Shanker: Pharmacol. Res. Commun. *19*, 617 (1987).

115	V. K. Srivastava, J. P. Singh, Shradha Singh, M. B. Gupta and K. Shanker: Indian J. Pharm. Sci. *48*, 133 (1986).

116	P. K. Naithani, G. Palit, V. K. Srivastava and K. Shanker: Indian J. Chem. *28*B, 745 (1989).

117	M. T. Bogert and J. Chambers: J. Am Chem. Soc. *27*, 649 (1905).

118	E. A. Zeller: Pharmacol. Rev. *11*, 387 (1959).

119	S. S. Parmar, K. Kishore, P. K. Seth and R. C. Arora: J. Med. Chem. *12*, 138 (1969).

120	S. S. Parmar, A. K. Chaturvedi and B. Ali: J. Prakt. Chemie *312*, 950 (1970).

121	S. Nagar and S. S. Parmar: Indian J. Pharm. *33*, 61 (1971).

122	S. S. Parmar, V. K. Rastogi and R. C. Arora: J. Prakt. Chemie *312*, 958 (1970).

123	S. S. Parmar, V. K. Rastogi, T. K. Gupta and R. C. Arora: Jap. J. Pharmacol. *20*, 325 (1970).

124	L. D. Joshi, R. C. Arora and S. S. Parmar: Indian J. Pharm. *33*, 80 (1971).

125	S. S. Parmar, A. K. Chaturvedi, A. Chaturvedi and S. J. Brumleve: J. Pharm. Sci. *63*, 356 (1974).

126	S. Nagar, K. Kishore, A. Chaudhari and S. S. Parmar: Indian J. Pharm. *4*, 13 (1972).

127	V. K. Rastogi, J. P. Barthwal and S. S. Parmar: J. Prakt. Chemie, *314*, 187 (1972).

128	R. C. Gupta, A. K. Saxena, K. Shanker and K. Kishor: Indian J. Pharm. *39*, 22 (1977).

129	G. Sathi, V. R. Gujarati, J. C. Agarwal, C. Nath, K. P. Bhargava and K. Shanker: Indian Drugs *18*, 90 (1980).

130	S. Bahadur, M. Saxena, J. C. Agarwal and K. Shanker: Indian J. Pharm. *45*, 121 (1983).

131	R. C. Saxena, N. S. Bhatnagar, S. C. Misra and K. P. Bhargava: Brit. J. Anaesth. *44*, 83 (1972).

132	D. J. Berry: J. Chromatogr. *42*, 39 (1969).

133	C. Cardini, Y. Quercia and A. Calo: J. Chromatogr. *37*, 190 (1968).

134	R. Nanikawa and S. Kotoku: Yonago Acta Med. *10*, 49 (1966); Chem. Abstr. *64*, 18223 g (1966).

135 S. J. Christenson: J. Psychedel. Drugs 5, 505 (1972).

136 R. W. Piepho and M. F. O'Connor: Res. Commun. Chem. Path. Pharmacol. 6, 101 (1973).

137 L. C. Weaver, W. R. Jones and T. L. Karley: Arch. Int. Pharmacodyn. Ther. 143, 119 (1963).

138 S. S. Brown and G. A. Smart: J. Pharm. Pharmacol. 21, 466 (1969).

139 S. Goenechea, S. S. Brown and M. M. Ferguson: "Jahrestagung der Deutschen Gesellschaft für Verkahrsmedizin e.v., Cologne, April, 1972".

140 G. A. Smart and S. S. Brown: Anal. Biochem. 35, 518 (1970).

141 W. L. F. Armarego: Quinozolines: in Brown, D. J. Editor: Fused pyramidines, New York, 1967, Interscience Publishers, Part 1, Chapter XI.

142 S. H. Prabhu and G. F. Shah: Indian J. Med. Sci. 21, 524 (1967).

143 D. S. Platt and B. L. Cockrill: Biochem. Pharmacol. 18, 459 (1969).

144 Y. Cohen, J. Wepierre, Y. F. du Picard and J. R. Boissier: Therapie 20, 101 (1965).

145 H. Eberhardt, K. J. Freundt and J. W. Langbein: Arzneim. Forsch. 12, 1087 (1962).

146 M. Akagi, Y. Oketani, M. Takada and T. Suga: Chem. Pharm. Bull. 11, 321 (1963).

147 M. Akagi, Y. Oketani and S. Yamane: Chem. Pharm. Bull. 11, 1216 (1963).

148 H. Nowak, G. Schorre and R. Struller: Arzneim. Forsch. 16, 407 (1966).

149 J. T. Allen, D. Fry and V. Marks: Lancet 1, 951 (1970).

150 M. M. Geldmacherv and U. Mang: Z. Klin. Chem. Klin. Biochem. 8, 259 (1970).

151 J. H. Goudie and D. Burnett: Clin. Chim. Acta 35, 133 (1971).

152 A. Heyndrickx and A. de Leenheer: Eur. J. Toxicol. 11, 56 (1969).

153 T. Murata and I. Yamamoto: Chem. Pharm. Bull. 18, 138 (1970).

154 T. Murata and I. Yamamoto: Chem. Pharm. Bull. 18, 138 (1970).

155 T. Murata and I. Yamamoto: Chem. Pharm. Bull. 18, 143 (1970).

156 S. Parmar and P. K. Seth: Can. J. Biochem. 43, 1179 (1965).

157 P. K. Seth, S. S. Parmar and K. Kishor: Biochem. Pharmacol. 13, 1362 (1964).

158 A. Soulairae and C. Gottesmann: Life Sci. 6, 1229 (1967).

159 C. C. Pfeiffer, L. Goldstein and H. B. Murphree: J. Clin. Pharmacol. 8, 235 (1968).

160 R. L. Willims and H. W. Agnew: Exp. Med. Surg. 27, 53 (1969).

161 L. Goldstein, N. W. Stoltzfus and R. R. Smith: Res. Commun. Chem. Pathol. Pharmacol. 2, 927 (1971).

162 K. Etzler, R. Hoenle, E. H. Joswig, C. Kohler and H. J. Mallach: Arzneim. Forsch. 19, 988 (1969).

163 R. Barcelo: Can. Med. Assoc. 85, 1305 (1961).

164 I. M. Baird and L. W. Buckler: Practitioner 188, 361 (1961).

165 T. T. Hohenthal: Arzneim. Forsch. 19, 1527 (1969).

166 N. E. Kullander: Arzneim. Forsch. 19, 1530 (1969).

167 J. S. Madden: Brit. Med. J. 1, 676 (1966).

168 K. H. Beyer: Arzneim. und gerichtliche Chemie Berlin Dtsch. Apoth. Ztg. 103, 967 (1963).

169 A. Schmitt: Nervenartz 33, 418 (1962).

170 P. Bunger, A. Donhardt, G. Laubinger and W. Nachtwey: Münch. Med. Wochenschr. 106, 2298 (1964).

171 K. Ibe: Arch. Toxicol. 21, 289 (1966).

172 H. Matthew, P. Roscoe and N. Wright: Practitioner 208, 254 (1972).

173 H. C. Searkoreugh: US 3,073,826 (1963).

174 K. N. Sareen, R. P. Kohli, L. M. Pandey, K. Kishore, M. K. P. Amma and M. L. Gujral: Indian J. Physiol. Pharmacol. *3*, 182 (1959).

175 C. Bianchi and A. David: J. Pharm. Pharmacol. *12*, 501 (1960).

176 B. L. Schaub, R. E. Joseph, J. P. McEvoy and J. H. Klilliams: J. Org. Chem. *17*, 148 (1952).

177 M. Koizumi, Y. Murakami and I. Matsuura: Jpn. 7751,378 (1977) Apr. 25; Chem. Abstr. *87*, 201571 g (1977).

178 M. Seth and N. M. Khanna: Indian J. Chem. *14*B, 536 (1976).

179 T. Oine, Y. Yamada, K. Ozaki and S. Wakamoto: Jpn. 77,153,983 (1977) Dec. 21; Chem. Abstr. *88*, 190882 b (1978).

180 T. Oine, Y. Yamada, K. Ozaki and S. Wakamoto: Jpn. 77,153,984 (1977) Dec. 21; Chem. Abstr. *88*, 190883 c (1978).

181 T. Oine, Y. Yamada, K. Ozaki and S. Wakamoto: Jpn. 77,153,982 (1977) Dec. 21; Chem. Abstr. *88*, 190881 a (1978).

182 M. Vansant: Jpn. 7729,315 (1977) Aug. 01; Chem. Abstr. *88*, 62409 r (1978).

183 K. Noda, A. Nakagama, S. Yamazaki, K. Noguchi, T. Hachitani and H. Ide: Jpn. 77,144,683 (1977) Dec. 02. Chem. Abstr. *88*, 136662 s (1978).

184 H. J. Schwarz: US 4,071,516 (1976) Aug. 20; Chem. Abstr. *88*, 170184 x (1978).

185 H. Yamamoto, T. Komatsu and H. Awata: Ger. Offen.. 2,637,914 (1977) Jan. 13; Chem. Abstr. *86*, 115372 r (1977).

186 M. Yamamoto, S. Katayana, M. Koshiba and H. Yamamoto: Ger. 2,647,853 (1977) May 05; Chem. Abstr. *87*, 85043 k (1977).

187 M. Yamamoto, S. Katayama, M. Koshiba and H. Yamamoto: Ger. Offen. 2,702,530 (1977) Jul. 28; Chem. Abstr. *87*, 152263 x (1977).

188 G. Gamboni, W. Schmid and A. Sutter: Ger. Offen. 2,753,970 (1978) Jun. 15; Chem. Abstr. *89*, 109565 b (1978).

189 M. Yamamoto, M. Koshiba and H. Yamamoto; Jpn. 7805,180 (1978) Jan. 18; Chem. Abstr. *89*, 434774 n (1978).

190 Y. Yanagi, H. Awata, Y. Koga, H. Kurokawa and T. Inukai: Nippon Yakurigaku Zasshi *74*,, 749 (1978); Chem. Abstr.*90*, 48363 f (1979).

191 Y. Koga, Y. Yanagi: Ensho *4*, 309 (1984).

192 G. E. Hardtmann, H. J. Schwarz and E. A. Papp: Ger. Offen. 2,809,210 (1978) Mar. 03; Chem. Abstr. *92*, 41989 x (1980).

193 H. Ott: Rom. 53,396 (1978) Jul. 06; Chem. Abstr. *92*, 41979 u (1980).

194 Roussel-UCLAF: Jpn. 8005,505 (1980) Feb. 07: Chem. Abstr. *93*, 204682 d (1980).

195 S. Inaba, K. Ishizumi, K. Mori, H. Yamamoto and M. Yamamoto: US 4,202,895 (1980) May 13; Chem Abstr. *93*, 186401 e (1980).

196 H. K. Bader: Ger. Offen. 3,041,678 (1981) May 27; Chem. Abstr *95*, 81017 x (1981).

197 K. Tsurumi, K. Kyuki, K. Yasudo and H. Fujimura: Oyo Yakuri *16*, 125 (1978).

198 M. Verma, J. N. Sinha, V. R. Gujrati, T. N. Bhalla, K. P. Bhargava and K. Shanker: Pharmacol. Res. Commun. *13*, 967 (1981).

199 I. P. Singh, A. K. Saxena, J. N. Sinha, K. P. Bhargava and K. Shanker: Indian J. Chem. *23*B, 592 (1984).

200 H. Ott: Scand. J. Rheumatol, Suppl. *21*, 5 (1978).

201 K. Ozaki, Y. Yamada, T. Oine, T. Ishizuka and Y. Iwasawa: J. Med. Chem. *28*, 568 (1985).

202   S. Plescia, M. L. Bajrdi, D. Raffa, G. Daidone, M. Matera: Eur. J. Med. Chem.-Chim. Ther. *21*, 291 (1986).

203   R. Agarwal, C. Singh and V. S. Misra: Indian Drugs *25*, 185 (1988).

204   A. M. Farghaly, I. Chaaban, M. A. Khalil and A. A. Bekhit: Arch. Pharm. *323*, 311 (1990).

205   A. M. Farghaly, I. Chaaban, M. A. Khalil and A. A. Bekhit: Arch. Pharm. *323*, 833 (1990).

206   A. M. Farghaly, I. Chaaban, M. A. Khalil and A. A. Bekhit: Alexandria J. Pharm. Sci. *4*, 52 (1990).

207   K. Pande, T. N. Bhalla, J. P. Barthwal, G. P. Gupta and S. S. Parmar: J. Pharm. Sci. *79*, 317 (1990).

208   N. I. Chernobrovin, Yu. V. Kozhevnikov, O. V. Bobrouskaya and B. Ya. Syropyatov: Khim.-Farm. Zh. *25*, 37 (1991).

209   S. Plescia, G. Daidone, D. Raffa and M. L. Bajardi: Farmaco. *47*, 465 (1992).

210   S. Saxena, M. Verma, A. K. Saxena and K. Shanker: Indian J. Pharm. Sci. *53*, 48 (1991).

211   H. J. Hess, J. H. Cronin and A. Senahins: J. Med. Chem. *11*, 130 (1968).

212   G. Heder and W. E. Siems: Ger. Offen. 225,131 (1985) Jul. 24; Chem. Abstr. *104*, 207299 r (1986).

213   M. A. Hussain, A. T. Chin, W. A. Price, P. B. Timmermans and E. Shefter: Pharm. Res. *5*, 242 (1988).

214   V. T. Bandurco and S. Levine: Ger. Offen. 2,949395 (1980) Jun. 19; Chem. Abstr. 93, 23944 j (1980).

215   V. T. Bandurco and S. Levine: Can. 1,125,170 (1982) Jun. 08; Chem. Abstr. *97*, 120488 q (1982).

216   V. T. Bandurco, C. F. Schwender, S. C. Bell, D. W. Combs, R. M. Kanojia, S. D. Levine, D. M. Mulvey, M. A. Appolina and M. S. Reed: J. Med. Chem. *30*, 1421 (1987).

217   V. T. Bandurco, S. C. Bell, R. Falotico, C. F. Schwender and A. J. Tobia: US 4,668,787 (1987) May 26; Chem. Abstr. *107*, 96733 t (1987).

218   M. Teranishi, N. Nakamizo, H. Obase, K. Kubo, H. Takai, Y. Kasuya: Eur. 29,707 (1981) Jun. 03; Chem. Abstr. *95*, 132947 k (1981).

219   H. Takai, H. Obase, N. Nakamizo, M. Teranishi, K. Kubo, K. Shuto, Y. Kasuya, K. Shigenobu, M. Hashikami and N. Karashima: Chem. Pharm. Bull. *33*, 1116 (1985).

220   H. Amschler, K. Klimn and W. Schoelensack: Ger. Offen. 2,027,645 (1971) Dec. 09.

221   M. Dubey, V. K. Verma, K. Shanker, J. N. Sinha, K. P. Bhargava and' K. Kishore: Pharmazie *34*, 18 (1979).

222   S. Sato and S. Vehida: Jpn. 63,198,670 (1987) Sep. 02; Chem. Abstr. *108*, 94581 p (1988).

223   M. Takebayashi, T. Ozeki, S. Sato, S. Uchida and S. Hagiwara: Jpn. 62,258,369 (1987) Nov. 10; Chem. Abstr. *109*, 149556 n (1988).

224   Botros and S. F. Saad: Eur. J. Med. Chem. *24*, 585 (1989).

225   J. C. Agarwal, Y. K. Gupta, J. N. Sinha, K. P. Bhargava and K. Shanker: Pharmacol. Res. Commun. *13*, 49 (1981).

226   D. Horii and A. Ishibashi: Tohoku J. Exp. Med. *150*, 101 (1986).

227   M. Hosono and N. Taira: J. Cardiovasc. Pharmacol. *9*, 633 (1986).

228   T. Sekiya, M. Tsutsui, D. Horii and A. Ishibashi: Jpn. 62,135,465 (1987) Jun. 18; Chem. Abstr. *107*, 198351 j (1987).

229   A. Kumar, S. Gurtu, J. N. Sinha, KP. Bhargava and K. Shanker: Eur. J. Med. Chem. Chim. Ther. *20*, 95 (1985).

230   K. C. Liu and M. K. Hu: T'ai-wan Yao Hsueh Tsa Chih *38*, 85 (1986); Chem. Abstr. *108*, 56048 n (1988).

231   W. B. Wright and A. S. Tomcufcik: US 4710,502 (1987) Dec. 01; Chem. Abstr. *108*, 112476 q (1991).

232   W. B. Wright, A. S. Tomcufcik, P. S. Chan, J. W. Marsico and J. B. Pess: J. Med. Chem. *30*, 2277 (1987).

233   Y. Nomoto, H. Takai, T. Ohno and K. Kubo: Eur. 326,307 (1988) Jan. 23; Chem. Abstr. *112*, 21004 a (1990).

234   A. Morimoto and K. Nishikawa: Eur. 445,211 (1991) Sep. 11; Chem. Abstr. *115*, 256219 a (1991).

235   S. P. Vishnoi, G. K. Patnaik, A. Shoeb and R. C. Srimal: Indian Drugs *28*, 537 (1991).

236   P. N. Bhargava and H. Singh: Ind. J. Pharm. *31*, 111 (1969).

237   A. M. Mahmood, H. A. H. El-Sherif, G. M. El-Naggar and A. E. Abdul-Rahman: Indian J. Chem. *22B*, 491 (1983).

238   R. Lakhan and B. J. Rai: J. Chem. Eng. Data *32*, 384 (1987).

239   M. M. Kamel, M. M. Ismail, B. Abd El-Fattah and N. A. Moneib: Egypt. J. Pharm. Sci. *32*, 191 (1991).

240   R. S. Varma: J. Indian Chem. Soc. *52*, 344 (1975).

241   Ram Prakash and R. S. Varma: Indian Drugs *23*, 142 (1985).

242   R. S. Varma, R. Prakash and M. M. A. A. Khan: Indian Drugs 23, 345 (1986).

243   W. Takahashi and H. Yamane: Jpn. 62,252,778 (1987) Nov. 04; Chem. Abstr. 108, 186763 c (1988).

244   W. Takahashi and H. Yamane: Jpn. 01,110,676 (1989) Apr. 27; Chem. Abstr. 112, 7504 g (1990).

245   G. Achaiah, Y. Jayamma and V. M. Reddy: Indian J. Heterocycl. Chem. 1, 39 (1991).

246   Yu. V. Kozhevnikov, O. E. Sattarova, V. S. Zalesov, I. I. Gradel and A. N. Plaksina: Khim. Farm. Zh. 16,. 1349 (1982).

247   D. E. Sattarova, Yu. V. Kozhevnikov, V. S. Zalesov and S. N. Nikulina: Khim. Farm. Zh. 18, 1208 (1984).

248   A. K. SenGupta and T. Bhattacharya: J. Indian Chem. Soc. 60, 373 (1983).

249   S. Bahadur and M. Saxena: Arch. Pharm. 316, 964 (1983).

250   C. R. Shanker, A. D. Rao, B. J. Reddy and V. M. Reddy: J. Indian Chem. Soc. 60, 61 (1983).

251   M. B. Devani, U. S. Pathak and D. G. Naik: Ind. J. Chem. 12, 905 (1974).

252   P. M. Parasharya and A. R. Parikh: Acta Cienc. Indica Chem.11, 71 (1985),

253   J. S. Shukla and M. Fadayan: Indian J. Pharm. Sci. 51, 5 (1989).

254   S. M. Rida, F. S. G. Soliman and El Sayed A. M. Badawy: Pharmazie 41, 563 (1986).

255   M. I. Husain and S. Shukla: Indian J. Chem. 25B, 552 (1986).

256   M. A. Khalil and N. S. Habib: Farmaco, Ed. Sci. 42, 973 (1987).

257   A. N. Ahmed, M. A. Abd-Alla and M. F. El-Zohry: J. Chem. Technol. Biotechnol. 43, 63 (1988).

258   I. M. Labouta, H. M. Salama, N. H. Eshba and E. El-Chrbini: Acta Pharm. Jugosl. 38, 189 (1988).

259   M. F. El-Zohry, Abd El Hamed N. Ahmed, E. A. Omar and M. A. Abd-Alla: J. Chem. Technol. Biotechnol. 53, 329 (1992).

260   G. Achaiah and V. M. Reddy: Indian J. Pharm. Sci. 53, 253 (1991).

261   H. Y. Hassan, A. A. Ismaiel and H. A. H. El-Sherief: Eur. J. Med. Chem. 26, 743 (1991).

262   Y. A. Ammar, A. M. S. El-Scharief, Y. A. Mohammed and H. A. Ahmed: J. Serb. Chem. Soc. 52, 633 (1987).

263   Y. A. Mohammed, Y. A. Ammar, A. M. S. El-Sharief and H. Ahmed: Proc. Indian Natl. Sci. Acad. 55A, 87 (1989).

264   Y. A. Mohammed, A. M. El-Sharief, Y. A. Ammar, N. E. Amir and M. M. Ghorab: J. Serb. Chem. Soc. 54, 179 (1989).

265   Y. A. Ammar, Y. A. Mohammed, N. E. Amir and M. M. Ghorab: Curr. Sci. 58, 1231 (1989).

266   Y. D. Kulkarni, S. M. Ali and S. Rowhani: Indian Drugs 25, 505 (1988).

267   Y. D. Kulkarni and R. Ali: J. Indian Chem. Soc. 67, 46 (1990).

268   A. Khan and R. K. Saxena: Pharmazie 43, 864 (1988).

269   Yu. V. Kozhevnikov, V. A. Skvortsov, N. I. Chernobrovin, Z. N. Semenova and B. Ya Syropyatov: USSR 1, 160,699 (1991) Jul. 30; Chem. Abstr. 116, 143834 z (1992).

270   N. I. Chernobrovin, Yu. V. Kozhevnikov, A. N. Plaksina, N. V. Semyakina and V. S. Zalesov: USSR 1,089,935 (1991) Sep. 15; Chem. Abstr. 116, 188057 q (1992).

271   P. N. Gupta and A. K. Shakya: J. Indian Chem. Soc. 68, 618 (1991).

272   G. A. Bullock and P. J. Sheeran: US 3,867,384 (1975) Feb. 18; Chem. Abstr. 82, 171037 q (1975).

273   M. S. El-Kerdawy, A. M. Samour and A. G. El-Agamey: Acta Farm. Jugosl. 26, 135 (1976).

274   P. C. Joshi and P. C. Joshi: J. Indian Chem. Soc. 55, 465 (1978).

275   R. C. Gupta, R. Nath, K. Shanker, K. P. Bhargava and K. Kishor: J. Indian Chem. soc. 56, 219 (1979).

276   Kh. M. Shakhidoyatov, S. Yangibaev, L. M. Yun and Ch. Sh. Kadyrov: Khim. Prir. Soedin. 112 (1982).

277   L. H. Edwords: US 4,652,558 (1987) Mar. 24; Chem. Abstr. 107, 23504 j (1987).

278   S. Andreae and E. Schmitz: Ger. 289,525 (1991) May 22; Chem. Abstr. 115, 232271 k (1991).

279   M. R. Chaurasia, S. K. Sharma and S. Kumar: Curr. Sci. 50, 841 (1981).

280   M. R. Chaurasia and A. K. Sharma: J. Nepal Chem. Soc. 2, 1 (1982).

281   M. R. Chaurasia and S. K. Sharma: J. Indian Chem. Soc. 59, 370 (1982).

282   M. R. Chaurasia and S. K. Sharma: J. Nepal Chem. Soc. 1, 11 (1981).

283   M. R. Chaurasia and A. K. Sharma: J. Indian Chem. Soc. 62, 308 (1985).

284   R. Lakhan and B. J. Rai: J. Chem. Eng. Data 31, 501 (1986).

285   B. Dash, P. K. Mahapatra and P. K. Mahapatra: J. Inst. Chem. 55, 216 (1983).

286   A. M. Reddy, Y. Jayamma, P. R. Reddy and V. M. Reddy: Indian Drugs 25, 182 (1988).

287   P. Mitra and A. S. Mitra: Acta Cienc. Indica Chem. 9, 109 (1983).

288   D. E. Green and A. Percival: Eur. 183,458 (1986) Jun 04; Chem. Abstr. 105, 97495 n (1986).

289   W. Gauss, H. J. Kabbe, W. Paulus, H. J. Rosslenbroich and W. Brandes: Ger. 3,412,080 (1985) Oct. 03; Chem. Abstr. 104, 64209 y (1986).

290   A. M. Reddy, R. R. Reddy and V. M. Reddy: Indian J. Pharm. Sci. 53, 229 (1991).

291   A. D. Rao, C. R. Shanker, P. B. Reddy and V. M. Reddy: J. Indian Chem. Soc. 62, 234 (1985).

292 P. B. Reddy, S. M. Reddy, K. L. Reddy and P. Lingaiah: Indian Phytopathol. 38, 361 (1985).

293 S. Sailaja, E. T. Rao, E. Rajanarendar and A. Krishnamurthy: J. Indian Chem. Soc. 65, 200 (1988).

294 M. Rawat: J. Inst. Chem. 60, 58 (1988).

295 M. Yamamoto, K. Ishizumi, S. Morooka, K. Mori and H. Noguchi: Ger. 2,242,375 (1973) Mar. 15; Chem. Abstr. 78, 159660 x (1973).

296 M. Yamamoto, S. Morooka, M. Koshiba, T. Komatsu, H. Noguchi, S. Inaba and H. Yamamoto: US 4,146,717 (1979) Mar. 27; Chem. Abstr. 91, 20538 p (1979).

297 S. K. Shukla, A. K. Agnihotri and B. L. Chowdhary: Indian Drugs 19, 59 (1981).

298 S. R. Nautiyal, V. R. Agarwal and S. K. Shukla: Indian Drugs 20, 94 (1982).

299 V. K. Pandey, D. Misra, M. N. Joshi and K. Chandra: Pharmacol. Res. Commun. 20, 153 (1988).

300 V. K. Pandey, R. P. Misra and B. L. Chowdhary: Indian Drugs 23, 269 (1986).

301 P. N. Bhargava and H. Singh: Indian J. Pharm. 31, 111 (1969).

302 K. S. L. Srivastava: Indian J. Pharm. 32, 97 (1970).

303 R. P. Rao, B. Shrama and N. Zaidi: Indian J. Chem. 16B, 1023 (1978).

304 N. B. Zaidi, R. P. Rao and B. Sharma: Acta Cienc. Indica Chem. 7, 63 (1981).

305 N. S. Habib and A. A. B. Hazzaa: Sci. Pharm. 49, 246 (1981).

306 P. Kumar, K. N. Dhawan, S. Vrat, K. P. Bhargava and K. K. Kishore: Arch. Pharm. 316, 759 (1983).

307 P. N. Bhargava and R. Shyam: Egypt. J. Chem. 18, 393 (1977).

308 G. Chen and X. Zhang: Yaoxue Xuebao 19, 796 (1984).

309 N. Singhal, I. S. Gupta and P. C. Bansal: J. Indian Chem. Soc. 61, 690 (1984).

310 J. S. Shukla and V. K. Agarwal: Indian J. Chem. 24B, 886 (1985).

311 R. Lakhan, O. P. Singh and R. L. Singh: J. Indian Chem. Soc. 64, 316 (1987).

312 G. P. Beardsley, E. C. Taylor, G. B. Grindey, R. G. Moran in: Chemistry and Biology of Pteridines; B. A. Copper, V. M. Whitehead, Eds. de Gruyter: Berlin 1986, p. 953.

313 D. W. Fry, R. C. Jackson: Cancer Metastasis Rev. 5, 251 (1987).

314 T. R. Jones, A. H. Calvert, A. L. Jackman, S. J. Brown, M. Jones and K. R. Harrap: Eur. J. Cancer 17, 11 (1981).

315 A. H. Calvert, D. L. Alison, S. J. Harland, B. A. Robinson, A. L. Jackson, T. R. Jones and D. R. Newell et al.: J. Clin. Oncol. 4, 1245 (1986).

316 B. M. J. Cantwell, M. Carnshaw and A. L. Harris: Cancer Treatment Rep. 70, 1335 (1986).

317 M. F. Bassendine, N. J. Curtin, H. Loose, A. L. Harris and O. F. W. James: J. Hepatol. 4, 349 (1987).

318 A. H. Calvert, D. R. Newell, A. L. Jackman, L. A. Gumbrell, E. Sikora, B. Grzelakowska-Sztabert, J. A. M. Bishop, I. R. Judson, S. J. Harland and K. R. Harrap: Natl. Cancer Inst. Monogr. 5, 213 (1987).

319 S. Vest, E. Bork and H. H. Hansen: Eur. J. Cancer Clin. Oncol. 24,, 201 (1988).

320 B. M. J. Cantwell, V. Macaulay, A. L. Harris, S. B. Kaye, I. E. Smith, R. A. V. Milsted and A. H. Calvert: Eur. J. Cancer Clin. Oncol. 24, 733 (1988).

321 C. Sessa, M. Zucchetti, M. Ginier, Y. Willems, M. D'Incalci and F. Cavalli: Eur. J. Cancer Clin. Oncol. 24, 769 (1988).

322 D. R. Newell, Z. H. Siddik, A. H. Calvert, A. L. Jackman, D. L. Alison, K. G. McGhee and K. R. Harrap: Proc. Am. Assoc. Cancer Res. 23, 181 (1982).

323   D. R. Newell, Z. H. Siddik, A. L. Jackman, P. M. O'Connor, K. G. McGhee, M. Radcic, A. H. Calvert and K. R. Harrap: Brit. J Cancer 48, 139 (1983).

324   T. R. Jones, A. H. Calvert, A. L. Jackman, M. A. Eakin, M. J. Smithers, R. F. Betteridge, D. R. Newell and A. J. Hayter et al.: J. Med. Chem. 28, 1468 (1985).

325   T. R. Jones, R. F. Betteridge, S. Neidle, A. L. Jackman and A. H. Calvert: Anti Cancer Drug Res. 3, 243 (1989).

326   T. R. Jones, M. J. Smithers, M. A. Taylor, A. L. Jackman, A. H. Calvert, S. J. Harland and K. R. Harrap: J. Med. Chem. 29, 468 (1986).

327   T. R. Jones, M. J. Smithers, R. F. Betteridge, M. A. Taylor, A. L. Jackman, A. H. Calvert, L. C. Davies and K. R. Harrap: J. Med. Chem. 29, 1114 (1986).

328   T. R. Jones, T. J. Thornton, A. Flinn, A. L. Jackman, D. R. Newell and A. H. Calvert: J. Med. Chem. 32, 847 (1989).

329   D. J. McNamara, E. M. Berman, D. W. Fry and L. M. Werbel: J. Med. Chem. 33, 2045 (1990).

330   G. M. F. Bisset, A. L. Jackman, B. O'Connor, T. R. Jones, A. H. Calvert and L. R. Hughes: Chem. Biol. Pteridines 1980 Proc. Int. Symp. Pteridines Folic Acid Deriv. 9th 1989 (Pub. 1990) 114; Chem. Abstr. 115, 92862 b (1991).

331   T. R. Jones, M. D. Varney, S. E. Webber, K. Appelt and G. Marzoni: Eur. 365,763 (1990). May 02; Chem. Abstr. 113, 191383 m (1990).

332   L. R. Hughes: Eur. 284,338 (1988) Sep. 28; Chem. Abstr. 110, 95797 s (1989).

333   L. R. Hughes: Eur. 239,362 (1987) Sep. 30; Chem. Abstr. 108, 205094 d (1988).

334   L. R. Hughes, J. Oldfield, S. J. Pegg, A. J. Barker and P. R. Marshan: Eur. 373,891 (1990) Jun. 20; Chem. Abstr. 114, 23978 m (1991).

335   E. M. Berman, L. M. Werbel, D. J. McNamara: Eur. 316,657 (1989) May 24; Chem. Abstr. 111, 214500 x (1989).

336   H. E. Kunzel, G. D. Wolf, R. Bierling, S. Peterson, G. Nischk and D. Steinnoff: US 3,932,409 (1976) Jan. 13.

337   P. Singh and I. S. Gupta: J. Indian Chem. Soc. 56, 77 (1979).

338   P. C. Joshi, M. M. Sah and K. C. Pant: J. Indian Chem. Soc. 68, 416 (1991).

339   J. B. Jiang, D. P. Hesson, B. A. Dusak, D. L. Dexter, G. J. Kang and E. Hamel: J. Med. Chem. 33, 1721 (1990).

340   M. Y. Ebeid, S. M. El-Moghazy, A. N. Mikhael and A. A. Eissa: Egypt. J. Pharm. Sci 33, 293 (1992).

341   N. P. Peet, L. E. Baugh, S. Sunder, J. E. Lewis, E. H. Matthews, E. L. Clderding and D. N. Shah: J. Med. Chem. 29, 2403 (1986).

342   A. P. Vinogroff: Eur. 161,661 (1985) Nov. 21: Chem. Abstr. 104, 129925 a (1986).

343   N. Chand, J. Pillar, W. Diamantis and R. D. Sofia: Agents Actions 16, 318 (1985).

344   S. Ollier, C. A. Gould and R. J. Davies: J. Allergy Clin. Pharmacol. 78, 358 (1986).

345   J. R. Prous ed: Annu. Drug Data Rep. 8, 1072 (1988).

346   J. W. Coates and L. I. Kruse: Eur. 371,731 (1990) Jun 06: Chem. Abstr. 113, 212006 h (1990).

347   I. Uedo and M. Kato: Eur. 129,891 (1985) Jan. 02; Chem. Abstr. 102, 203981 t (1985).

348   H. Amschler, K. Klemm and W. Schoetensack: Ger. 2,027,645 (1971) Dec. 09; Chem. Abstr. 76, 85842 t (1972).

349   G. E. Hardtman: US 3,936,453 (1976) Feb. 03; Chem. Abstr. 84, 164832 h (1976).

350   S. Buyuktimkin, A. Buschaver and W. Schunack: Arch. Pharm. 324, 291 (1991).

351   F. E. Janssens, G. M. Diels and F. M. Sommen: PCT Int. Appl. Wo 9206,086 (1990) Oct. 01; Chem. Abstr. 117, 111638 t (1992).

352   A. Koda, H. Nagai, H. Mori, N. Inagaki and M. Mihara: Arzneim. Forsch. 36, 1609 (1986).

353   S. W. Kohno, T. Murata, T. Kinoshita and K. Ohata: Arzneim. Forsch. 36, 1619 (1986).

354   K. Tsurumi, K. Kyuki, M. Niwa, J. Haregawa, K. Fujimura: Arzneim. Forsch. 36, 1637 (1986).

355   Y. Yanagihara and T. Shida: Arzneim. Forsch. 36, 1627 (1986).

356   G. J. Durant, J. C. Emmett, C. R. Ganellin, P. D. Miles, M. E. Parson, H. D. Prain and C. R. White: J. Med. Chem. 20, 901 (1971).

357   T. H. Brown and Y. C. Yound: Drugs of Future 10, 51 (1985).

358   M. Oshita, K. Morikawa, T. Aratani, H. Kato and Y. Ito: Jap. J. Pharmacol. 42, 229 (1986).

359   N. Dgawa, T. Yoshida, T. Aratani, E. Koshinaka, H. Kato and Y. Ito: Chem. Pharm. Bull. 36, 2955 (l98a).

360   C. R. Ganellin: "Quantitative Approaches to Drug Design" ed. by J. C. Dearden, Elsevier Science Publisher B.V. Amesterdam 1983, p. 239.

361   T. Takahashi, T. Haraguchi, K. Nakamura and Y. Suzuki: Eur. 276,825 (1988) Aug. 03; Chem. Abstr. 109, 190443 m (1988).

362   T. Takahashi, T. Haraguchi, K. Nakamura and Y. Suzuki: Eur. 276,826 (1988). Aug. 03; Chem. Abstr. 109, 170453 m (1988).

363   M. J. Yu, J. R. Mecowan, R. Jefferson and K. J. Thrasher: US 5075,313 (1991) Dec. 24; Chem. Abstr. 116, 128964 y (1992).

364   G. Doria, C. Passarotti, R. Magrini, R. Sala and R. Castello: Farmaco. Ed. Sci. 39, 968 (1984).

365   Y. Ito, H. Kato, E. Etsuchu, N. Ogawa and T. Suzuki: Jpn. 61,115,072 (1986) Jun. 02; Chem. Abstr. 105, 208918 z (1986).

366   Y. Ito, H. Kato, E. Etsuchu, N. Ogawa and T. Yoshida: Jpn. 6205,969 (1987) Jan. 12; Chem. Abstr. 107, 77825 h (1987).

367   C. M. Gupta, S. T. Husain, A. P. Bhaduri, N. M. Khanna and S. K. Mukherjee: Nature 223, 524 (1969).

368   M. Koizumi: Jpn. 77,07,978 (1977) Jan. 21; Chem. Abstr. 87, 53366 k (1977).

369   M. Yamamoto, M. Koshiba and H. Yamamoto: Jpn. 7805,180 (1976) Jul. 01; Chem. Abstr. 89, 43474 n (1978).

370   M. I. Husain and G. C. Srivastava: Indian J. Chem. 19B, 916 (1980).

371   M. I. Husain and K. B. Gupta: Indian J. Pharm. Sci. 44, 37 (1982).

372   M. I. Husain and V. P. Srivastava: Acta Pharm. Jugosl. 34, 31 (1984).

373   M. I. Husain and M. R. Jamali: Indian J. Chem. 27B, 43 (1988).

374   V. R. Agarwal, S. R. Nautiyal and D. D. Mukerjee: Indian Drugs 23, 458 (1986).

Progress in Drug Research, Vol. 43 (E. Jucker, Ed.)
© 1994 Birkhäuser Verlag, Basel (Switzerland)

Production and action of interferons: New insights into molecular mechanisms of gene regulation and expression

By Mark P. Hayes and Kathryn C. Zoon

Center for Biologics Evaluation and Research, Food and Drug Administration, Bethesda, MD 20892, USA

1   Interferons as therapeutics and bio-active mediators

The discovery of interferon (IFN) by Isaacs and Lindenmann [1] almost 40 years ago initiated a long and arduous course of scientific investigation that has culminated in its therapeutic use today for a variety of diseases. IFN, originally described on the basis of its capacity for inducing in cells a relatively nonspecific resistance to viruses, is now known to be composed of a large family of related proteins with similarities in structure and/or biological activity. Members of this family were initially distinguished on the basis of reactivity with specific antibodies, by their susceptibility to acid treatment, and by their cellular origin [2–5]. cDNA and genomic cloning of the IFN genes revealed the existence of a complex superfamily composed of numerous genes and pseudogenes [6, 7]. The most current classification of IFNs defines an IFN-alpha (IFN-α) family of at least 13 functional genes, unique genes for IFN-beta (IFN-β) and IFN-gamma (IFN-γ), one functional IFN-omega (IFN-ω), also referred to as IFN-$\alpha_{\parallel}1$) gene, a number of pseudogenes placed in the α or ω families, and a few unclassified pseudogenes [7]. Emphasis in this review will be placed on human IFN-α and IFN-γ, with references to the others as necessary. The reader is also referred to many excellent reviews of the subject [6, 8–10].

IFNs were the original members of the continually expanding class of proteins termed cytokines, which are loosely defined as biologically active mediators of cell-cell communication involved in such functions as proliferation, differentiation, and host defense. In the last two decades, cytokines have been the subject of intense interest both for their therapeutic potential and for the revelations that their study has provided with respect to basic principles of cell biology and immunology. As IFNs led the way toward the discovery of other cytokines, they were also pioneers into the clinical use of cytokines. *A priori,* it has been difficult to predict the capacity of cytokines, and IFNs in particular, to be efficacious in the treatment of various human diseases. Even if much is known about the *in vitro* activities of these proteins, understanding their potential and actual *in vivo* activities involves additional complex factors. These are, after all, proteins that are normally produced endogenously in response to a variety of stimuli, and they are under the control of highly regulated networks that often involve other cytokines.

IFNs were initially shown to have antiviral and antiproliferative properties on a number of different cell types. It seemed appropriate, therefore, to test IFNs clinically in diseases that were: 1) thought to be of viral etiology, or

2) disorders of cell proliferation, such as cancer. Later, when the immuno-modulating properties of IFNs, particularly IFN-γ, were revealed, an additional rationale for clinical use became available. While the overall clinical success of interferons was initially somewhat disappointing, there have been some successes which have led to licensure of several IFNs for clinical use in the United States by the Food and Drug Administration [reviewed in 11–14]. IFN-α has been used successfully to treat chronic viral hepatitis B [15] and hepatitis C [16, 17], condyloma acuminata [18, 19], hairy cell leukemia, and AIDS-related Kaposi's sarcoma [both reviewed in 20]. IFN-γ was shown to restore defective function in monocytes and neutrophils from patients with chronic granulomatous disease (CGD) of childhood [21, 22], which led to clinical trials that demonstrated efficacy of this IFN in CGD [23]. The most recent licensure for an IFN was for IFN-β in the treatment of multiple sclerosis [24–26].

The therapeutic use of IFNs and other more recently discovered cytokines has been restricted by a number of factors. In spite of their high potency and specific activity, the *in vivo* activity of these agents is limited by their rapid clearance from the circulation and brief biological half-life. As a result, these drugs are typically administered at extremely high non-physiologic doses in the hope of stimulating an appropriate response. What is perhaps a more important limitation on the effective use of IFNs and other cytokines is our lack of understanding of the molecular mechanisms by which these mediators act at the cellular level. In addition, control of the endogenous production of cytokines under physiological conditions is still poorly understood. A better understanding of how IFN production is normally regulated would be of value in establishing a rationale for its use *in vivo*, and could yield alternative approaches for therapy by way of endogenous induction of IFNs or, conversely, suppression of undesirable IFN production that may exist in various pathological states.

This review will focus on recent advances in the understanding of IFN production and action. Substantial progress has been made in the past few years in the elucidation of molecular events by which IFN and IFN-induced genes are regulated. The identification and cloning of receptors for IFN-γ and IFN-α represented significant accomplishments, but ultimately served only to reveal the complexities involved in IFN recognition and intracellular signalling [27, 28]. Important advances were also made in the area of transcriptional control of IFN and IFN-induced genes, with the identification of transcription factors that appear to bridge the gap between extracellular signalling and the induction of gene transcription and the dissection of potential regulatory controls over the activity and localization of those factors. However, these discoveries have only begun to scratch the surface of the complex series of events leading to activation of these genes.

2   Regulation of interferon production

2.1   The interferon alpha/beta gene family

Studies on the expression of IFN-α genes are complicated by the existence of so many distinct genes, each of which is likely to be subject to independent regulation. As with most cytokines, IFN was originally discovered and described based upon its biological activity [1]. The progression of IFN research led to the determination that IFNs could be distinguished on the basis of their pH stability, antigenicity, and cellular origin. Wheelock discovered an IFN-like activity in leukocyte cultures stimulated with mitogen which could be distinguished from other IFNs by virtue of its acid lability [2]. Youngner and Salvin proposed that IFNs be classified as Type I and Type II, based on a number of distinctive properties [3]. Type I IFN was induced by non-specific stimuli such as virus or bacterial lipopolysaccharide (LPS), was acid-stable, and active on heterologous species. Type II IFN was induced by specific antigen, was acid-labile, and species-specific. Furthermore, antibodies made to Type I IFN would not neutralize Type II IFN [3]. Havell et al. further distinguished IFNs from leukocyte versus fibroblast sources, using specific antibodies, that were later shown to be IFN-α and IFN-β, respectively [4]. In 1980, an IFN nomenclature committee classified the three types of IFN known at that time as IFN-α (leukocyte-derived, acid-stable), IFN-β (fibroblast-derived, acid-stable), and IFN-γ (T lymphocyte-derived, antigen- or mitogen-induced, acid-labile) [5].

In the late 1970s and early 80s, purification of IFN proteins and the subsequent cloning of IFN genes ultimately revealed the large number of IFN components that are now known to exist [7]. In the human, IFN-β and IFN-γ are represented by single genes. The original IFN-α family, however, consists of at least 14 functional genes and 12 pseudogenes. That family has now been split into the IFN-α family that contains all but one of the functional IFN-α genes, and the IFN-ω family, of which there is only one functional member (formerly known as IFN-$\alpha_{\parallel}1$) [7]. A protein with substantial sequence homology to IFN-ω, designated trophoblast IFN (IFN-τ), has been identified in the preimplantation conceptus of sheep [29]. While a human counterpart has yet to be identified, this gene is of considerable interest since it is involved in reproductive functions and is not apparently regulated by viral induction [30].

Extensive purification and characterization of natural IFN-α proteins has revealed the presence of sequences that are not found in known IFN genes, raising the possibility that this family is even larger than originally predicted. In lymphoblastoid IFN preparations, for example, there are at least 22 biochemically separable components, among which there are several unique amino-terminal sequences [31]. There are distinct patterns of biological activities for each of these IFN-α components, which may provide a rationale for the existence of so many different IFNs [31–34].

The induction of IFN-α synthesis and secretion occurs in response to a wide variety of stimuli, such as viruses, double-stranded RNA (dsRNA, usually in the form of poly-I,C), bacterial products (e.g. LPS), and other microbial products [9]. Most cell types that have been tested are capable of producing IFN-α or -β. Many, but not all, viruses probably induce IFN through the intermediate presentation of double-stranded viral RNA [35, 36]. The type of IFN induced is dependent upon both the inducer and the cell type being induced [37, 38]. The original designation of IFN-α as a leukocyte-derived product and IFN-β as a fibroblast product is usually appropriate, but there are exceptions; both IFN subtypes are often produced concurrently [39–41]. In another example of the difficulty of predicting the *in vivo* situation from *in vitro* observations, Tovey et al. have shown that IFN-α mRNA appears constitutively in "normal" human tissues [42]. While this does not imply that the IFN proteins are necessarily being produced in these tissues, it suggests that as yet uncharacterized elements may control *in vivo* interferon production under normal physiological conditions.

2.2   Transcription of IFN-α, β genes

The expression of IFN genes can potentially be controlled at many levels, including transcription, mRNA metabolism, translation, and secretion. Considerable effort has been expended on the regulation of IFN-α transcription. Weidle and Weissmann concluded that the human IFNα-1 gene was transcriptionally regulated, based on the behavior of IFN-α/β-globin constructs in transfected cells [43]. The primary focus on transcriptional regulation has been the identification of 1) 5' promoter regions required for transcriptional activation with virus or dsRNA and 2) the transcription factors that bind to these regions in some functional manner [44]. The original observations that the 5' promoter region was necessary and sufficient for transcriptional activation of IFN-α/β genes [45–47] led to a search for specific cis-acting elements that were required for transcriptional induction in response to known stimuli. The boundaries for these elements were defined through deletion analysis of promoter constructs from both IFN-α and -β genes [48–50]. A schematic summary of some of these elements is provided in Figure 1 for reference.

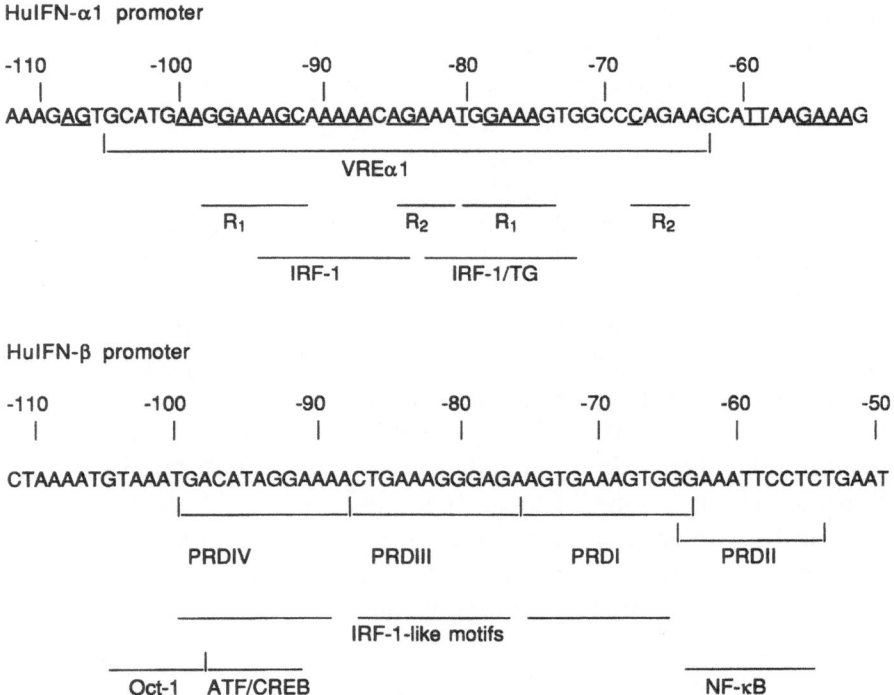

Figure 1.
Schematic representation of the human IFN-α and IFN-β promoters. Nucleotide numbering is relative to the transcription start sites. The IFN-α promoter is from the IFN-α1 sequence; bases homologous to all IFN-α genes are underlined. The virus-responsive element (VREα1) was described in [55]. The octameric (R_1) and pentameric (R_2) repeats were delineated in [48]. Sites labelled with IRF-1 are potential interferon regulatory factor binding sites, and the TG element, whose physiological functions are uncertain, were described in [59]. The positive regulatory domains (PRDI-IV), Oct-1, ATF-CREB (activating transcription factor/cAMP response element binding protein), and NF-κB elements of the IFN-β promoter were as described by Maniatis and colleagues [58].

In the case of the human IFN-α1 gene, the minimal requirement for viral inducibility occurred between position -109 to -64 [50]. Further analysis of IFN-α and IFN-β promoters indicated that, while there are some similarities between them, there are distinctive functional elements which may serve to explain the differential expression of these genes. For example, the IFN-β promoter contains a functional NF-κB consensus sequence not found in IFN-α promoters [51–54]. The 46-bp sequence in the human IFN-α1 gene promoter required for virus inducibility has been termed the virus-responsive element [VRE]. This VRE is composed of two imperfect repeats, called repA and repB. A tetrameric repeat of repA, like the VRE, conferred virus inducibility upon reporter constructs [55]. The virus-responsive element of the human IFN-β gene, alternatively referred to as the VREβ or IRE [interferon response element] was initially dissected into three distinct regulatory elements: PRDI and PRDII [positive response elements] and NRDI [a negative response element] [56, 57], and more recently into four positive regulatory elements (PRDI through IV) and two negative regulatory elements (NRDI and II) [reviewed in 58]. Using multimerized repeats of the sequence GAAANN, MacDonald et al. [59] delineated three distinct elements that could mediate virus inducibility, two of which were represented in IFN-β promoter (which could bind IRF-1-like and NF-κB-like elements, respectively) and one in the IFN-α1 promoter (called the TG sequence).

Following identification of the *cis* sequences required for virus inducibility, there remained the challenge of characterizing the *trans* elements that interact with those sequences in a functionally meaningful way. Taniguchi and colleagues identified and cloned a factor termed interferon regulatory factor 1 (IRF-1), which bound to sequences found in the VREs of both IFN-α and IFN-β promoters [60, 61]. A homologous factor, was subsequently isolated, termed IRF-2, which bound to the same regions with similar affinity [62]. Initial evidence favored a functional role for these factors in IFN gene expression. Over-expression of IRF-1 in COS cells was shown to induce moderate expression of IFN-α and IFN-β genes [63], and IRF-2 repressed IRF-1-induced IFN expression when co-transfected into embryonal carcinoma cells that express neither IRFs nor IFNs endogenously. IRF-1 and IRF-2 expression were induced with kinetics that were consistent with a role in IFN induction following viral infection [62]. In addition, induction of IRF-1 mRNA correlated with induction of IFN-α under a variety of alternative stimulus conditions [64].

While it was clear that IRFs bound to and were capable of activating or repressing IFN promoters, and that their expression was commensurate with that function, other data suggested that IRF-1 was neither necessary nor sufficient for IFN-β induction, in response to poly-I,C and cyclohex- imide [65]. Analysis of factors that interacted with the PRDI element of the IFN-β promoter revealed that there were multiple complexes formed under various induction conditions [66]. Components of some of these complexes appeared to be related to IRFs, but no detectable IRF-1 was observed in the absence of protein synthesis, while IFN-β induction clearly takes place under such conditions. IRF knockout mice provided interesting insights into IFN gene induction [67]. IRF-1-deficient cells failed to produce IFN in response to poly-I,C, but responded normally to viral stimulation (New- castle disease virus). However, IRF-2-deficient cells produced more IFN in response to NDV but were normal in their response to poly-I,C. Stably expressed IRF-1 caused substantially higher expression of IFN-β in re- sponse to viral induction, while IRF-1 antisense constructs completely abolished IFN-β induction [68]. What these experiments ultimately demon- strated was the complex nature of DNA:protein interactions that can occur during IFN-β induction, without taking into account factors that interact with the other regulatory elements of this promoter (see below). IRFs appear to play an important role in the regulation of IFN expression, but are clearly not the only factors involved. The situation is additionally complicated by the variables of the inducing stimulus and pathways of induction, as suggested by the results with the knockout mice.

There are additional factors which interact with IFN promoters and may be active in influencing transcription. Convincing evidence supported a role for NF-κB in IFN-β induction following its interaction with the PRDII element [51–54]. More recently, it was demonstrated that viral induction of IFN-β requires not only NF-κB, but the high mobility group protein HMG I(Y), and that both act through binding to the PRDII element [69]. An additional complex involved in IFN-β induction was defined which acted through the PRDIV element, which interacts with at least one member of the activating transcription factor/cAMP response element (ATF/CREB) family [70]. Other candidate transcription factors have been partially characterized that interact with IFN promoters. One of the binding sites for IRFs is the PRDI element of the IFN-β promoter [62]. cDNAs encoding other PRDI-binding proteins have been cloned. One of these, a zinc finger protein termed PRDI-BF1 (PRDI-binding factor), appeared to act as a repressor of IFN-β transcription [71]. The other, the interferon consensus sequence binding protein (ICSBP), is restricted in its expression to certain cell types (see below), and has been implicated in IFN-induced gene expression [72]. It is unclear what role, if any, it might play in IFN gene regulation. Two other factors that bound to the PRDI sequence, called PRDI-BFc (constitutive) and PRDI-BFi (inducible) were identified as IRF-2 and a truncated form of IRF-2 created by an inducible proteolytic event. The truncated IRF-2 lost repressor activity even though it retained a similar binding affinity for the PRDI element [73]. Activation of IRF-1 has been shown to require a post-translational event that could occur in the presence of cycloheximide, and the IRF-1 protein is apparently much more labile ($T_{1/2} < 30$ minutes) than IRF-2 ($T_{1/2} > 8$ hr) [74]. These observations raised new issues as to how IRFs could be regulated other than by *de novo* induction.

The promoters of IFN-α genes are less well-characterized than the IFN-β promoter. The TG factor identified by MacDonald et al. has not yet been identified or cloned [59]. In the murine system, Pitha and colleagues have shown that different IFN-α genes are transcribed at different rates, implying that the individual promoters differ in their activity depending on the cell type and inducing stimulus [75]. They have characterized two overlapping sites as virus-induction elements in the IFN-α promoter. One binds IRF-1 or an IRF-1-like factor. The other was termed the αF1 site, and formed a complex with at least two proteins of 68 and 96 kDa. Results from binding and transfection studies suggested that viral induction involves cooperative binding of transcription factors to both of these sites, and that cell-specific IFN-α subtype expression is related to cell-specific repressors that affect these interactions [76]. The elucidation of mechanisms by which specific expression of individual IFNα genes occur may provide some insights into how large, seemingly redundant gene families are regulated.

2.3   Post-transcriptional regulation of IFN-α, β genes

While considerable effort has gone into analyzing transcriptional regulation of IFN genes, far less attention has been given to posttranscriptional mechanisms that affect IFN expression. One of the hallmarks of IFN induction is that, like most cytokines, IFN mRNAs are expressed only transiently. The transient nature of the mRNA accumulation is a function of both transcriptional and posttranscriptional effects [77]. IFN mRNA accumulation is enhanced and prolonged when cells are induced in the presence of metabolic inhibitors (of protein or RNA synthesis); this phenomenon has been referred to as superinduction [78–81]. Recent insights into the molecular mechanisms of superinduction have been provided. One potential contributory factor is the post-induction repression of IFN tran-scription. Whittemore and Maniatis reported that this repression is depend-ent on protein synthesis and on the presence of two of the regulatory elements that were also required for transcriptional induction (PRDI and PRDII), implying the existence of virus-inducible repressors that are syn-thesized *de novo* following induction [82, 83]. Another hypothesis for explaining superinduction was the existence of a labile factor(s) that medi-ated mRNA degradation. Cycloheximide would prevent mRNA decay by suppressing the synthesis of this factor, thereby leading to enhanced mRNA accumulation. Both IFN-β and the IFN-α family have sequences that appear to target their mRNA for rapid degradation [82, 84, 85]. One of these sequences is the 3' AU-rich motif which has been associated with mRNA instability and is present in many cytokine and other inducible mRNAs [86, 87]. The AU-rich sequences have also been shown to affect translatability of mRNA [88]. Another mRNA destabilizing region has also been described that is within the coding sequence for IFN-β [82]. This region has been localized to the carboxyl-terminal end of the coding region and was termed the coding region instability domain (CRID) [89].

There is some controversy as to whether IFN mRNA stability is regulated with induction, and that may depend on the conditions of stimulation [77, 82, 90, 91]. Treatment of cells with glucocorticoids was found to increase IFN-β mRNA turnover [92]. Some, but not all, of the cytokine mRNAs containing instability sequences were found to be more unstable following inhibition of protein kinase C, suggesting that mRNA degradation was a kinase-regulated event [93]. Considerable effort has been devoted to iden-tifying *trans* factors that interact with mRNAs and are involved in their metabolism. Several laboratories have identified factors that bind to the AU-rich sequences [reviewed in 94]. Some of these factors possess varying degrees of specificity for particular mRNAs [95]. Raj and Pitha identified a 65-kDa protein in cell extracts that binds to three relatively homologous regions in the human IFN-β mRNA that correspond to the CRID and the AU-rich regions of this message [89]. Interestingly, this protein was de-tected only in fibroblasts, but not in T cells, where IFN-β is not inducible. Further efforts in this area should help to clarify the role of mRNA stability and translatability in IFN induction. The identification and characterization of intracellular factors involved in mRNA metabolism will undoubtedly provide additional insight into this important mechanism for control of pro-inflammatory gene expression.

2.4   Transcription of IFN-γ

The induction of IFN-γ differs from IFN-α, β with respect to both the stimuli that induce its production and the specific cell types that produce it. The only cell types known to produce IFN-γ are T lymphocytes and large granular lymphocytes [96], although there are exceptions [97]. There are a number of stimuli that have been shown to induce IFN-γ expression, alone or in combination. These include interleukin-2 [98, 99], stimulation of the T cell receptor [100] or CD16 [101], lectins [102], phorbol esters [103], and Ca++ ionophores [104]. Most of these are also signals for T cell activation in general, and it is difficult to separate IFN-γ induction from other aspects of the immune response of T cells. However, there are conditions that can segregate IFN-γ induction from other T cell responses (e.g. stimulation with natural killer cell stimulatory factor or NKSF/IL12) [105].

As with IFN-α, β, the primary mechanism governing IFN-γ induction appears to be transcriptional [106], although some recent data suggests that post-transcriptional regulation is active under certain conditions [107]. Other aspects of IFN-γ regulation that are shared with IFN-α, β include lack of a requirement for protein synthesis, the capacity for superinduction, and the presence of the destabilizing AU-rich sequence in IFN-γ mRNA. The regulatory elements governing IFN-γ transcription not only affect induction, but tissue-specific regulation of expression. All of the elements necessary for tissue-specific induction are present within 2.7 kb of the 5' end and 1 kb of the 3' end of the gene, as judged by expression in transgenic mice [108]. Two T cell-specific DNAase I hypersensitivity sites were identified in the 5' flanking region and first intron, respectively, along with a third inducible site in the 5' end [109, 110]. The intronic regulatory region has been shown to act as an enhancer and as a binding site for the c-rel protooncogene product [111]. Transfection experiments confirmed and localized regulatory elements near the hypersensitivity sites between -540 and -47 bp from the 5' start site [112, 113]. Further localization of critical sites for tissue-specific inducible IFN-γ expression was recently achieved [114]. Within 108 bp of the transcription start site, two highly conserved promoter elements were identified. The distal element, bp -96 to -80, included a consensus GATA motif [also found in the promoters of T cell receptor genes] and a sequence homologous to critical elements found in the granulocyte macrophage colony stimulating factor (GM-CSF) and macrophage inflammatory protein (MIP-1α/β) promoters. The proximal element, bp -73 to -48, was homologous to the NFIL-2A element of the IL-2 promoter. *Trans* factors that bound to these elements were detected in extracts from Jurkat T cells that were not present in myeloid cell lines. The nuclear factor GATA-3 binds to the distal element, but its functional role is uncertain. The NFIL-2A (nuclear factor, IL-2) element of the IL-2 promoter binds the Oct-1 transcription factor, but this factor was not recognized by the IFN-γ proximal element. Other more distal sequences in the IFN-γ promoter affected expression moderately in transfectants and may play important roles in IFN-γ expression, but they are not absolutely required for the tissue-specific inducible expression seen with the elements described above [114]. Methylation of critical promoter sites may also be an important determinant of the tissue specificity of IFN-γ expression [97]. Future efforts should definitively identify important transcription factors involved in activation of the IFN-γ gene, and will also provide important insights into the more complex issues of lymphokine expression and T lymphocyte function.

3   Interferon action: opening the black box of intracellular signalling

3.1   Interferon alpha-beta receptors

Although IFNs have been the subject of research for more than 30 years, it was only recently that substantial progress was made in the characterization of IFN receptors. A key element to this progress was the cloning of a cDNA encoding a functional human IFN-α receptor [115]. Historically, binding data have indicated that all IFN-αs, IFN-β, and IFN-ω bind to the same receptor, while IFN-γ binds to a distinct receptor [116]. The latter was not surprising based upon the structure of IFNs; IFN-γ is not structurally related to the other IFNs, in spite of its capacity to induce some similar biological responses. There may be other elements involved in signalling which provide an explanation for these common (e.g. antiviral) responses (see Section 3.5). Recent evidence, however, has indicated that the nature of the IFN-α receptor is more complex. There may be more than one human IFN-α binding site, and the receptor may consist of more than one component. This is consistent with the multiplicity of ligands that it must recognize.

The cloned IFN-α receptor cDNA did not offer any direct insights into intracellular signalling mechanisms by IFNs; there were no sequence motifs reminiscent of kinases or other modifying enzymes. The genomic sequences surrounding the IFN-α receptor gene have been analyzed. The gene is composed of 11 exons and 10 introns on chromosome 21 [117]. The most interesting feature of this gene product was that, upon transfection into heterologous cells, it failed to bind or confer biological responsiveness to all IFN subtypes. The cDNA was originally isolated by an expression cloning technique using responsiveness to human IFN-αB (also called IFN-α8 or IFNA8), since this subtype possesses a greater degree of species specificity than other IFN-αs. It encodes a protein of 557 amino acids with a single predicted 21-AA transmembrane domain, a 27-AA signal sequence, and an intracellular domain of 100 amino acids [115]. It was initially shown to confer responsiveness to IFN-αB, but to only marginally enhance the response to IFN-β or IFN-αA (the latter is also known as IFN-α2 or IFNA2) [115]. Therefore, it was hypothesized that accessory proteins were required for functionally effective binding of other IFNs to human cells. This was supported by the ability to dissociate IFN-α and IFN-β sensitivity in mutant cell lines that had been selected for alterations in IFN sensitivity [118], and by early biochemical analysis suggesting the existence of larger receptor complexes [119, 120]. Antibodies generated against recombinant receptor transfectants were able to neutralize the activity of several human IFNs on human cells, including IFN-β and IFN-αA (IFNA2), suggesting that the immunogen was at least part of the accessible IFN receptor complex on the cell surface [121]. Monoclonal antibodies have been generated to an engineered soluble form of the cloned receptor protein. One of these antibodies was able to neutralize the activity of several IFN subtypes, including α2, αB, β, ω, and purified natural IFN-α preparations [122]. Further insight into the specificity of the cloned receptor protein came from the cloning of its murine counterpart and subsequent transfection experiments. When the murine receptor was transfected into human cells, those cells responded to only certain murine IFN-α subtypes. However, the murine receptor cDNA completely restored responsiveness to all IFN-α/β subtypes in a previously unresponsive mutant murine cell line, suggesting that response specificity depended on host accessory factors that also interact with the receptor protein [123]. An extension of this same approach was used with the cloning of the bovine IFN-α receptor cDNA. The bovine receptor, transfected into human cells, conferred high sensitivity to human IFN-D, a subtype that normally has higher specific activity on bovine than on human cells [124]. The results suggested that IFN subtype recognition was mediated by this gene product, supporting the accessory factor hypothesis presented previously.

252   Mark P. Hayes and Kathryn C. Zoon

In an extension of the direct biochemical approach in the study of IFN receptor structure, monoclonal antibodies have been generated following immunization with a human myeloma cell line (U-266) that expressed relatively high numbers of IFN-α2 binding sites. These antibodies were able to immunoprecipitate ^{125}I-IFN-α2 complexes following cross-linking from human cells of 130 and 210 kDa and detected a 110-kDa protein on Western blots or from surface iodinated cells [125]. The recognized protein was referred to as the a subunit of the IFN-α receptor. This protein was found to be tyrosine phosphorylated following IFN-α treatment [126]. An additional monoclonal antibody has been reported, using the same immunogen [U-266 cells] that blocks binding and activity of several IFN subtypes (including IFN-β and IFN-γ). Both this antibody and the original antibodies described above were found to recognize gene products mapping to chromosome 21 [127]. These antibodies apparently do not recognize the cloned IFN-α receptor. The purification and cloning of these gene products should provide invaluable information regarding the role of these proteins in IFN-α recognition and signalling.

The question of receptor recognition of distinct IFN-α subtypes has been raised in binding studies as well. IFN-αD (also known as IFN-α1) did not compete for IFN-α2 binding to Daudi cells, although they displayed similar antiproliferative activities on the same cells [128]. More recently, it was found that certain natural lymphoblastoid IFN-α components did not compete for IFN-α2 binding in a manner that correlated with their specific activities [33]. These data suggested the existence of more than one IFN-α binding site, perhaps in the context of a multi-component receptor. Future efforts will hopefully identify critical determinants on individual IFN-α proteins that determine receptor specificity. At the same time, further clarification of the nature of the IFN-α, β receptor(s) structure should help to resolve the questions about recognition of different members of the IFN-α family.

3.2   The interferon gamma receptor

The successful cloning and expression of the human IFN-γ receptor revealed a paradox similar in some ways to that of the IFN-α receptor [27]. Upon transfection into heterologous cells, the cloned cDNA conferred binding of IFN-γ, but failed to result in any biological responsiveness. The biological response (in this case, induction of class I MHC antigens) was later shown to require complementation by an unknown element[s] encoded on human chromosome 21 [129]. The isolated cDNA encoded a protein of 489 amino acids containing a 14-AA predicted signal sequence and a 21-AA putative transmembrane sequence. The intracellular domain of the protein was quite large (223 amino acids), and has been scrutinized for its potential role in signal transduction, though no obvious role could be gleaned from its sequence [27]. The gene was localized to human chromosome 6, consistent with previous results showing that chromosome 6 could confer IFN-γ binding in hamster-human hybrids [130]. The requirement for chromosome 21 for a biological response was confirmed by stable transfection of the human receptor into hamster cells containing the long arm of this chromosome [131].

Further analysis of the cloned human IFN-γ receptor demonstrated that at least two regions (membrane-proximal and carboxy-terminal) of the intracellular domain were required for biological activity in murine transfectants. These constructs also distinguished between sequence requirements for receptor-mediated IFN-γ processing and biologic responses [132]. Hybrid murine-human IFN-γ receptor molecules were utilized to show that only the extracellular domain of the receptor was required for interaction with the chromosome 21 accessory factor[s] to provide a functional response [133]. The only requirement for full function was that both the extracellular domain and the accessory factor[s] were derived from the same species [134, 135]. Mutational analysis of the intracellular domain of the receptor has yielded some information on the regions of absolute functional importance. There is a 5-amino acid segment [YDKPH] in this domain that is absolutely conserved between mouse, rat, and human receptors which was absolutely required for biological activity of the receptor, as measured by induction of MHC class I antigens, IRF-1 expression, and nitric oxide synthase, and protection against encephalomyocarditis virus (EMCV) [136, 137]. Three of these amino acids were shown to be critical (Tyr, Asp, and His) [137]. Interestingly, no protection was afforded against vesicular stomatitis virus (VSV) in transfectants containing both the human receptor and chromosome 21, indicating the existence of another accessory factor required for more specific VSV resistance [136]. A 540-kb yeast artificial chromosome (YAC) clone has been isolated which contains the accessory factor(s) from human chromosome 21 that conferred inducibility of class I antigens, but not IFN-γ-induced resistance to EMCV, implying the existence of yet another required accessory factor; this factor is apparently encoded on chromosome 21 [138]. The authors proposed that a family of accessory factors exists which may be expressed in different cells under various conditions, and may offer an explanation for tissue-specific responses to IFN-γ. The specificity of IFN-induced gene products in mediating the antiviral response is the subject of a recent review [139]. cDNA clones encoding accessory factors have recently been isolated that reconstitute both human [140] and mouse IFN-γ responsiveness [141]. The human protein, termed AF-1 (accessory factor 1) permits responses for induction of class I antigens and incomplete protection against EMCV. AF-1 is a putative transmembrane protein that displays some homology to other members of the class 2 cytokine receptor family (which includes the IFN receptors) [140].

A mutant mouse strain has been developed that lacks the IFN-γ receptor gene to assess its *in vivo* functions. Surprisingly, the effects of this deletion on the development of the immune system were not obviously detrimental. However, these mice had decreased resistance to *Listeria monocytogenes* and vaccinia virus, and had some reduction in the IgG2a response [142]. In addition, these mice had increased lethality to Bacillus Calmette-Guérin infection, and decreased lethality to endotoxin following BCG inoculation; the latter correlated with cytokine (TNF, IL-1, IL-6) serum levels [143]. Examination of macrophage function from these mice indicated the expected loss of IFN-γ-dependent functions involved in class II antigen expression and nitric oxide production [144]. These mice should provide substantial useful information with regard to the *in vivo* functional roles of IFN-γ.

3.3   Interferon alpha intracellular signalling

Most, if not all, of the biological responses of cells to IFNs are mediated by the expression of a large number of proteins that are synthesized *de novo*. The expression of these new proteins typically involves the induction of transcription of the genes encoding them. A substantial research effort has been invested into dissecting the molecular control of IFN-induced gene expression, with emphasis on the regulation of transcription of these genes. Overlapping sets of genes are induced by IFN-α, β and IFN-γ, and other genes are down-regulated by IFNs as well [reviewed in 145]. For a recent excellent review of interferon signalling and transcription factor activation, see also David [146] and refer to Figure 2 (reprinted from [146]).

IFN-α and -β specifically induce the transcription of a subset of genes in a rapid, protein synthesis-independent manner [147–151]. There were no immediately identifiable second messengers that were candidates for me-

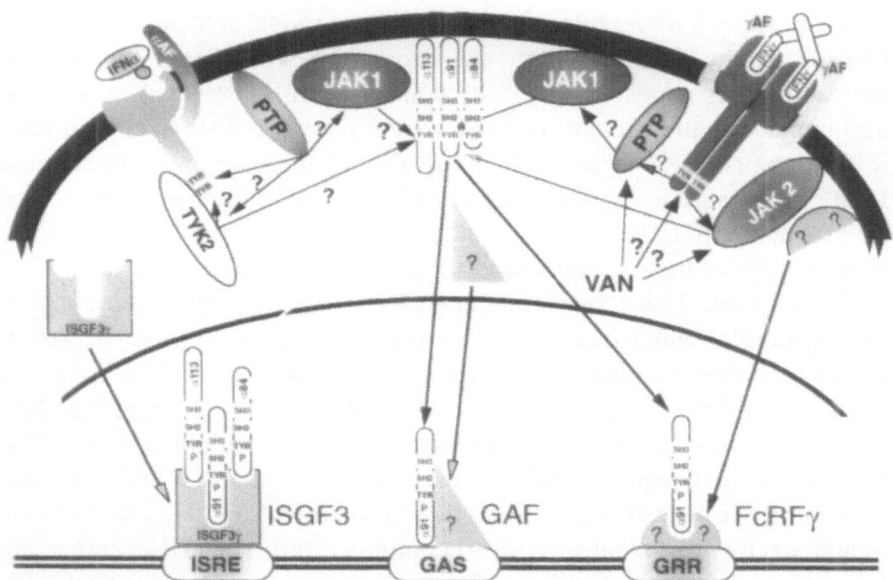

Figure 2.
Elements involved in intracellular signalling and transcription factor activation in response to IFNs [reprinted from 146]. IFN-α and IFN-γ receptors are depicted on the left and right, respectively. αAF and γAF are the accessory factors required for IFN responsiveness to the respective transfected receptors. TYK2, JAK1, and JAK2 refer to kinases known to be required for IFN signalling (see text for details). PTPs are as yet undefined protein tyrosine phosphatases. VAN refers to sodium vanadate. ISGF3 is the interferon-stimulated gene factor activated in response to IFN-α. GAF (IFN-gamma-activated factor) and FcRFγ (FcγRI DNA-binding factor, IFN-γ induced) are activated in response to IFN-γ. ISRE (interferon-stimulated response element), GAS (IFN-gamma activation sequence), and GRR (IFNgamma response region) are the *cis* elements recognized by the transcription factors. α84, α91, and α113 are the polypeptides originally described as components of ISGF3α.

diating these early transcriptional responses [152]. Examination of IFN-inducible genes revealed the presence of a 5' flanking sequence, termed the interferon-stimulated response element (ISRE), which was identified by deletion and mutation analysis to be required for IFN-induced transcriptional responses [149, 153–155]. This sequence has been conserved in most, if not all, genes that are directly inducible by IFN. Gel retardation experiments have shown that the ISRE forms complexes with both pre-existing and inducible cellular factors [155, 156]. The presence of a factor that resulted in one of these complexes, called ISGF-3 (interferon-stimulated gene factor 3), correlated well with the induction of gene expression, suggesting that it represented a primary transcriptional activator [155, 157]. Clues as to how ISGF-3 was activated came from experiments showing that the factor first appeared in the cytoplasm of IFN-α-treated cells, then accumulated in the nucleus, and required at least two distinct components to form the active complex [158, 159]. One of these components, termed ISGF-3γ (because it accumulated in IFN-γ-treated cells), was distinguished by its sensitivity to N-ethylmaleimide [NEM]. The other, which accumulated in IFN-α-treated cells, was termed ISGF3α, and its activity was NEM-resistant. These two components combined stoichiometrically to form a complex which then translocated to the nucleus [158]. The activation of this factor (also called the E factor) could be induced by the stimulation of nuclei-free cytoplasts, but not in nucleoplasts, with IFN-α [159]. Subsequent purification of ISGF-3 revealed that it was actually a complex of four distinct polypeptides: the original ISGF-3γ, which is a DNA-binding protein of Mr 48,000 daltons, and three proteins of 84, 91, and 113 kDa which together formed the ISGF-3α complex [160]. The cDNAs encoding all of these proteins have been cloned and sequenced. The 48-kDa ISGFγ displayed significant homology with the murine interferon regulatory factor proteins (IRF-1 and -2) and the interferon consensus sequence binding protein (ICSBP), all of which are capable of binding to a core sequence within the ISRE [161]. The 84-kDa and 91-kDa proteins are derived from the same gene by alternative splicing of the C-terminus [162]. The 113-kDa is a distinct gene product, but shows 42% homology to the 91, 84-kDa proteins. Other remarkable features of these proteins are the presence of heptad leucine repeats and a region conserved in all three proteins resembling SH2 and SH3 (src homology) domains found in tyrosine kinases and their substrates [163].

The availability of antibodies to the ISGF3 proteins allowed further examination of their functional responses to IFN stimulation. Several laboratories demonstrated that ISGF3α proteins were tyrosine phosphorylated upon stimulation of cells with IFN-α, and that these phosphorylations were required for the formation of the active transcription complex [164–167]. At the same time, one of these proteins, the 91-kDa factor, was shown to be tyrosine phosphorylated in response to IFN-γ [165, 168]. Utilizing subcellular fractions from homogenates of IFN-responsive cells, it was shown that IFN-α could be incubated with a plasma membrane-enriched fraction to activate ISGF3α, which could then be combined with a cytosolic source of ISGF3γ to form an active complex. This suggested that the latent

ISGF3α proteins were membrane-associated and that the activation event [i.e. phosphorylation] took place in the same membrane fraction [169]. Using this same cell-free system, David et al. [167] provided evidence that activation of ISGF3 required the sequential activity of a tyrosine phosphatase and a tyrosine kinase, ultimately leading to activation of the transcription complex. A tyrosine kinase that appears to mediate the phosphorylation of ISGF3 proteins in response to IFN-α has been identified as tyk2 (a non-receptor kinase of previously unknown function) by virtue of its ability to complement an IFN-α-unresponsive mutant cell line [170], although it is still not certain that this kinase is responsible for the direct phosphorylation of these substrates.

The revelations of the IFN-α signalling pathway have provided a new model for activation of gene expression in other systems, including responses to IFN-γ (see below) and many other polypeptide ligands such as cytokines and growth factors. These findings are remarkable because they have filled in many of the previously unknown gaps in our knowledge of how signals can be transmitted from receptors to inducible genes in a manner that maintains specificity while allowing for common responses such as the induction of antiviral or antiproliferative activities.

3.4   Interferon gamma intracellular signalling

In contrast to the early research on IFN-α signalling, evidence has been reported for the potential involvement of known second messengers in IFN-γ signalling. In murine macrophages, IFN-γ was shown to rapidly activate the Na+/H+ antiporter, and that inhibition of that antiporter with amiloride could block the expression of certain IFN-induced genes [171]. Several studies have implicated a role for Ca++ and/or protein kinase C in IFN-γ responses [172–177]. The purification and cDNA cloning of the IFN-γ receptor led to experiments showing that the receptor is phosphorylated on serine/threonine residues following its interaction with the ligand [178]. The degree of phosphorylation correlated with the biological response (HLA-DR induction) and was dependent on functionally active receptors [179]. However, these phosphorylation events occurred at a much slower rate than more recently defined signalling events that are involved in transcription factor activation (see below). It is still unclear what role, if any, the phosphorylation of the IFN-γ receptor plays in intracellular signalling. This issue may be clarified upon identification of the kinases involved in these reactions. The absolute conservation of a critical tyrosine residue at the carboxy-terminus of the IFN-γ receptor may be relevant to phosphorylation events in response to IFN-γ (see Section 3.2).

The elucidation of the activation pathway of IFN-α-induced gene expression has expanded into analogous systems, including the induction of genes by IFN-γ. Some, but not all, genes induced by IFN-γ are activated directly, without a requirement for protein synthesis. A subset of these genes are directly induced by both IFN-γ and IFN-α. The induction of these genes has been used to explore early signalling events following IFN-γ stimulation.

The guanylate-binding protein (GBP) is a cytoplasmic protein that is rapidly induced by IFN-γ and IFN-α [180, 181]. However, the promoter sequences required for induction by either IFN are not the same. The GBP promoter contains an ISRE, which appears to mediate the IFN-α response. An additional overlapping sequence, termed the gamma interferon activation site (GAS), was found to be required for the IFN-γ response [181]. An inducible factor which interacts with this sequence was detected using an exonuclease III protection assay and was called the gamma interferon activation factor (GAF) [182]. The GAF, located in the cytoplasm, was activated and bound to the GAS following IFN-γ stimulation of whole cells or cytoplasts [182]. Characterization of GAF revealed that it contains the 91-kDa protein previously identified as part of the ISGF3 complex. Furthermore, its activation involved tyrosine phosphorylation which was specific for the p91; other ISGF3α proteins were not phosphorylated in response to IFN-γ [168, 183]. Using a cell-free system [169], Igarashi et al. [168] presented evidence that GAF activation was mediated by tyrosine kinase activity, and that pre-treatment [before IFN-γ] of homogenates with tyrosine phosphatase inhibitors also prevented GAF complex formation. These data suggested that a tyrosine phosphatase/kinase cascade was active in this system similar to that described for IFN-α signalling [167].

The high affinity Fc receptor for IgG (FcγRI) is also directly induced by IFN-γ, but not IFN-α, treatment of cells of the myelomonocytic lineage. Analysis of its promoter also revealed a sequence that was necessary and sufficient for IFN-γ inducibility. This sequence was termed the IFN-γ response region (GRR); the GRR displayed significant homology to similar elements previously identified in other IFN-γ-inducible genes [184]. Factors binding to the GRR, termed FcRFγ (FcγRI DNA-binding factor, IFN-γ induced) were observed following IFN-γ stimulation of human monocytes, and the activation of these factors was inhibited by staurosporine and phenyl arsine oxide, implying a role for kinase and phosphatase activities in this response [185]. Further studies of the FcRFγ demonstrated that it was composed of at least two polypeptides, the ISGF3 p91 protein and an unidentified 43-kDa component. The activation of the complex occurred in a membrane-enriched fraction from mono-cytes. This complex was sensitive to tyrosine phosphatase treatment, and a tyrosine phosphatase inhibitor, sodium vanadate, was able to induce the activated complex in the absence of IFN-γ stimulation [186]. Vanadate also induced the expression of some IFN-γ-inducible genes, although the FcR gene was not one of them. In separate studies, an inducible GRR complex called GIRE-BP (gamma IFN response element binding protein) was characterized in different cell types. GIRE-BP complex formation was inhibited by an antibody to p91 of the ISGF3 family, implying that p91 is present in this complex. The GRR is not sufficient for tissue-specific expression of the FcR; that restriction is mediated by an upstream element termed the myeloid activating transcriptional element (MATE) [187]. More detailed analysis of the GRR element revealed a GAS-like core region which is critical, but not sufficient, for optimal inducibility. Examination of complexes that formed with this core region as well as the intact GRR indicated that the ISGF3 protein p91 was part of two types of interaction: 1) binding to the GAS core region, and 2) binding to the intact GRR. Both are induced specifically by IFN-γ [188].

3.5   Common elements in interferon signalling

The involvement of ISGF3 p91 in both IFN-γ and IFN-α signalling fore-shadowed its role in signalling for other stimuli. The tyrosine phosphory-lation and activation of p91 also occurred in response to epidermal growth factor (EGF), platelet-derived growth factor (PDGF), colony stimulating factor-1 (CSF-1), and interleukin-10 (IL-10) [189–192]. In monocytes and basophils, IFN-γ and IL-10 induced GRR-binding complexes that contained tyrosine-phosphorylated p91, while other cytokines (IL-3, IL-5, GM-CSF) induced GRR complexes containing an undefined 80-kDa protein (also tyrosine-phosphorylated). Only the stimuli that induced p91 activation also induced the appearance of FcγRI mRNA [189]. Tyrosine-phosphorylated p91 also bound to the sis-inducible element [SIE] of the c-fos promoter in response to both IFN-γ and growth factors [190, 191]. Sadowski et al. [192] distinguished three complexes with the SIE of the c-fos promoter (SIF-A, B, and C). SIF-A lacked p91, SIF-C was identified as GAF or p91 alone, and SIF-B contained p91 in combination with other unknown factors. These experiments addressed the issue of specificity by showing that different stimuli (IFN-γ, EGF, IL-6) preferentially induce different complexes, although many of these complexes bind to the same or similar promoter/enhancer sites.

A new nomenclature has been proposed for these transcription factors. p91 is now referred to as Stat91 (signal transducer and activator of transcription). Peptide mapping demonstrated that a single tyrosine residue was phosphorylated on Stat91 (Tyr^{701}), and that this phosphorylation was required for the nuclear localization and transcriptional induction activities of Stat91. Although its truncated form, Stat84, was also phosphorylated and bound to DNA, Stat84 did not mediate transcriptional induction [193]. A wealth of evidence has supported the requirement for tyrosine phosphorylation of transcription factors such as Stat91 for their translocation and activity. Recently, evidence was presented for the existence of a nuclear tyrosine phosphatase which acts to de-activate these factors and results in the decline of transcription of previously induced genes [194]. Recent work has shown that the tyrosine phosphorylation of Stat91 results in its dimerization via SH2-phosphotyrosine interactions, and that the dimeric form is what binds to DNA promoter elements [195].

The tyrosine kinase involved in the selective phosphorylation of Stat91 in response to IFN-γ has not been definitively identified. However, attention has been focussed on other members of the non-receptor tyrosine kinase family to which Tyk2 belongs [196]. The development of mutant cell lines that have lost responsiveness to IFNs has been invaluable in establishing a role for these kinases in IFN signalling [reviewed in 197]. A cell line defective in its response to IFN-γ (but which responds normally to IFN-α) was complemented by the expression of the tyrosine kinase JAK2. In addition, JAK2 was tyrosine phosphorylated and activated in normal cells in response to IFN-γ, but not IFN-α [198].

Another cell line which was defective in responses to both IFN-α and IFN-γ was shown to lack the JAK1 kinase, and could be complemented by transfection with the JAK1 gene [199, 200]. These results, combined with earlier results on IFN-α signalling [170], indicated that the three known tyrosine kinases of the JAK family are all involved in IFN responses: JAK 1 was required for both IFN-α and IFN-γ, Tyk2 was required only for IFN-α, and JAK2 was required only for IFN-γ signal transduction. It is not yet known whether the JAK family kinases are directly responsible for phosphorylating the ISGF3 factors following IFN stimulation or are simply part of a signalling cascade that results in the relevant phosphorylations. In an attempt to address these questions, Shuai et al. [201] examined patterns of phosphorylation in response to IFN-α, -γ, and EGF. All three stimuli resulted in the phosphorylation of Stat91 (at Tyr^{701}) and all three induced the phosphorylation of JAK1, even though other kinases were independently phosphorylated, leading to the hypothesis that JAK1 was responsible for the Stat91 phosphorylation on Tyr^{701}. Further support for this hypothesis came from the observation that over-expression of JAK1 resulted in Stat91 activation, although JAK2 over-expression also had the same effect. The issue is complicated by the fact that these kinases were able to trans-activate each other [202]. Therefore, it is still uncertain which of these enzymes, if any, represents the physiological kinase for Stat91. The definitive identification of the substrates for these kinases will clarify their functional roles in responses to IFNs and other ligands known to activate them (the list of which is getting longer every day). The current model for elements involved in early interferon signalling events and and activation of transcription factors is summarized in Figure 2 (reprinted from [146]).

Gene promoters have recently been described which contain GAS-like elements and respond to both IFN-α and IFN-γ by the interaction of Stat91 with the same element. Interestingly, one of these genes is the interferon regulatory factor (IRF-1 or ISGF2), whose involvement in IFN and IFN-stimulated gene expression is still unclear, but plays a potentially important role in cellular growth regulation [203]. Common elements also may be involved in repression of transcription by IFN-α and IFN-γ. Both interferon regulatory factor 2 (IRF-2) and the interferon consensus sequence-binding protein (ICSBP) repressed transcription of a reporter driven by the MHC class I promoter acting through indistinguishable sites [204]. The ICSBP, however, is more tissue-restricted in its expression than IRF-2, which may be pertinent for its *in vivo* role.

4   Conclusions

The recent explosion of information regarding the regulation of IFN and IFN-induced genes has led to new insights about intracellular signalling that have rapidly expanded into other systems of gene regulation. The IFN system has provided a model system for the study of cytokines and the regulation of gene expression. Understanding the stringent controls governing the production and action of cytokines is critical to our ability to utilize these agents effectively in the clinic. One hope for the future will be to develop ways to affect the endogenous expression of these potent mediators rather than administering them systemically in large doses in an effort to induce some biological effect. This can only be accomplished by the development of detailed knowledge about how cytokine networks interact and how the expression of physiologically important genes is regulated at every possible level.

We have come a long way in our understanding of factors affecting IFN production and action, as well as interferon structure-function relationships. The identification of DNA and RNA sequence elements that are crucial for positive and negative gene regulation was quickly followed by the detailed characterization of transcription factors and intracellular signal transduction pathways that are responsible for the cascade of effects that IFNs induce. Not surprisingly, as is so often the case in basic science research, we are left with more questions than answers as we gather more information about these intracellular events. For example, why has nature provided us, paradoxically, with over twenty different variations of IFN-α, while using a single intracellular factor such as Stat91 in responses to so many different stimuli? There are many levels at which potential therapeutic intervention could occur that have not been explored due to our lack of knowledge about IFN regulation specifically and cytokine regulation in general. However, the foundation has been laid for future investigation that should ultimately lead to a more complete understanding of how these important molecules perform their appropriate functions.

5   Notes added in proof

Following submission of this manuscript, numerous further contributions to the field appeared in publication. Additional members of the signal transducers and activators of transcription (STAT) family have been identified [205]. Under the current proposed nomenclature, the original Stat91 and Stat84 of the ISGF3-α complex are called Stat1α and Stat1β, respectively; Stat113 becomes Stat2. Stat3 is activated by EGF or IL-6, but not IFN-γ [205, 206], and Stat4 has no known function [205, 207]. Improta, et al. [208] have shown that the phosphorylation of Stat113 (Stat2) occurs independently of Stat91 (Stat1α) phosphorylation, but appears to depend upon Stat91 for its transport into the nucleus. They had also previously shown that Stat91 and Stat84 are interchangeable for transcriptional function [209].

An additional, novel receptor for IFN-α,β has been cloned by Novick, et al. [210] which interacts with several IFN-αs and IFN-β. This receptor was cloned following its identification as a soluble receptor in human serum and urine [211]. The receptor protein is a 331-amino acid which exists as a disulfide-linked homodimer of 51 kD subunits, and is physically associated with the JAK1 kinase [210].

References

1   A. Isaacs and J. Lindenmann: Proc. R. Soc. Lond. (Biol) *147*, 258 (1957).
2   E. F. Wheelock: Science *149*, 310 (1965).
3   J. S. Youngner and S. B. Salvin: J. Immunol. *111*, 1914 (1973).
4   E. A. Havell, B. Berman, C. Ogburn, K. Berg, K. Paucker, and J. Vilcek: Proc. Natl. Acad. Sci. USA *72*, 2185 (1975).
5   Interferon Nomenclature. Nature *286*, 110 (1980).
6   C. Weissmann and H. Weber: Prog. Nucl. Acid Res. Mol. Biol. *33*, 251 (1986).
7   Nomenclature of the Human Interferon Genes. J. Interferon Res. *13*, 243 (1993).
8   J. Vilcek in: Peptide Growth Factors and Their Receptors. Vol II. M. Sporn and A. B. Roberts, Eds. Springer-Verlag, Berlin, Germany 1990, p. 3.
9   E. DeMaeyer and J. DeMaeyer-Guignard, Eds.: Interferons and Other Regulatory Cytokines. Wiley, New York, 1988.
10   S. Pestka, J. A. Langer, K. C. Zoon, and C. E. Samuel: Ann. Rev. Biochem. *56*, 727 (1987).
11   S. Baron, S. K. Tyring, W. R. Fleischmann, and others: JAMA *266*, 1375 (1991).
12   W. N. Katkov and J. L. Dienstag: Semin. Liver Dis. *11*, 165 (1991).
13   R. T. Dorr: Drugs *45*, 177 (1993).
14   J. U. Gutterman: Proc. Natl. Acad. Sci. USA *91*, 1198 (1994).
15   R. P. Perrillo, E. R. Schiff, G. L. Davis, and others: N. Engl. J. Med. *323*, 295 (1990).
16   A. M. Di Bisceglie, P. Martin, C. Kassianides, M. Lisker-Melman, L. Murray, et al.: New Engl. J. Med. *321*, 1506 (1989).
17   G. L. Davis, L. A. Balart, E. R. Schiff, K. Lindsay, H. C. Bodenheimer, Jr., R. P. Perillo, W. Carey, I. M. Jacobson, J. Payne, J. L. Dienstag, D. H. VanThiel, G. Tamburro, J. Lefkowitch, J. Albrecht, C. Meschievitz, T. J. Ortego, A. Gibas, and the Hepatitis Interventional Therapy Group: N. Engl. J. Med. *321*, 1501 (1989).
18   R. C. Reichman, D. Oakes, W. Bonnez, et al.: Ann. Intern. Med. *108*, 675 (1988).
19   R. C. Reichman, D. Oakes, W. Bonnez, et al.: J. Infect. Dis. *162*, 1270 (1 990).
20   S. E. Krown in: Biologic therapy of cancer, V. T. DeVita, S. Hellman, and S. A. Rosenberg, Eds. J. B. Lippincott, Philadelphia, 1991, p. 346.
21   R. A. B. Ezekowitz, S. H. Orkin, and P. E. Newberger: J. Clin. Invest. *80*, 1009 (1987).
22   J. M. G. Sechler, H. L. Malech, C. J. White, and J. I. Gallin: Proc. Natl. Acad. Sci. USA *85*, 4874 (1988).
23   International Chronic Granulomatous Disease Cooperative Study Group: New Engl. J. Med. *324*, 509 (1991).
24   H. S. Panitch and C. T. Bever, Jr.: J. Neuroimmunol. 46, 155 (1993).

25   D. W. Paty, D. K. Li, the UBC MS/MRI Study Group, and the IFNB Multiple Sclerosis
      Study Group: Neurology *43*, 662 (1993).
26   The IFNB Multiple Sclerosis Study Group: Neurology *43*, 655 (1993).
27   M. Aguet, Z. Dembic, and G. Merlin: Cell *55*, 273 (1988).
28   G. Uzé, G. Lutfalla, and I. Gresser: Cell *60*, 225 (1990).
29   J. Cross and R. Roberts: Proc. Natl. Acad. Sci. USA *88*, 3817 (1991).
30   R. Roberts, J. Cross, and D. Leaman: J. Interferon Res. *11*, S66 (1991).
31   K. C. Zoon, D. Miller, J. Bekisz, D. zur Nedden, J. C. Enterline, N. Y. Nguyen, and
      R.-Q. Hu: J. Biol. Chem. *267*, 15210 (1992).
32   K. C. Zoon, D. L. zur Nedden, J. C. Enterline, J. F. Manischewitz, D. R. Dyer, R. A.
      Boykins, J. Bekisz, and T. L. Gerrard in: The Biology of the Interferon System 1986,
      K. Cantell and H. Schellekens, Eds. Martinus Nijhoff, Dordrecht, The Netherlands,
      1987, p.567.
33   R.-Q. Hu, Y. Gan, J. Liu, D. Miller, and K. C. Zoon: J. Biol. Chem. *268*, 12591 (1993).
34   D. S. A. Webb, D. L. zur Nedden, D. M. Miller, K. C. Zoon, and T. L. Gerrard: Cell.
      Immunol. *124*, 158 (1989).
35   L. A. Clavell and M. A. Bratt: J. Virol. *8*, 500 (1971).
36   M. H. T. Lai and K. Joklik: Virology *51*, 191 (1973).
37   J. Hiscott, J. Ryals, P. Dierks, V. Hofmann, and C. Weissmann: Philos. Trans. R. Soc.
      Lond. (Biol) *307,* 217 (1984).
38   J. Hiscott, K. Cantell, and C. Weissmann: Nucl. Acids Res. *12*, 3727 (1984).
39   E. A. Havell, Y. K. Yip, and J. Vilcek: J. Gen. Virol. *38*, 51 (1978).
40   T. G. Hayes, Y. K. Yip, and J. Vilcek: Virology *98,* 351 (1979).
41   G. Allen and K. H. Fantes: Nature *287*, 408 (1980).
42   M. G. Tovey, M. Streuli, I. Gresser, J. Gugenheim, B. Blanchard, J. Guymarho,
      F. Vignaux, and M. Gigou: Proc. Natl. Acad. Sci. USA *84,* 5038 (1987).
43   U. Weidle and C. Weissmann: Nature *303*, 442 (1983).
44   N. Tanaka and T. Taniguchi: Adv. Immunol. *52,* 263 (1992).
45   H. Ragg and C. Weissmann: Nature *303,* 439 (1983).
46   S. Ohno and T. Taniguchi: Nucl. Acids Res. *11*, 5403 (1983).
47   K. A. Zinn, D. Dimaio, and T. Maniatis: Cell *34*, 865 (1983).
48   J. Ryals, P. Dierks, H. Ragg, and C. Weissmann: Cell *41*, 497 (1985).
49   T. Fujita, S. Ohno, H. Yasumitsu, and T. Taniguchi: Cell *41*, 489 (1985).
50   S. Goodbourne, K. Zinn, and T. Maniatis: Cell *41*, 509 (1985).
51   M. J. Lenardo, C.-M. Fan, T. Maniatis, and D. Baltimore: Cell *57*, 287 (1989).
52   K. V. Visvanathan and S. Goodbourne: EMBO J. *8,* 1129 (1989).
53   T. Fujita, M. Miyamoto, Y. Kimura, J. Hammer, and T. Taniguchi: Nucl. Acids Res.
      17, 3335 (1989).
54   J. Hiscott, D. Alper, L. Cohen, J. F. LeBlanc, L. Sportza, A. Wong, and S. Xanthoudakis:
      J. Virol. *63*, 2557 (1989).
55   D. Kuhl, J. de la Fuente, M. Chaturvedi, S. Parimoo, J. Ryals, F. Meyer, and C.
      Weissmann: Cell *50,* 1057 (1987).
56   S. Goodbourne and T. Maniatis: Proc. Natl. Acad. Sci. USA *85*, 1447 (1988).
57   C.-M. Fan and T. Maniatis: EMBO J. *8,* 101 (1989).
58   T. Maniatis, L. A. Whittemore, W. Du, C.-M. Fan, A. D. Keller, V. J. Palombella, and
      D. N. Thanos in: Transcriptional Regulation, S. McKnight and K. Yamamoto, Eds.
      Cold Spring Harbor Laboratory Press, Cold Spring Harbor, New York (1992).

59   N. J. MacDonald, D. Kuhl, D. Maguire, D. Näf, P. Gallant, A. Goswamy, H. Hug, H.
      Büeler, M. Chaturvedi, J. de la Fuente, H. Ruffner, F. Meyer, and C. Weissmann: Cell
      60, 767 (1990).
60   T. Fujita, J. Sakakibara, Y. Sudo, M. Miyamoto, Y. Kimura, and T. Taniguchi: EMBO
      J. *7*, 3397 (1988).
61   M. Miyamoto, T. Fujita, Y. Kimura, M. Maruyama, H. Harada, Y. Sudo, T. Miyata, and
      T. Taniguchi: Cell *54*, 903 (1988).
62   H. Harada, T. Fujita, M. Miyamoto, Y. Kimura, M. Maruyama, A. Furia, T. Miyata,
      and T. Taniguchi: Cell *58*, 729 (1989).
63   T. Fujita, Y. Kimura, M. Miyamoto, E. L. Barsoumian, and T. Taniguchi: Nature *337*,
      270 (1989).
64   T. Fujita, L. F. L. Reis, N. Watanabe, Y. Kimura, T. Taniguchi, and J. Vilcek: Proc. Natl.
      Acad. Sci. USA *86*, 9936 (1989).
65   R. Pine, T. Decker, D. S. Kessler, D. E. Levy, and J. E. Darnell, Jr.: Mol. Cell. Biol.
      10, 2448 (1990).
66   S. T. Whiteside, K. V. Visvanathan, and S. Goodbourne: Nucl. Acids Res. *20*, 1531
      (1992).
67   T. Matsuyama, T. Kimura, M. Kitagawa, K. Pfeffer, T. Kawakami, N. Watanabe, T. M.
      Kündig, R. Amakawa, K. Kishihara, A. Wakeham, J. Potter, C. L. Furlonger, A.
      Narendran, H. Suzuki, P. S. Ohashi, C. J. Paige, T. Taniguchi, and T. W. Mak: Cell *75*,
      83 (1993).
68   L. Reis, H. Harada, J. D. Wolchok, T. Taniguchi, and J. Vilcek: EMBO J. *11*, 185 (1992).
69   D. Thanos and T. Maniatis: Cell *71*, 777 (1992).
70   W. Du and T. Maniatis: Proc. Natl. Acad. Sci. USA *89*, 2150 (1992).
71   A. D. Keller and T. Maniatis: Genes Dev. *5*, 868 (1991).
72   P. H. Driggers, D. L. Ennist, S. L. Gleason, W. H. Mak, M. S. Marks, B. Z. Levi, J. R.
      Flanagan, E. Appella, and K. Ozato: Proc. Natl. Acad. Sci. USA *87*, 3743 (1990).
73   V. J. Palombella and T. Maniatis: Mol. Cell. Biol. *12*, 3325 (1992).
74   N. Watanabe, J. Sakakibara, A. G. Hovanessian, T. Taniguchi, and T. Fujita: Nucl. Acids
      Res. *19*, 4421 (1991).
75   F. Bisat, N. B. K. Raj, and P. M. Pitha: Nucl. Acids Res. *16*, 6067 (1988).
76   W.-C. Au, Y. Su, N. B. K. Raj, and P. M. Pitha: J. Biol. Chem. *268*, 24032 (1993).
77   N. B. K. Raj and P. M. Pitha: Proc. Natl. Acad. Sci. USA *80*, 3923 (1983).
78   J. Vilcek, E. A. Havell, and M. Kohase: J. Infect. Dis. *133* Suppl., A22 (1976).
79   N. B. K. Raj and P. M. Pitha: Proc. Natl. Acad. Sci. USA *78*, 7426 (1981).
80   R. L. Cavalieri, E. A. Havell, J. Vilcek, and S. Pestka: Proc. Natl. Acad. Sci. USA *74*,
      4415 (1977).
81   P. B. Sehgal and I. Tamm: Virology *92*, 240 (1979).
82   L. A. Whittemore and T. Maniatis: Mol. Cell. Biol. *64*, 1329 (1990).
83   L. A. Whittemore and T. Maniatis: Proc. Natl. Acad. Sci. USA *87*, 7799 (1990).
84   M. van Heuvel, I. J. Bosveld, W. Luyten, J. Trapman, and E. C. Zwarthoff: Gene *45*,
      159 (1986).
85   K. Peppel and C. Baglioni: J. Biol. Chem. *266*, 6663 (1991).
86   G. Shaw and R. Kamen: Cell *46*, 659 (1986).
87   D. Caput, B. Beutler, K. Hartog, R. Thayer, S. Brown-Shimer, and A. Cerami: Proc.
      Natl. Acad. Sci. USA *83*, 1670 (1986).
88   V. Kruys, B. Beutler, and G. Huez: Enzyme *44*, 193 (1990).

89   N. B. K. Raj and P. M. Pitha: FASEB J. *7*, 702 (1993).

90   J. D. Mosca, P. M. Pitha, and G. S. Hayward: J. Virol. *66*, 3811 (1992).

91   M. P. Hayes and K. C. Zoon: Infect. Immun. *61*, 3222 (1993).

92   K. Peppel, J. M. Vinci, and C. Baglioni: J. Exp. Med. *173*, 349 (1991).

93   A. P. Lieberman, P. M. Pitha, and M. L. Shin: J. Biol. Chem. *267*, 2123 (1992).

94   A. B. Sachs: Cell *74*, 413 (1993).

95   P. R. Bohjanen, B. Petryniak, C. H. June, C. B. Thompson, and T. Lindsten: J. Biol. Chem. *267*, 6302 (1992).

96   H. A. Young and K. J. Hardy: Pharmacol. Ther. *45*, 137 (1990).

97   Y. Pang, Y. Norihisa, D. Benjamin, R. R. S. Kantor, and H. A. Young: Blood *80*, 724 (1992).

98   G. Trinchieri, M. Matsumoto-Kobayashi, S. C. Clark, J. Sheehra, L. London, and B. Perussia: J. Exp. Med. *160*, 1147 (1984).

99   K. Handa, R. Suzuki, H. Matsui, Y. Shimizu, and K. Kumagai: J. Immunol. *130*, 988 (1983).

100 H. Bhayani and R. Falcoff: Cell. Immunol. *94*, 536 (1985).

101 I. Anegón, M. C. Cuturi, G. Trinchieri, and B. Perussia: J. Exp. Med. *167*, 452 (1988).

102 S. Efrat, S. Pilo, and R. Kaempfer: Nature *297*, 236 (1982).

103 H. M. Johnson and B. A. Torres: Infect. Immun. *36*, 911 (1982).

104 H. M. Johnson, T. Vassollo, and B. A. Torres: J. Immunol. *134*, 967 (1985).

105 S. H. Chan, B. Perussia, J. W. Gupta, M. Kobayashi, M. Pospisil, H. A. Young, S. F. Wolf, D. Young, S. C. Clark, and G. Trinchieri: J. Exp. Med. *173*, 869 (1991).

106 K. J. Hardy and H. A. Young in: Interferon Principles and Medical Applications, S. Baron, D. H. Coppenhaver, F. Dianzani, W. R. Fleischmann, T. K. Hughs, Jr., G. R. Klimpel, D. W. Niesel, G. J. Stanton, and S. K. Tyring, Eds. Univ. Texas Medical Branch, Galveston, TX (1992), p. 47.

107 S. H. Chan, M. Kobayashi, D. Santoli, B. Perussia, and G. Trinchieri: J. Immunol. *148*, 92 (1992).

108 H. A. Young, K. L. Komschlies, V. Ciccarone, M. Beckwith, M. Rosenberg, N. A. Jenkins, N. G. Copeland, and S. K. Durum: J. Immunol. *143*, 2389 (1989).

109 K. J. Hardy, R. E. Peterlin, R. F. Atchison, and J. P. Stobo: Proc. Natl. Acad. Sci. USA *82*, 8173 (1985).

110 K. J. Hardy, B. Manger, M. Newton, and J. D. Stobo: J. Immunol. *138*, 2353 (1987).

111 A. Sica, T. H. Tan, N. Rice, M. Kretzschmar, P. Ghosh, and H. A. Young: Proc Natl. Acad. Sci. USA *89*, 1740 (1992).

112 V. C. Ciccarone, J. Chrivia, K. J. Hardy, and H. A. Young: J. Immunol. *144*, 725 (1990).

113 J. C. Chrivia, T. Wedrychowics, H. A. Young, and K. J. Hardy: J. Exp. Med. *172*, 661 (1990).

114 L. Penix, W. M. Weaver, Y. Pang, H. A. Young, and C. B. Wilson: J. Exp. Med. *178*, 1483 (1993).

115 G. Uzé, G. Lutfalla, and I. Gresser: Cell *60*, 225 (1990).

116 G. Merlin, E. Falcoff, and M. Aguet: J. Gen. Virol. *66*, 1149 (1985).

117 G. Lutfalla, K. Gardiner, D. Proudhon, E. Vielh, and G. Uzé: J. Biol. Chem. *267*, 2802 (1992).

118 S. Pellegrini, J. John, M. Shearer, I. M. Kerr, and G. R. Stark: Mol. Cell. Biol. *9*, 4605 (1989).

119 C. Vanden Broeke, and L. M. Pfeffer: J. Interferon Res. *8*, 803 (1988).

120   P. Eid and K. Mogensen: Biochem. Biophys. Acta *1034,* 114 (1990).
121   G. Uzé, G. Lutfalla, P. Eid, C. Maury, M.-T. Bandu, I. Gresser, and K. Mogensen: Eur. J. Immunol. *21,* 447 (1991).
122   P. Benoit, D. Maguire, I. Plavec, H. Kocher, M. Tovey, and F. Meyer: J. Immunol. *150,* 707 (1993).
123   G. Uzé, G. Lutfalla, M.-T. Bandu, D. Proudhon, and K. Mogensen: Proc. Natl. Acad. Sci. USA *89,* 4774 (1992).
124   E. Mouchel-Vielh, G. Lutfalla, K. E. Mogensen, and G. Uzé: FEBS Lett. *313,* 255 (1992).
125   O. R. Colamonici, F. D'Alessandro, M. O. Diaz, S. A. Gregory, L. M. Neckers, and R. Nordan: Proc. Natl. Acad. Sci. USA *87,* 7230 (1990).
126   L. C. Platanias and O. R. Colamonici: J. Biol. Chem. *267,* 24053 (1992).
127   O. R. Colamonici and P. Domanski: J. Biol. Chem. *268,* 10895 (1993).
128   G. E. Hannigan, D. R. Gewert, E. N. Fish, S. E. Read, and B. R. Williams: Biochem. Biophys. Res. Comm. *110,* 537 (1983).
129   V. Jung, A. Rashidbaigi, C. Jones, J. A. Tischfield, T. B. Shows, and S. Pestka: Proc. Natl. Acad. Sci. USA *84,* 4151 (1987).
130   A. Rashidbaigi, J. A. Langer, V. Jung, C. Jones, H. G. Morse, J. A. Tischfield, J. S. Trill, A. Kung, and S. Pestka: Proc. Natl. Acad. Sci. USA *83,* 384 (1986).
131   V. Jung, C. Jones, C. S. Kumar, S. Stefanos, S. O'Connell, and S. Pestka: J. Biol. Chem. *265,* 1827 (1990).
132   M. A. Farrar, J. Fernandez-Luna, and R. D. Schreiber: J. Biol. Chem. *266,* 19626 (1991).
133   V. C. Gibbs, S. R. Williams, P. W. Gray, R. D. Schreiber, D. Pennica, G. Rice, and D. V. Goeddel: Mol. Cell. Biol. *11,* 5860 (1991).
134   Y. Hibino, C. S. Kumar, T. M. Mariano, D. Lai, and S. Pestka: J. Biol. Chem. *267,* 3741 (1992).
135   S. Hemmi, G. Merlin, and M. Aguet: Proc. Natl. Acad. Sci. USA *89,* 2737 (1992).
136   J. R. Cook, V. Jung, B. Schwartz, P. Wang, and S. Pestka: Proc. Natl. Acad. Sci. USA *89,* 11317 (1992).
137   M. A. Farrar, J. D. Campbell, and R. D. Schreiber: Proc. Natl. Acad. Sci. USA *89,* 11706 (1992).
138   J. Soh, R. J. Donnelly, T. M. Mariano, J. R. Cook, B. Schwartz, and S. Pestka: Proc. Natl. Acad. Sci. USA *90,* 8737 (1993).
139   C. E. Samuel: Virology *183,* 1 (1991).
140   J. Soh, R. J. Donnelly, S. Kotenko, T. M. Mariano, J. R. Cook, N. Wang, S. Emanuel, B. Schwartz, T. Miki, and S. Pestka: Cell *76.* 793 (1994).
141   S. Hemmi, R. Böhni, G. Stark, F. DiMarco, and M. Aguet: Cell *76,* 803 (1994).
142   S. Huang, W. Hendriks, A. Althage, S. Hemmi, H. Bluethmann, R. Kamijo, J. Vilcek, R. M. Zinkernagel, and M. Aguet: Science *259,* 1742 (1993).
143   R. Kamijo, J. Le, D. Shapiro, E. A. Havell, S. Huang, M. Aguet, M. Bosland, and J. Vilcek: J. Exp. Med. *178,* 1435 (1993).
144   R. Kamijo, D. Shapiro, J. Le, S. Huang, M. Aguet, and J. Vilcek: Proc. Natl. Acad. Sci. USA *90,* 6626 (1993).
145   P. Staeheli: Adv. Virus Res. *38,* 147 (1990).
146   M. David: Pharmacol. Ther. *in press* (1994).

147 A. C. Larner, G. Jonak, Y.-S. E. Cheng, B. Korant, E. Knight, and J. E. Darnell, Jr.: Proc. Natl. Acad. Sci. USA *81*, 6733 (1984).
148 R. L. Friedman, S. P. Manly, M. McMahon, I. M. Kerr, and G. R. Stark: Cell *38*, 745 (1984).
149 R. L. Friedman and G. R. Stark: Nature *314*, 637 (1985).
150 A. C. Larner, A. Chaudhuri, and J. E. Darnell, Jr.: J. Biol. Chem. *261*, 453 (1986).
151 D. E. Levy, A. C. Larner, A. Chaudhuri, L. E. Babiss, and J. E. Darnell, Jr.: Proc. Natl. Acad. Sci. USA *83*, 8929 (1986).
152 I. Tamm, S. L. Lin, L. M. Pfeffer, and P. B. Sehgal: Interferon *9*, 13 (1987).
153 N. Reich, B. Evans, D. E. Levy, D. Fahey, E. Knight, and J. E. Darnell, Jr.: Proc. Natl. Acad. Sci. USA *84*, 6394 (1987).
154 P. Benech, M. Vigneron, D. Peretz, M. Revel, and J. Chebath: Mol. Cell. Biol. *7*, 4498 (1987).
155 D. E. Levy, D. S. Kessler, R. Pine, N. Reich, and J. E. Darnell, Jr.: Genes Dev. *2*, 383 (1988).
156 T. C. Dale, J. M. Rosen, M. J. Guille, A. R. Lewin, A. C. G. Porter, I. M. Kerr, and G. R. Stark: EMBO J. *8*, 831 (1989).
157 D. S. Kessler, R. Pine, L. M. Pfeffer, D. E. Levy, and J. E. Darnell, Jr.: EMBO J. *7*, 3779 (1988).
158 D. E. Levy, D. S. Kessler, R. Pine, and J. E. Darnell, Jr.: Genes Dev. *3*, 1362 (1989).
159 T. C. Dale, A. M. Ali Imam, I. M. Kerr, and G. R. Stark: Proc. Natl. Acad. Sci. USA *86*, 1203 (1989).
160 X.-Y. Fu, D. S. Kessler, S. A. Veals, D. E. Levy, and J. E. Darnell, Jr.: Proc. Natl. Acad. Sci. USA *87*, 8555 (1990).
161 S. A. Veals, C. Schindler, D. Leonard, X.-Y. Fu, R. Aebersold, J. E. Darnell, Jr., and D. E. Levy: Mol. Cell. Biol. *12*, 3315 (1992).
162 C. Schindler, X.-Y. Fu, T. Improta, R. H. Aebersold, and J. E. Darnell, Jr.: Proc. Natl. Acad. Sci. USA *89*, 7836 (1992).
163 X.-Y. Fu, C. Schindler, T. Improta, R. H. Aebersold, and J. E. Darnell, Jr.: Proc. Natl. Acad. Sci. USA *89*, 7840 (1992).
164 X.-Y. Fu: Cell *70*, 323 (1992).
165 C. Schindler, K. Shuai, V. R. Prezioso, and J. E. Darnell, Jr.: Science *257*, 809 (1992).
166 M. J. Gutch, C. Daly, and N. C. Reich: Proc. Natl. Acad. Sci. USA *89*, 11411 (1992).
167 M. David, G. Romero, Z.-Y. Zhang, J. E. Dixon, and A. C. Larner: J. Biol. Chem. *268*, 6593 (1993).
168 K. Igarashi, M. David, D. S. Finbloom, and A. C. Larner: Mol. Cell. Biol. *13*, 1634 (1993).
169 M. David and A. C. Larner: Science *257*, 813 (1992).
170 L. Velasquez, M. Fellous, G. R. Stark, and S. Pellegrini: Cell *70*, 313 (1992).
171 V. Prpic, S. Yu, F. Figueiredo, P. W. Hollenbach, G. Gawdi, B. Herman, R. J. Uhing, and D. O. Adams: Science *244*, 469 (1989).
172 H. M. Johnson and B. A. Torres: Proc. Natl. Acad. Sci. USA *82*, 5959 (1985).
173 T. A. Hamilton, D. L. Becton, S. D. Somers, P. W. Gray, and D. O. Adams: J. Biol. Chem. *260*, 1378 (1985).
174 A. Celada and R. D. Schreiber: J. Immunol. *137*, 2373 (1986).
175 S. D. Somers, J. E. Weiel, T. A. Hamilton, and D. O. Adams: J. Immunol. *136*, 4199 (1986).

176   D. Fan, M. Goldberg, and B. R. Bloom: Proc. Natl. Acad. Sci. USA *85*, 5122 (1988).

177   Y. Koide, Y. Ina, N. Nezu, and T. O. Yoshida: Proc. Natl. Acad. Sci. USA *85*, 3120 (1988).

178   C. Mao, G. Merlin, R. Ballotti, M. Metzler, and M. Aguet: J. Immunol. *145*, 4257 (1990).

179   G. K. Khurana Hershey, D. W. McCourt, and R. D. Schreiber: J. Biol. Chem. *265*, 17868 (1990).

180   T. Decker, D. J. Lew, Y. S. Cheng, D. E. Levy, and J. E. Darnell, Jr.: EMBO J. *8*, 2009 (1989).

181   D. J. Lew, T. Decker, I. Strehlow, and J. E. Darnell, Jr.: Mol. Cell. Biol. *11*, 182 (1991).

182   T. Decker, D. J. Lew, J. Mirkovitch, and J. E. Darnell, Jr.: EMBO J. *10*, 927 (1991).

183   K. Shuai, C. Schindler, V. R. Prezioso, and J. E. Darnell, Jr.: Science *258*, 1808 (1992).

184   R. N. Pearse, R. Feinman, and J. V. Ravetch: Proc. Natl. Acad. Sci. USA *88*, 11305 (1991).

185   K. C. Wilson and D. S. Finbloom: Proc. Natl. Acad. Sci. USA *89*, 11964 (1992).

186   K. Igarashi, M. David, A. C. Larner, and D. S. Finbloom: Mol. Cell. Biol. *13*, 3984 (1993).

187   C. Perez, J. Wietzerbin, and P. D. Benech: Mol. Cell. Biol. *13*, 2182 (1993).

188   R. N. Pearse, R. Feinman, K. Shuai, J. E. Darnell, Jr., and J. V. Ravetch: Proc. Natl. Acad. Sci. USA *90*, 4314 (1993).

189   A. C. Larner, M. David, G. M. Feldman, K. Igarashi, R. H. Hackett, D. S. A. Webb, S. M. Sweitzer, E. F. Petricoin III, and D. S. Finbloom: Science *261*, 1730 (1 993).

190   S. Ruff-Jamison, K. Chen, and S. Cohen: Science *261*, 1733 (1993).

191   O. Silvennoinen, C. Schindler, J. Schlessinger, and D. E. Levy: Science *261*, 1736 (1993).

192   H. B. Sadowski, K. Shuai, J. E. Darnell, Jr., and M. Z. Gilman: Science *261*, 1739 (1993).

193   K. Shuai, G. R. Stark, I. M. Kerr, and J. E. Darnell, Jr.: Science *261*, 1744 (1993).

194   M. David, P. M. Grimley, D. S. Finbloom, and A. C. Larner: Mol. Cell. Biol. *13*, 7515 (1993).

195   K. Shuai, C. M. Horvath, L. H. T. Huang, S. A. Qureshi, D. Cowburn, and J. E. Darnell, Jr.: Cell *76*, 821 (1994).

196   I. Firmbach-Kraft, M. Byers, T. Shows, R. Dalla-Favera, and J. J. Krolewski: Oncogene *5*, 1329 (1990).

197   T. Hunter: Nature *366*, 114 (1993).

198   D. Watling, D. Guschin, M. Müller, O. Silvennoinen, B. A. Witthuhn, F. W. Quelle, N. C. Rogers, C. Schindler, G. R. Stark, J. N. Ihle, and I. M. Kerr: Nature *366*, 166 (1993).

199   M. Müller, J. Briscoe, C. Laxton, D. Guschin, A. Ziemiecki, O. Silvennoinen, A. G. Harpur, G. Barbieri, B. A. Witthuhn, C. Schindler, S. Pellegrini, A. F. Wilks, J. N. Ihle, G. R. Stark, and I. M. Kerr: Nature *366*, 129 (1993).

200   J. E. Loh, C. Schindler, A. Ziemiecki, A. G. Harpur, A. F. Wilks, and R. A. Flavell: Mol. Cell. Biol. *14*, 2170 (1994).

201   K. Shuai, A. Ziemiecki, A. F. Wilks, A. G. Harpur, H. B. Sadowski, M. Z. Gilman, and J. E. Darnell, Jr.: Nature *366*, 580 (1993).

202   O. Silvennoinen, J. N. Ihle, J. Schlessinger, and D. E. Levy: Nature *366*, 583 (1 993).

203   R. Pine, A. Canova, and C. Schindler: EMBO J. *13*, 158 (1994).

204   N. Nelson, M. S. Marks, P. H. Driggers, and K. Ozato: Mol. Cell. Biol. *13*, 588 (1993).

205   Z. Zhong, Z. Wen, and J. E. Darnell, Jr.: Proc. Natl. Acad. Sci. USA *91*, 4806 (1994).
206   Z. Zhong, Z. Wen, and J. E. Darnell, Jr.: Science, in press (1994).
207   K. Yamamoto, F. W. Quelle, W. E. Thierfelder, B. L. Kreider, D. J. Gilbert, N. A. Jenkins, N. G. Copeland, O. Silvennoinen, and J. N. Ihle: Mol. Cell, Biol. *14*, in press (1994).
208   T. Improta, C. Schindler, C. M. Horvath, I. M. Kerr, G. R. Stark, and J. E. Darnell, Jr.: Proc. Natl. Acad. Sci USA *91*, 4776 (1994).
209   M. Muller, C. Laxton, J. Briscoe, C. Schindler, T. Improta, J. E. Darnell, Jr., G. R. Stark, and I. M. Kerr: EMBO J. *12*, 4221 (1993).
210   D. Novick, B. Cohen, and M. Rubinstein: Cell *77*, 391 (1994).
211   D. Novick, B. Cohen, and M. Rubinstein: FEBS Lett. *314*, 445 (1992).

The authors gratefully acknowledge Drs. Andrew C. Larner and David S. Finbloom for their critical review of the manuscript.

Progress in Drug Research, Vol. 43 (E. Jucker, Ed.)
© 1994 Birkhäuser Verlag, Basel (Switzerland)

Addendum

The formula CXXIV–CCXVII are to be inserted in the article "Natural products as anticancer agents" in PDR 42, page 116.

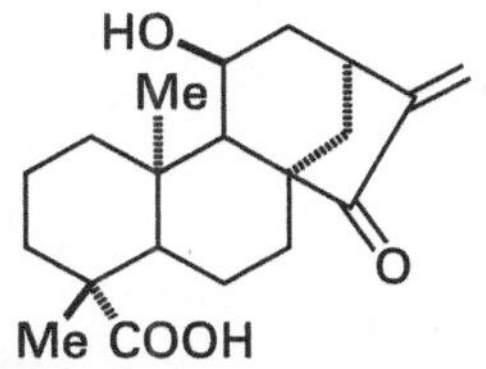

CXXIV

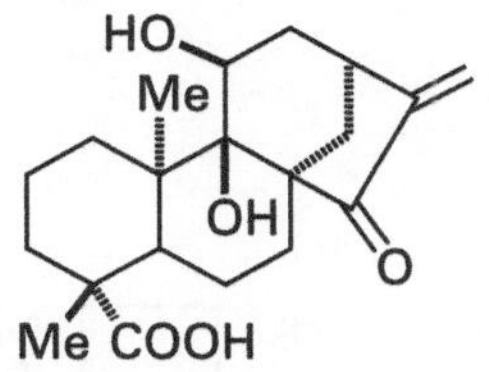

CXXV

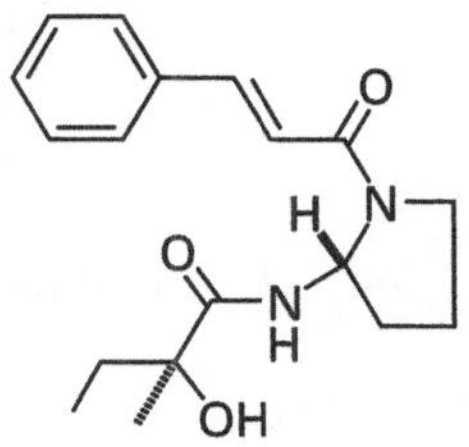

CXXVI

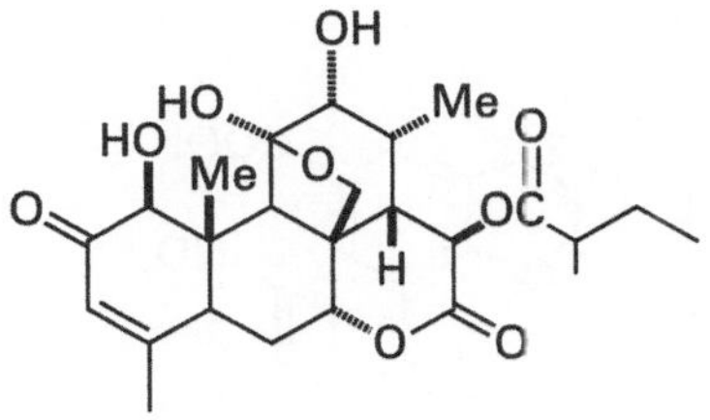

CXXVII

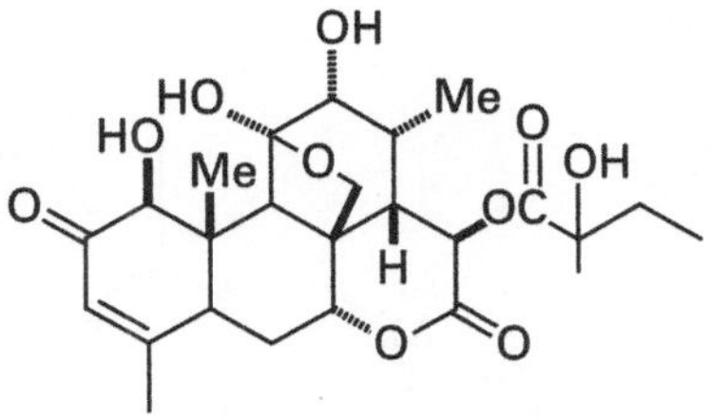

CXXVIII

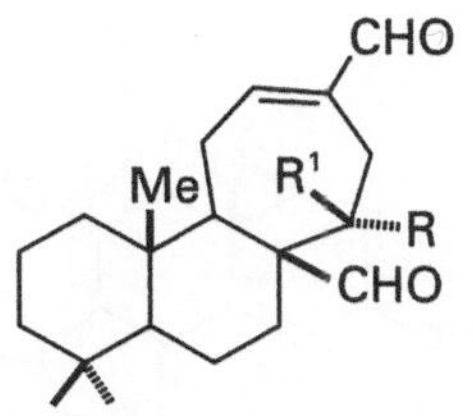

CXXIX R = OH, R^1 = H
CXXX   R = H, R^1 = OH

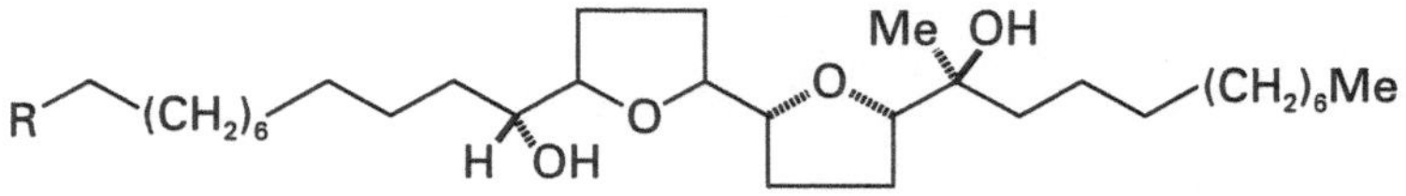

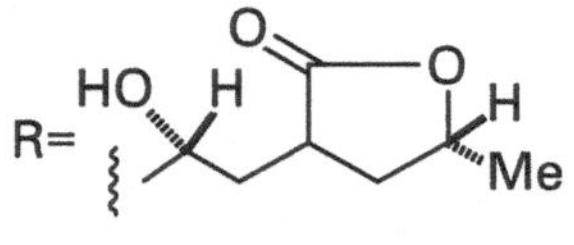

R—(CH₂)₆ ... (CH₂)₆Me structure with Me OH, H OH, O

R—$(CH_2)_6$ ... $(CH_2)_6Me$

Me OH
H OH

R= (HO H) ... Me

CXXXI

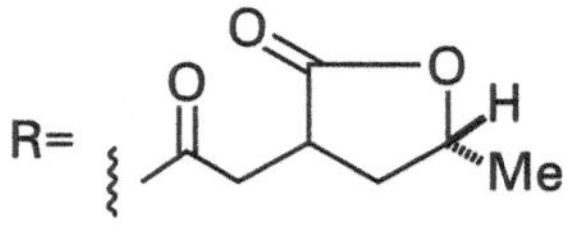

R= ... Me

CXXXXII

HO   OH   OH   OH   OH
$Me(CH_2)_mHC$ ... $CH(CH_2)_n CH(CH_2)_4 CH(CH_2)_3-CHCH_2$ ... Me

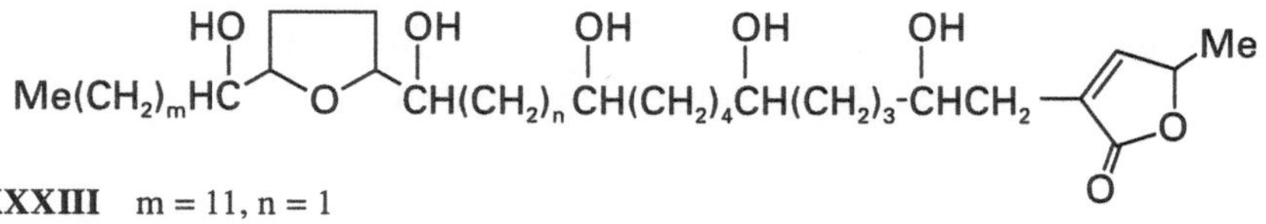

CXXXIII   m = 11, n = 1
CXXXIV   m = 9, n = 5

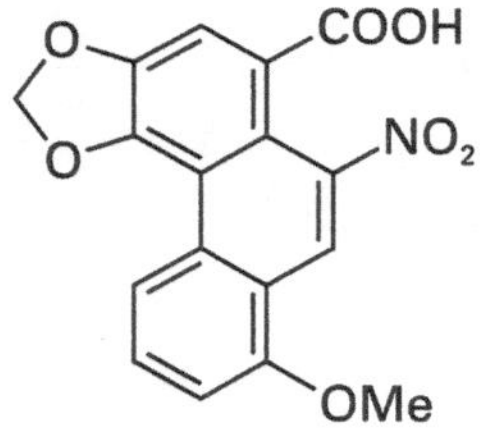

COOH
NO₂
OMe

CXXXV

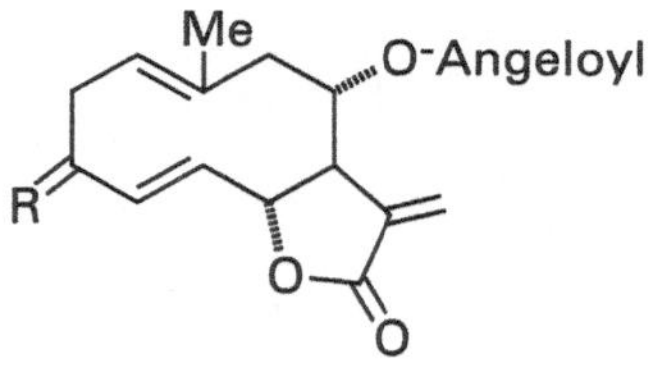

Me   O-Angeloyl
R

CXXXVI   R = OH, H
CXXXVII R = O

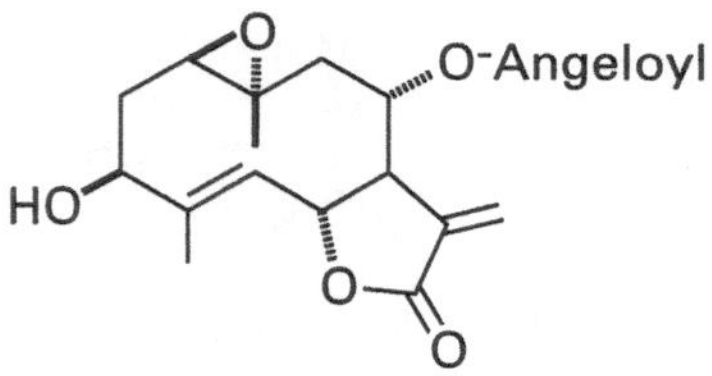

O-Angeloyl
HO

CXXXVIII

Me
Me
OH
R

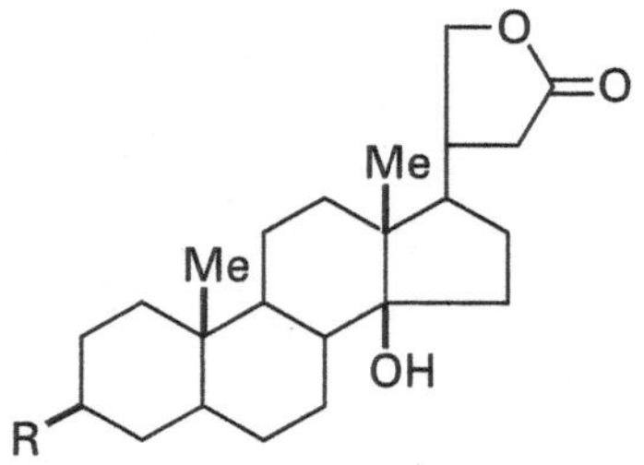

CXXXIX R = Glu(4—1)Glu

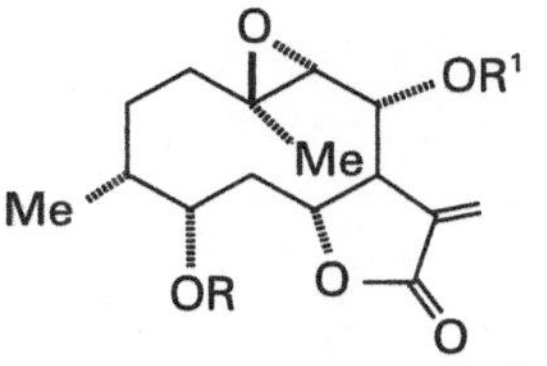

CXL   R = H, R^1 = COC(Me)=CHMe
CXLI   R = H, R^1 = COCH=CMe$_2$
CXLII R = Ac, R^1 = H

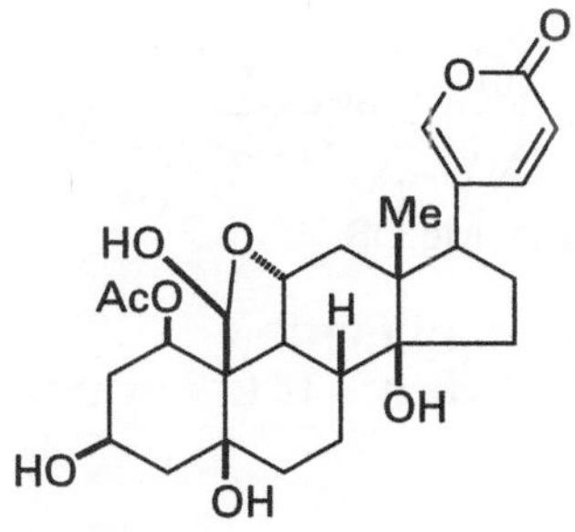

CXLIII

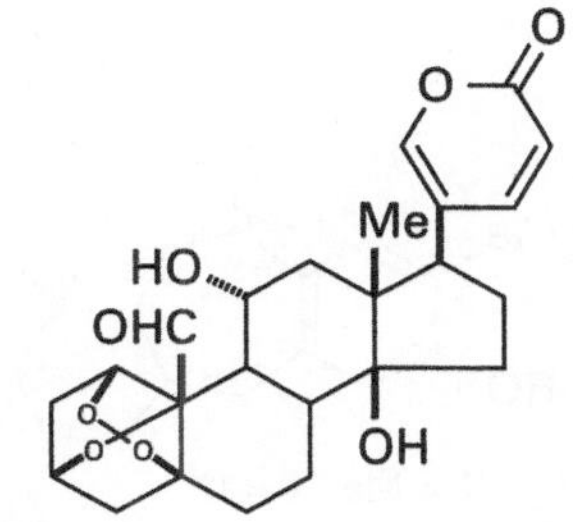

CXLIV

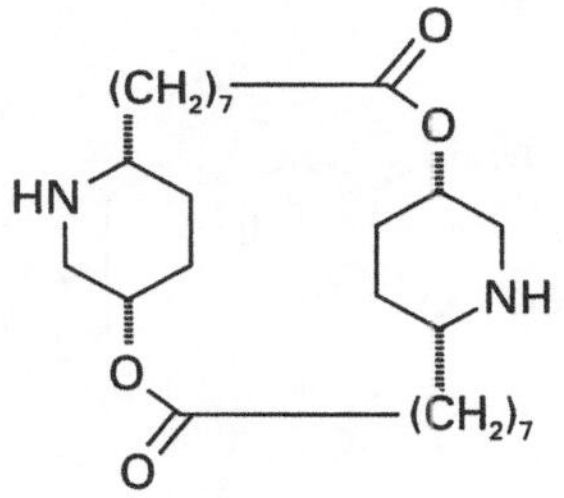

CXLV

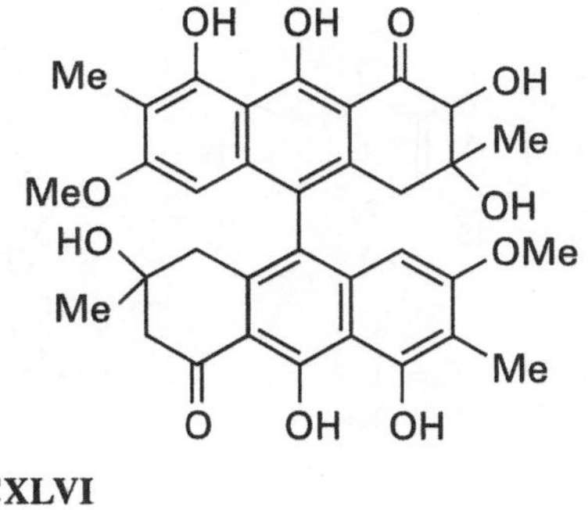

CXLVI

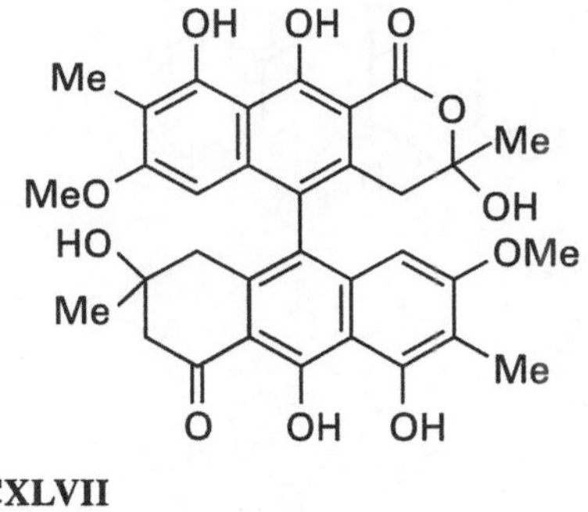

CXLVII

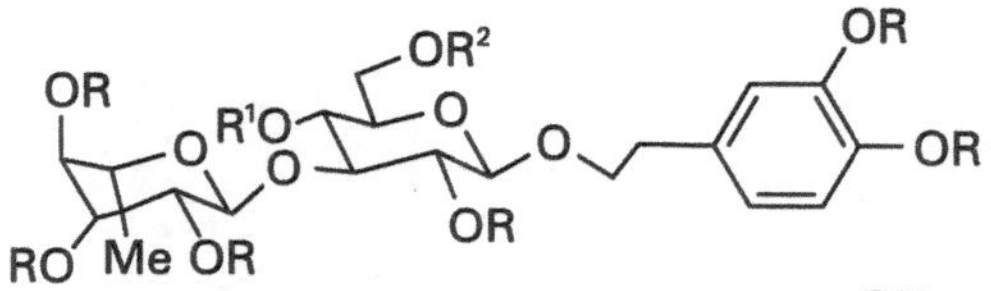

CXLVIII
R, R² = H, R¹ = COCH=CH—

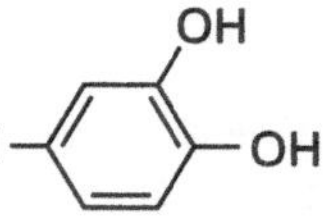

CXLIX
R, R¹ = H, R² = COCH=CH—

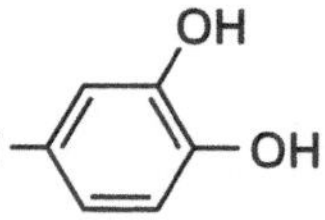

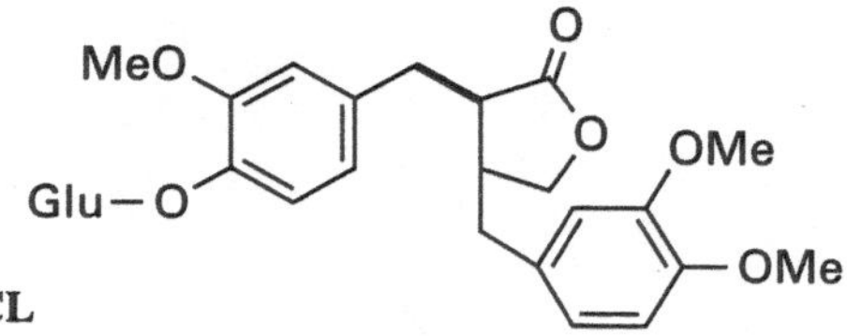

CL

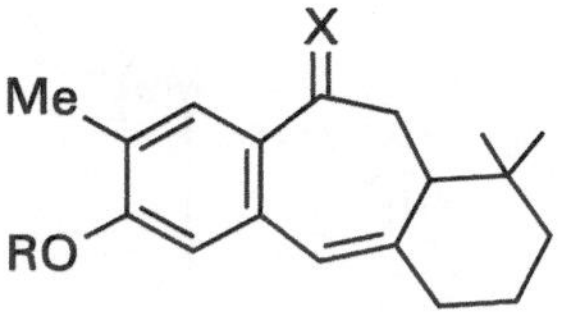

CLI   R = Me, X = O
CLII R = H, X = O
CLIII R = H, X = H,H

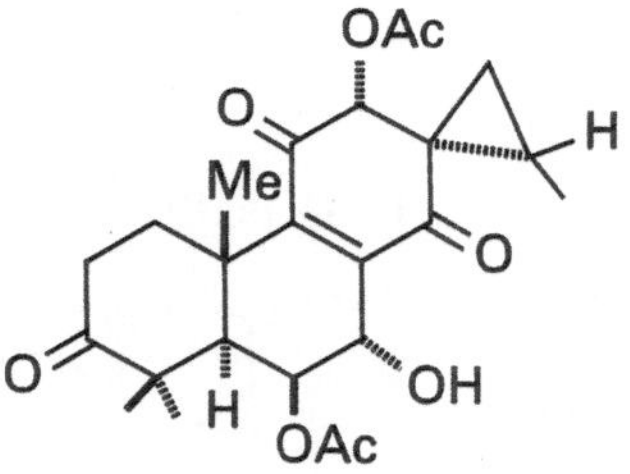

CLIV

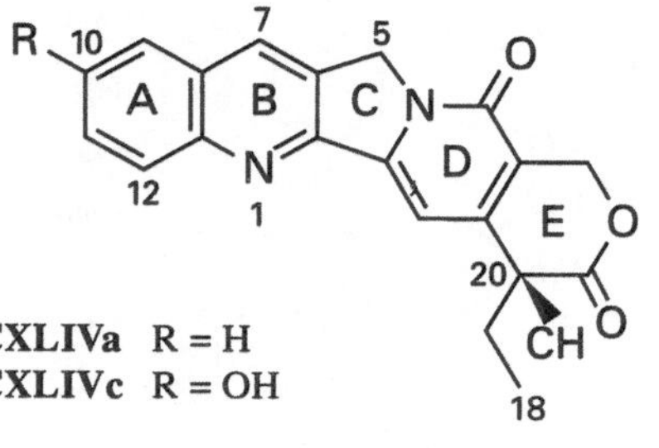

CXLIVa R = H
CXLIVc R = OH

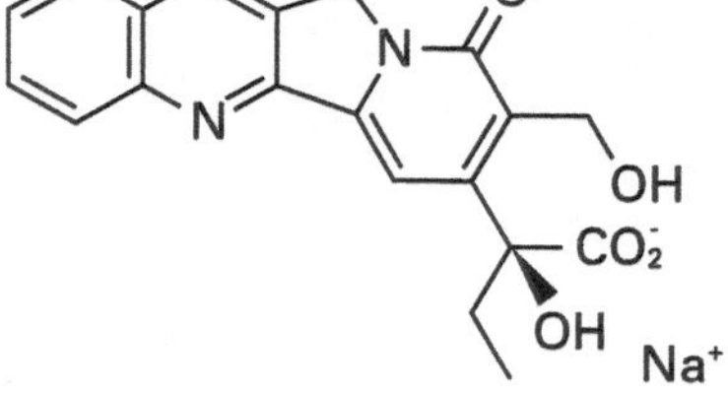

CXLIVb

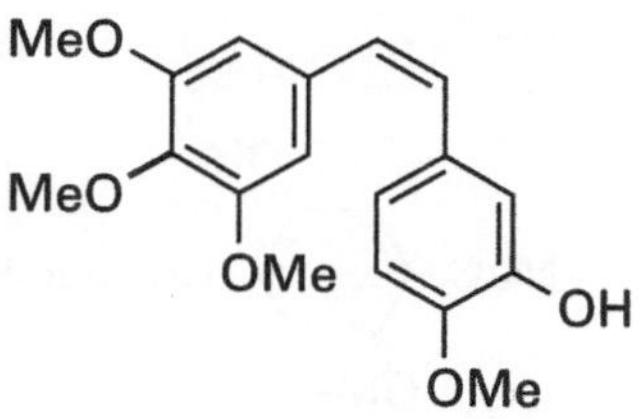

CLV

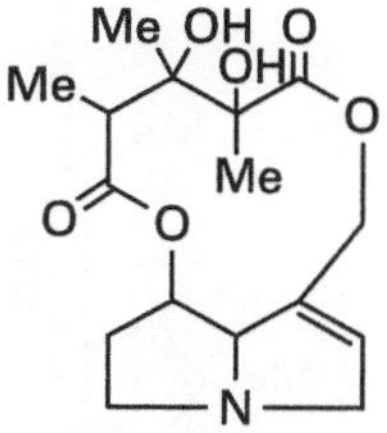

CLVI

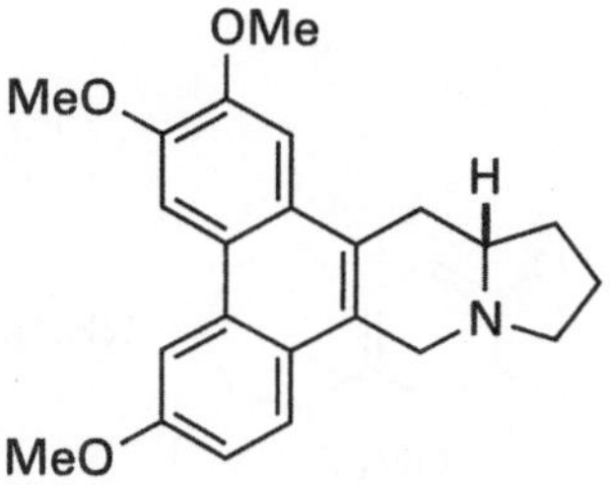

CLVII

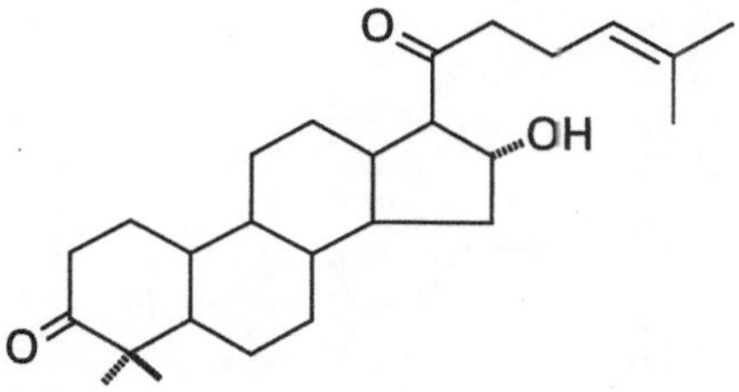

CLVIII

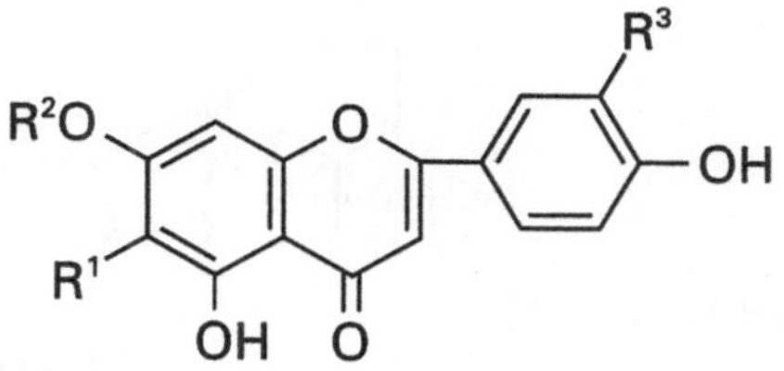

CLIX $R^1 = OMe, R^2 = Me, R^3 = H$
CLX $R^1 = R^2 = H, R^3 = OMe$

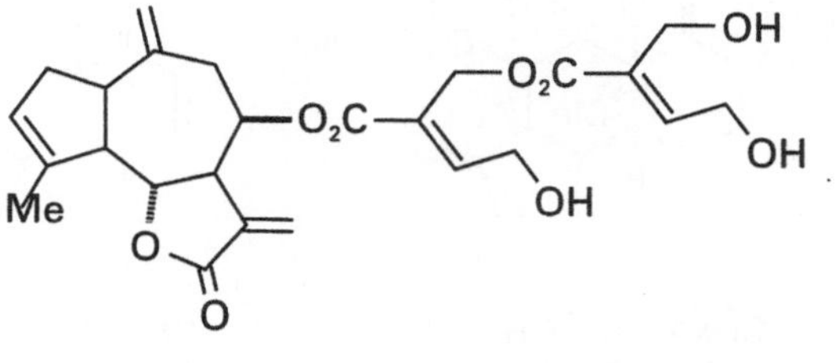

CLXI

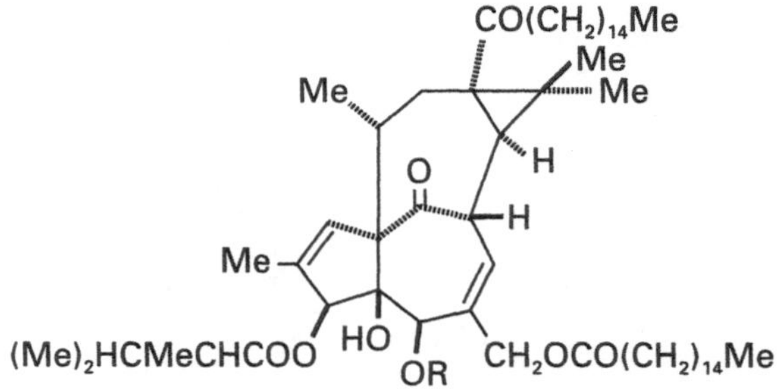

CLXII R = H
CLXIII R = Ac

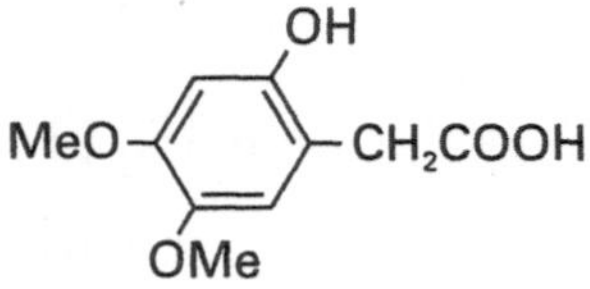

CLXV

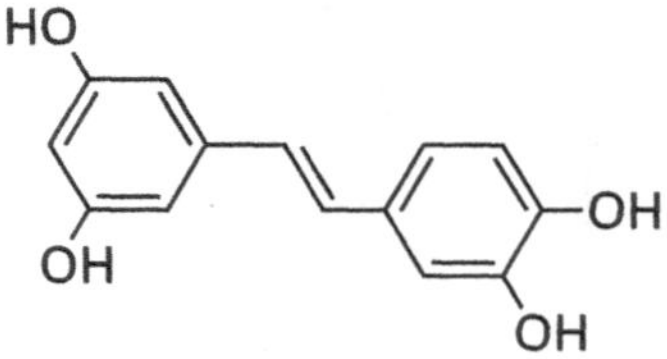

CLXIV

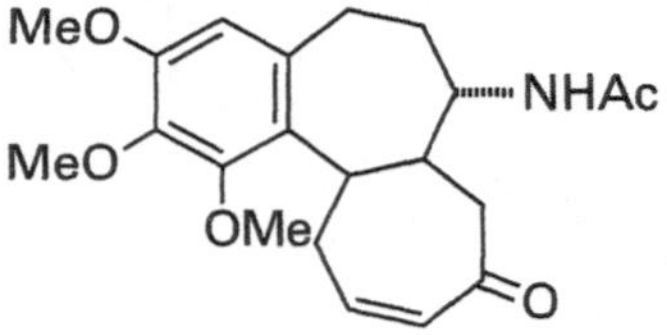

CLXVI

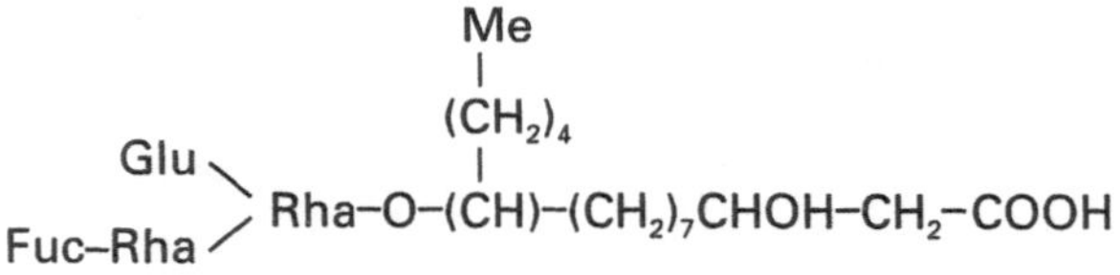

CLXVII

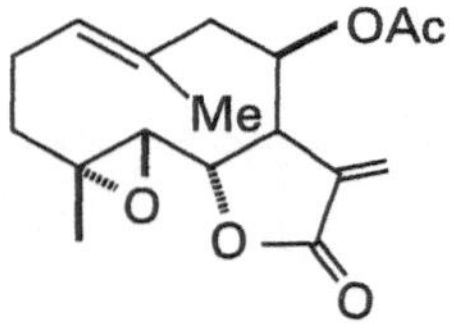

CLXVIII

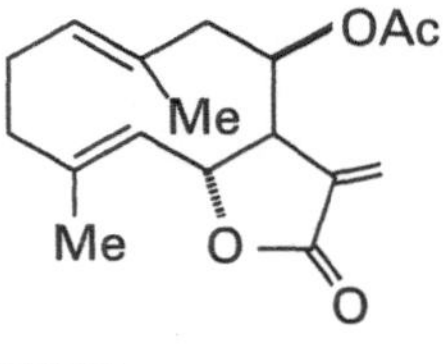

CLXIX

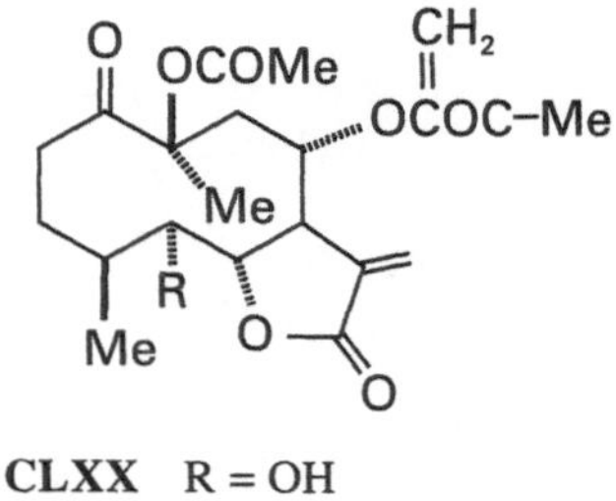

CLXX   R = OH
CLXXI R = H

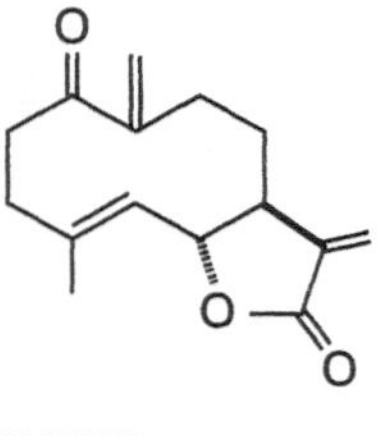

CLXXII

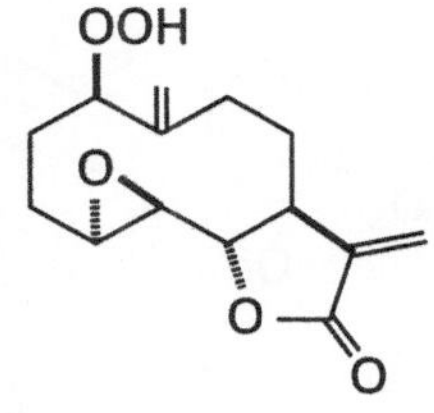

CLXXIII

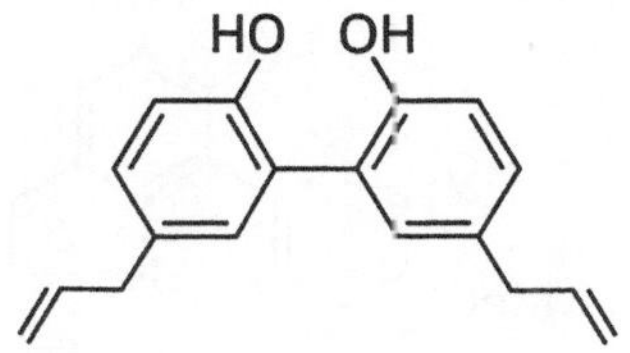

CLXXIV

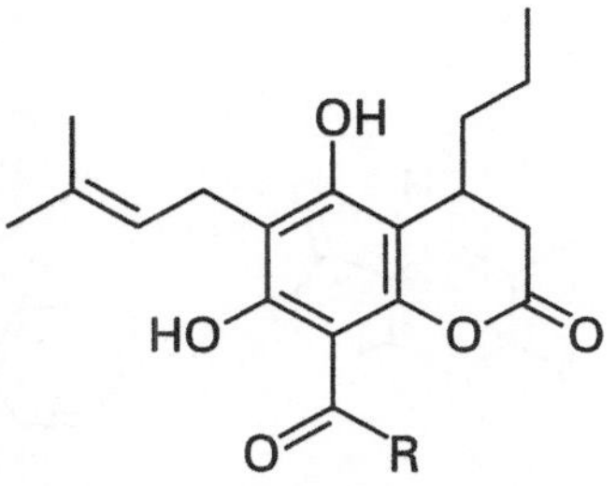

CLXXVI

CLXXV   R = Isobutyl

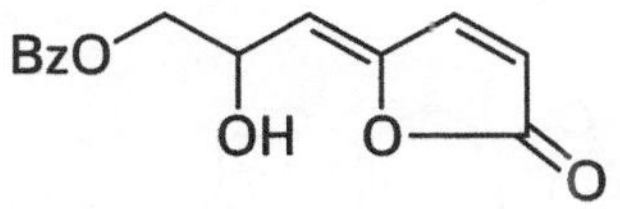

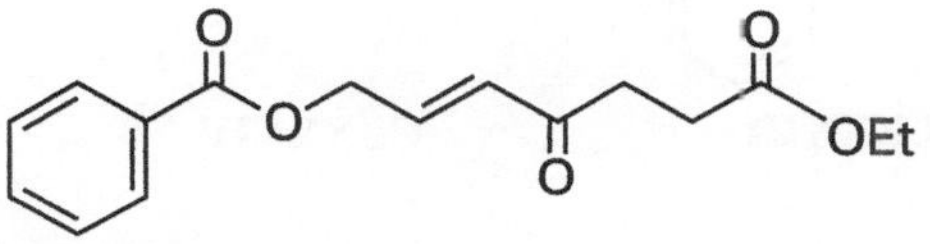

CLXXVII

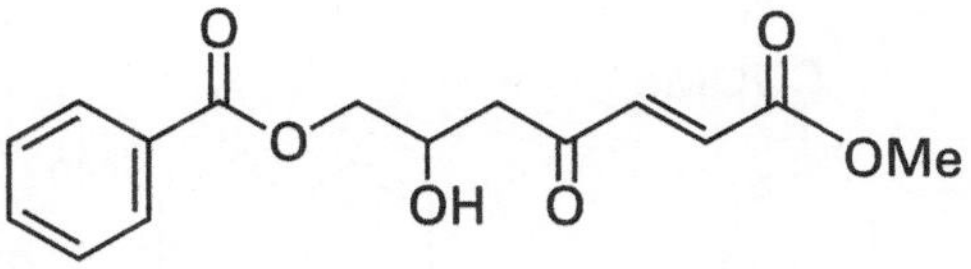

CLXXVIII

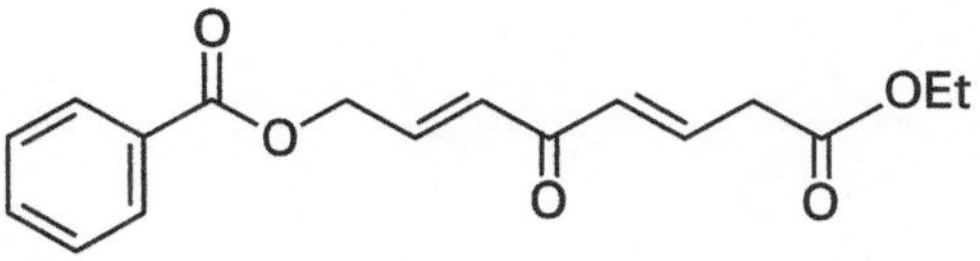

CLXXIX

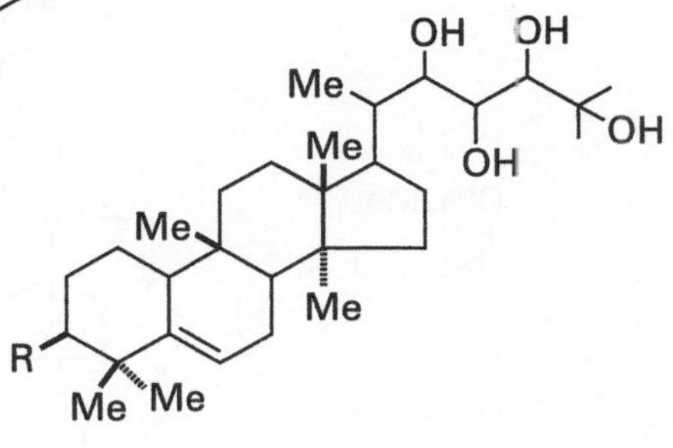

CLXXX

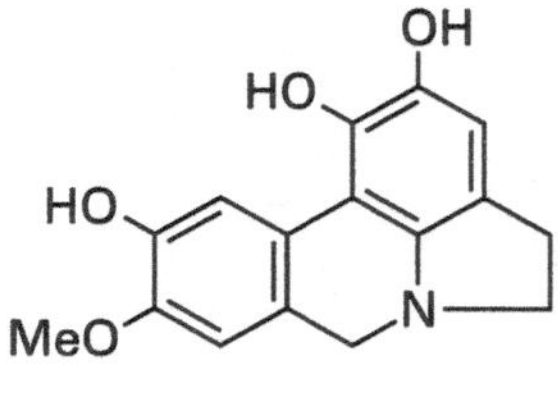

CLXXXI

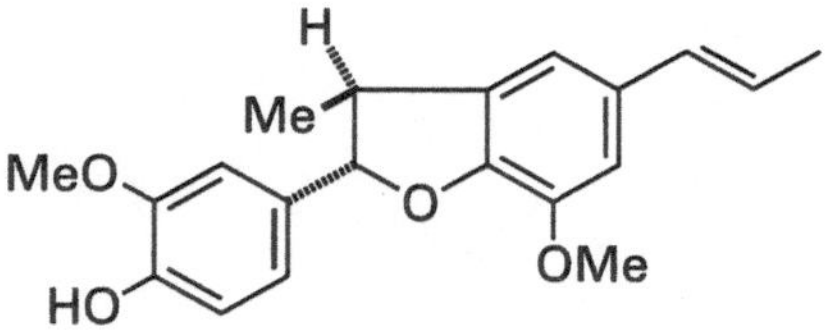

CLXXXII

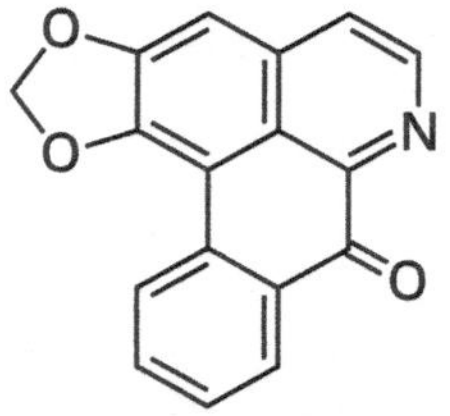

CLXXXIII

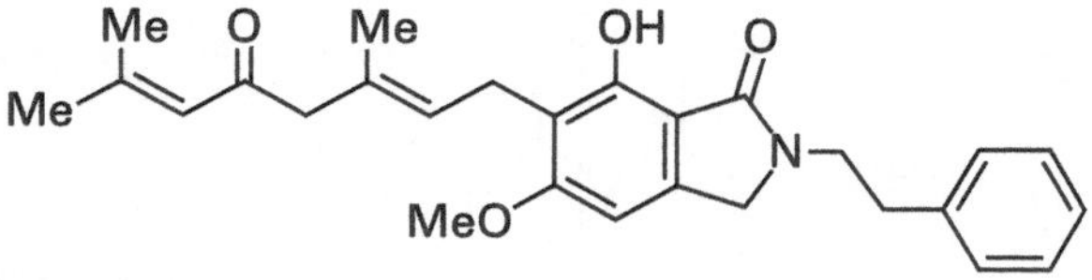

CLXXXIV

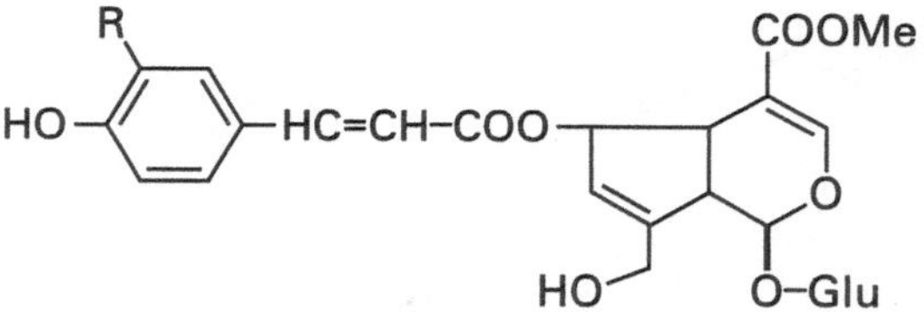

CLXXXV   R = H
CLXXXVI R = OMe

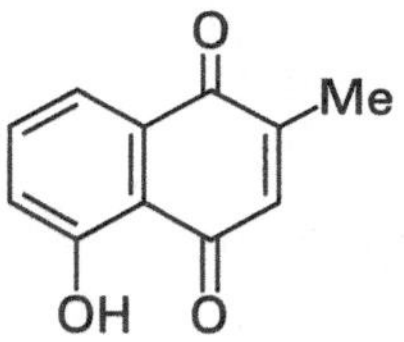

CLXXXVII

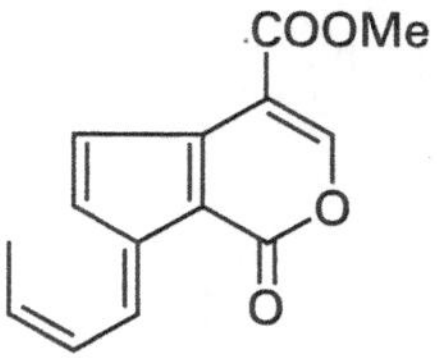

CLXXXVIII

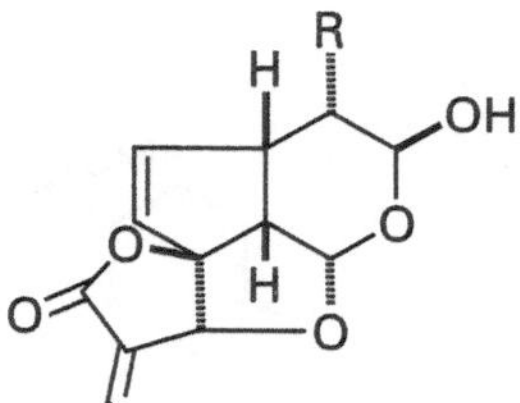

CLXXXIX R = H
XCC   R = COOMe

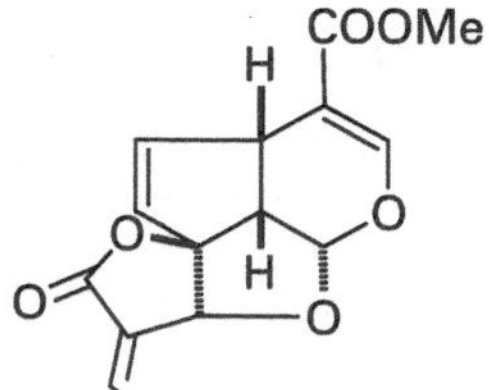

XCCI

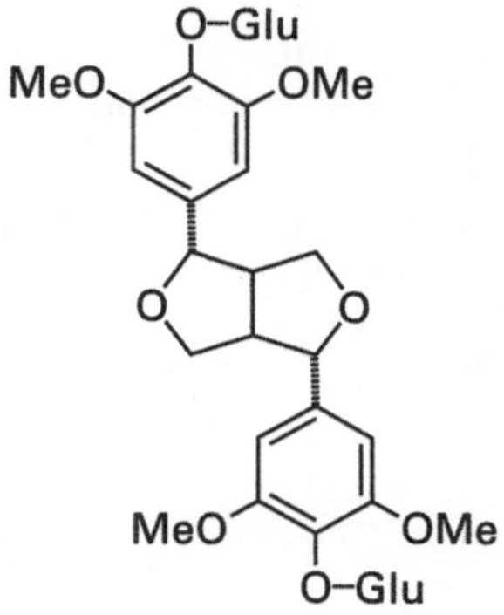

XCCII

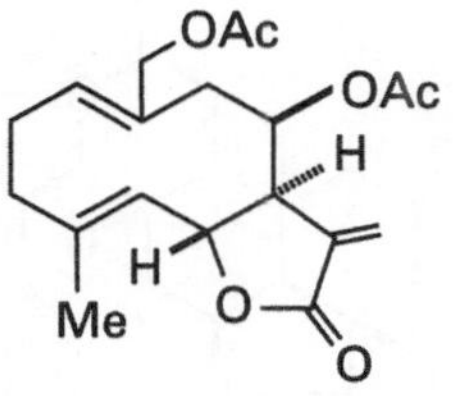

XCCIII

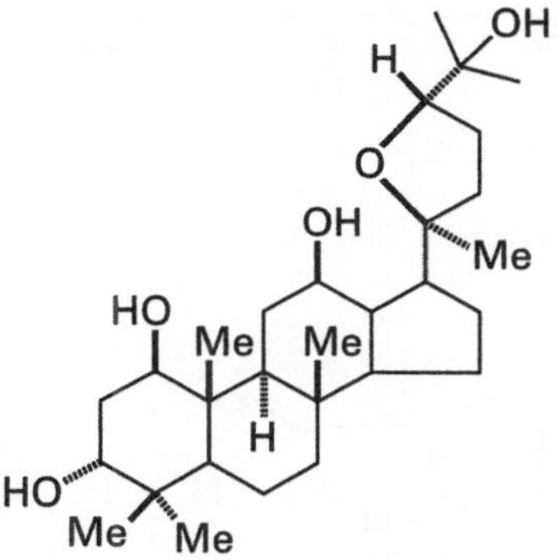

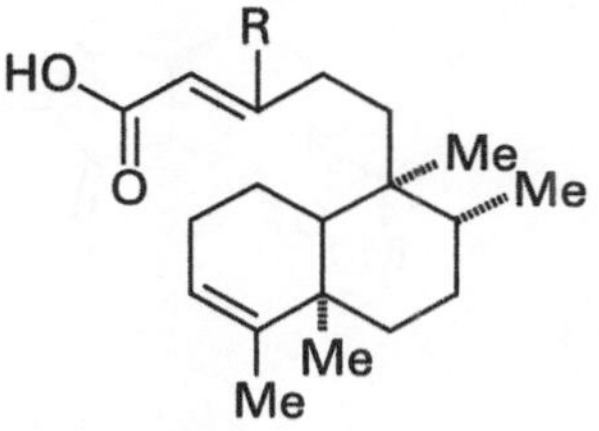

XCCV R = CHO
XCCVI R = Me

XCCIV

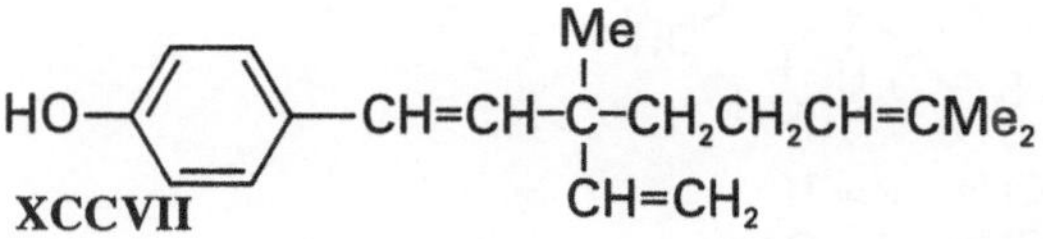

XCCVII

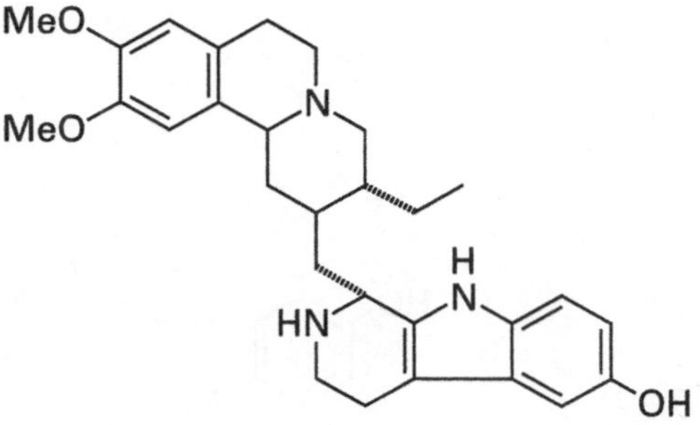

XCCVIII

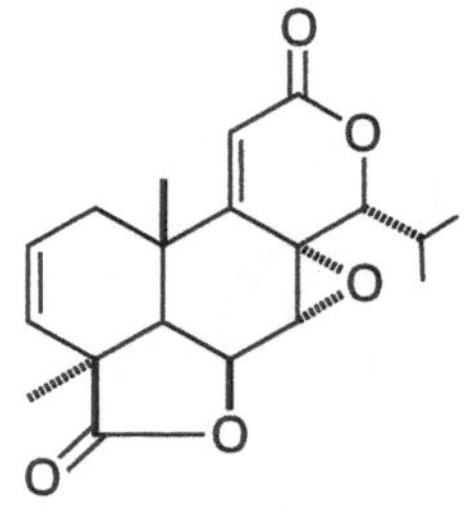

XCCIX

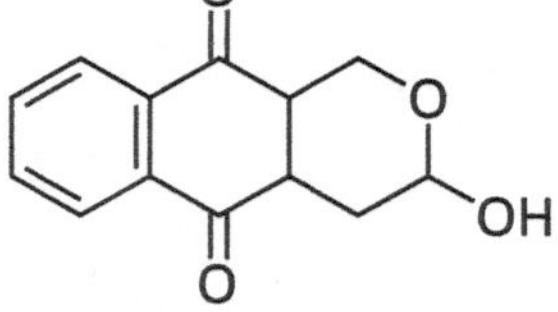

CC

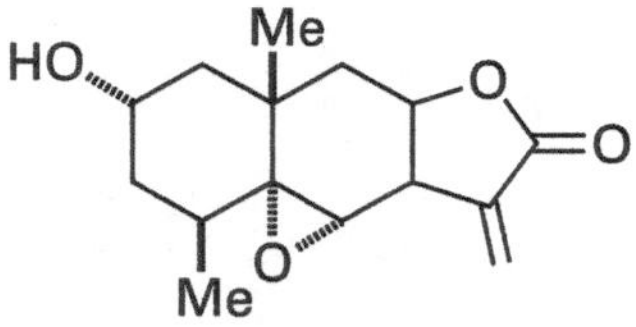

CCI

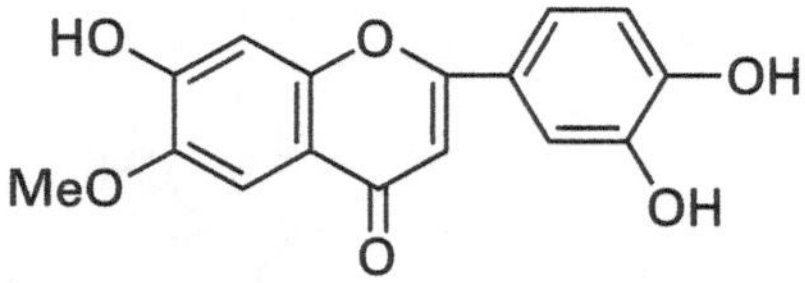

CCII

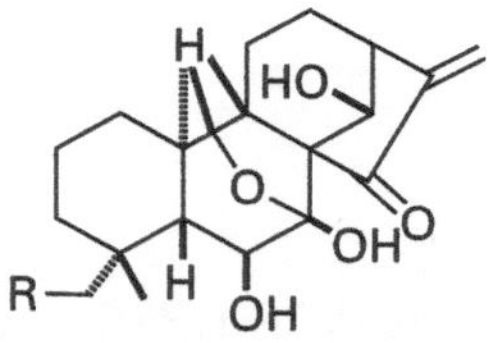

CCIIa   R = H
CCIIb   R = OAc

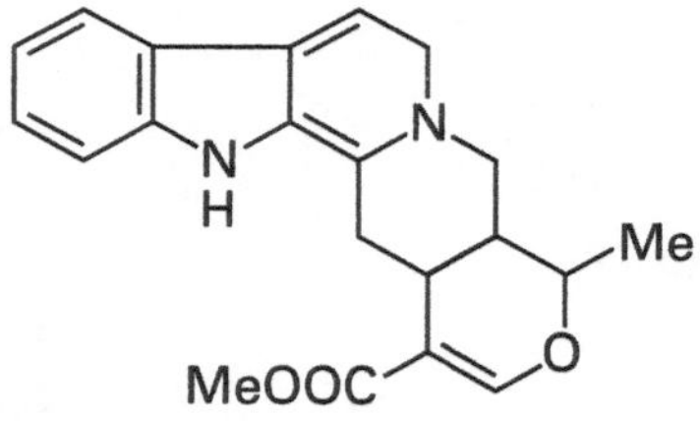

CCIII

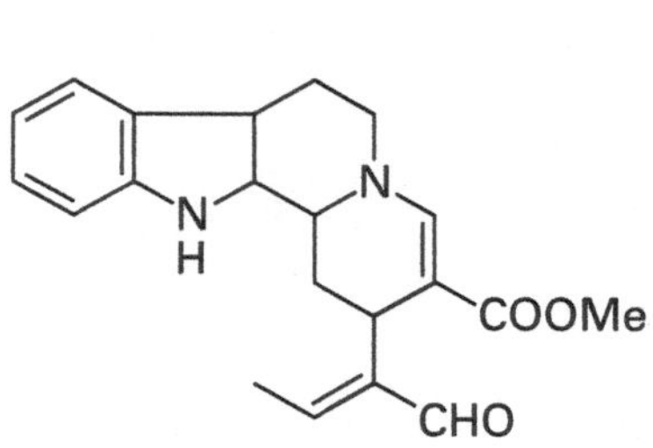

CCIV

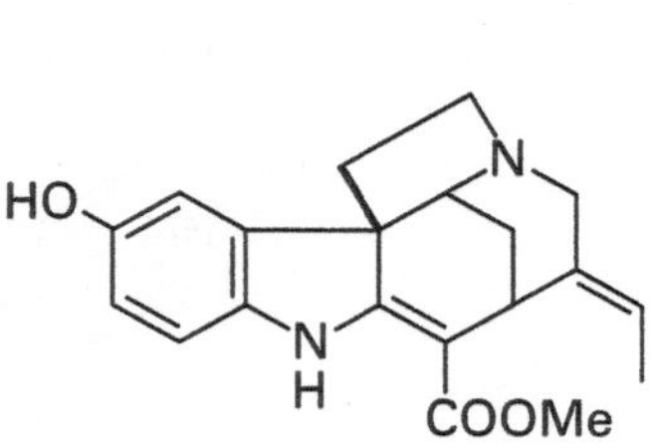

CCV

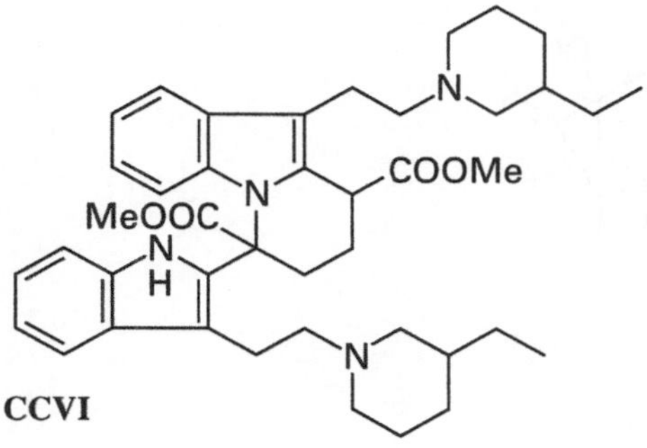

CCVI

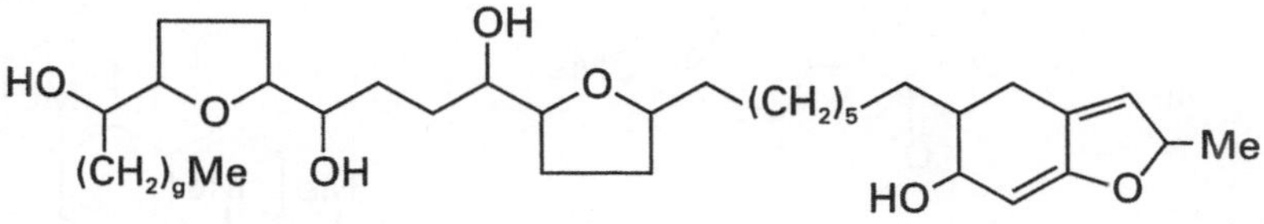

CCVIIa

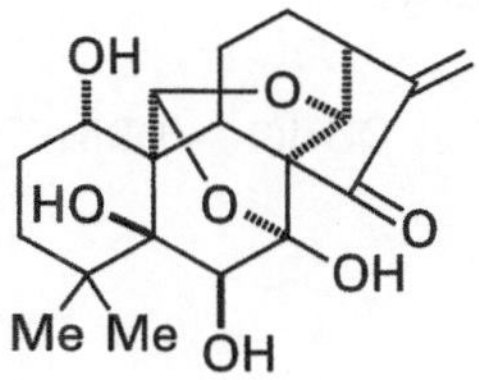

CCVIIb

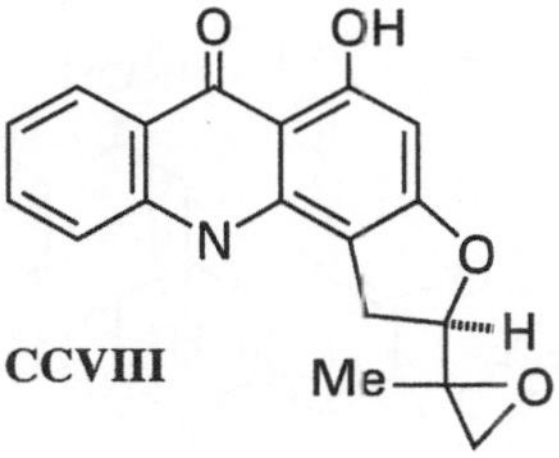

CCVIII

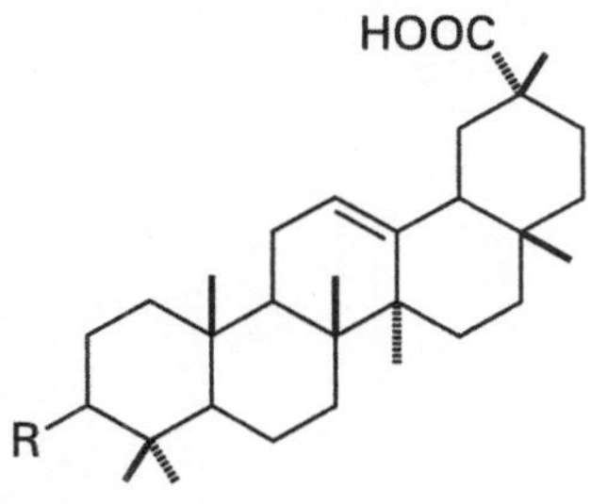

CCIX   R = O
CCX   R = OH

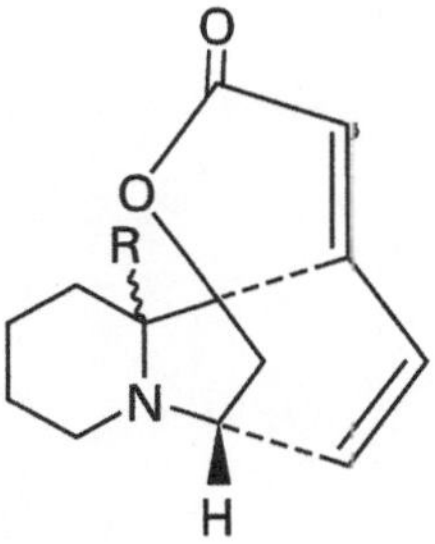

CCXI   R = α-H
CCXII   R = β-H

$H_2C=CH-CH(OH) \rightarrow C\equiv C-C\equiv C-CH=CH-CH(OH)(CH_2)_6-Me$

CCXIII

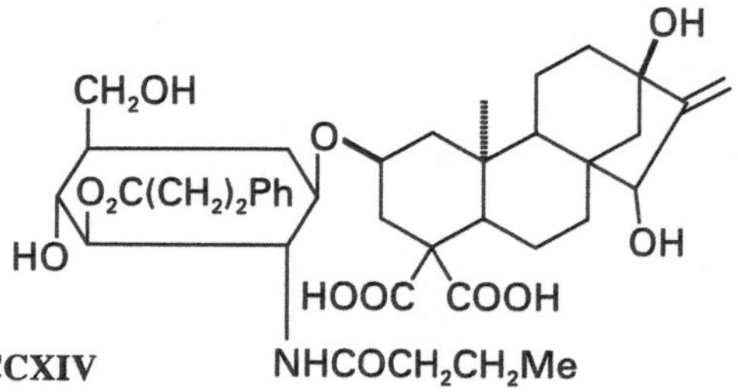

CCXIV

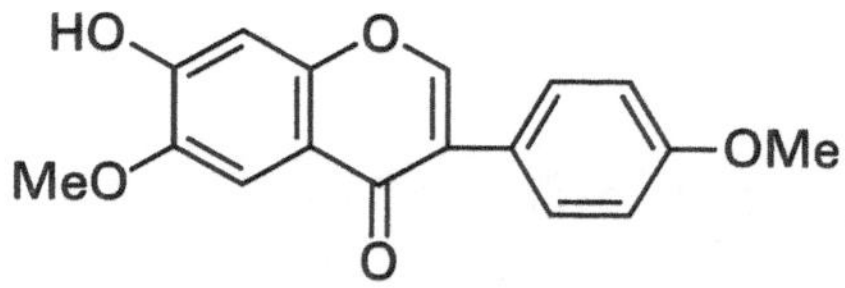

CH$_2$OH

O$_2$C(CH$_2$)$_2$Ph

HO

OH

OH

HOOC COOH

NHCOCH$_2$CH$_2$Me

CCXV

HO

MeO

OMe

O

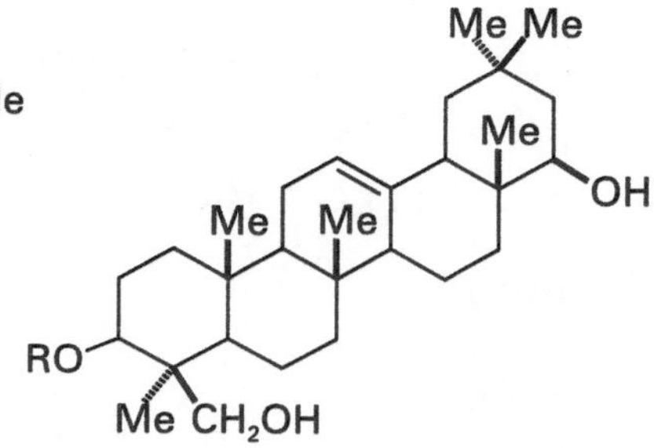

CCXVI
R = Gluc.acid(2 → 1)Gal(2 → 1)Rha

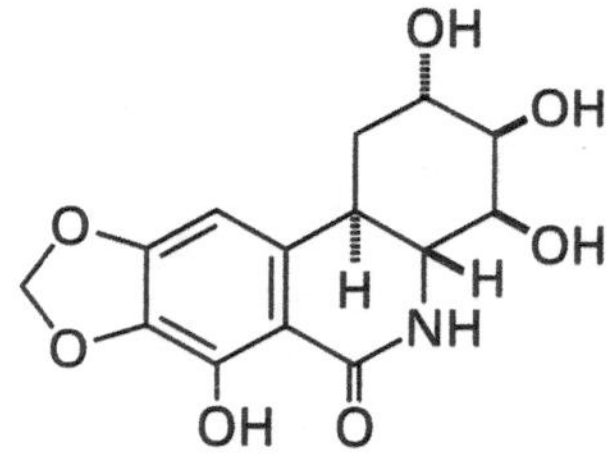

Me Me

Me

Me   Me

OH

RO

Me CH$_2$OH

CCXVII

OH

OH

OH

O

O

OH

H   NH

O

Index Vol. 43

The references of the Subject Index are given in the language of the respective contribution.
Die Stichworte des Sachregisters sind in der jeweiligen Sprache der einzelnen Beiträge aufgeführt.
Les termes repris dans la Table des Matières sind données selon la langue dans laquelle l'ouvrage est écrit.

Index of titles
Verzeichnis der Titel
Index des titres
Vol. 1–43 (1959–1994)

Author and paper index
Autoren- und Artikelindex
Index des auteurs et des articles
Vol. 1–43 (1959–1994)

Analysis of symptoms and signs related with intestinal parasitosis in 5,215 cases *19*, 10 (1975)	F. Biagi R. López J. Viso
Untersuchungen zur Biochemie und Pharmacologie der Thymoleptika *11*, 121 (1968)	M. H. Bickel
The role of adipose tissue in the distribution and storage of drugs *28*, 273 (1984)	M. H. Bickel
The β-adrenergic-blocking agents, pharmacology, and structure-activity relationships *10*, 46 (1966)	J. H. Biel B. K. B. Lum
Prostaglandins *17*, 410 (1973)	J. S. Bindra R. Bindra
In vitro models for the study of antibiotic activities *31*, 349 (1987)	J. Blaser S. H. Zinner
The red blood cell membrane as a model for targets of drug action *17*, 59 (1973)	L. Bolis
Epidemiology and public health. Importance of intestinal nematode infections in Latin America *19*, 28 (1975)	D. Botero
Clinical importance of cardiovascular drug interactions *25*, 133 (1981) Serum electrolyte abnormalities caused by drugs *30*, 9 (1986)	D. Craig Brater
Update of cardiovascular drug interactions *29*, 9 (1985)	D. Craig Brater Michael R. Vasko
Some practical problems of the epidemiology of leprosy in the Indian context *18*, 25 (1974)	S. G. Browne
Brain neurotransmitters and the development and maintenance of experimental hypertension *30*, 127 (1986)	Jerry J. Buccafusco Henry E. Brezenoff

Die Ionenaustauscher und ihre Anwendung in der Pharmazie und Medizin *1*, 11 (1959) Wert und Bewertung der Arzneimittel *10*, 90 (1966)	J. Büchi
Cyclopropane compounds of biological interest *15*, 227 (1971) The state of medicinal science *20*, 9 (1976) Isosterism and bioisosterism in drug design *37*, 287 (1991)	A. Burger
Human and veterinary anthelmintics (1965–1971) *17*, 108 (1973)	R. B. Burrows
The antibody basis of local immunity to experimental cholera infection in the rabbit ileal loop *19*, 471 (1975)	W. Burrows J. Kaur
Les dérivés organiques du fluor d'intérêt pharmacologique *3*, 9 (1961)	N. P. Buu-Hoï
Teaching tropical medicine *18*, 35 (1974)	K. M. Cahill
Anabolic steroids *2*, 71 (1960)	B. Camerino G. Sala
Immunosuppression agents, procedures, speculations and prognosis *16*, 67 (1972)	G. W. Camiener W. J. Wechter
Dopamine agonists: Structure-activity relationships *29*, 303 (1985)	Joseph G. Cannon
Analgesics and their antagonists: Recent developments *22*, 149 (1978)	A. F. Casy
Chemical nature and pharmacological actions of quaternary ammonium salts *2*, 135 (1960)	C. J. Cavallito A. P. Gray

Bioactive peptide analogs: In vivo and in vitro production *34*, 287 (1990)	Horst Kleinkauf Hans von Doehren
Opiate receptors: Search for new drugs *36*, 49 (1991)	Vera M. Kolb
Luteinizing hormone regulators: Luteinizing hormone releasing hormone analogs, estrogens, opiates, and estrogen-opiate hybrids *42*, 39 (1994)	Vera M. Kolb
Experimental evaluation of antituberculous compounds, with special reference to the effect of combined treatment *18*, 211 (1974)	F. Kradolfer
The oxidative metabolism of drugs and other foreign compounds *17*, 488 (1973)	F. Kratz
Die Amidinstruktur in der Arzneistofforschung *11*, 356 (1968)	A. Kreutzberger
Present data on the pathogenesis of tetanus *19*, 301 (1975) Tetanus: general and pathophysiological aspects: Achievement, failures, perspectives of elaboration of the problem *19*, 314 (1975)	G. N. Kryzhanovsky
Lipophilicity and drug activity *23*, 97 (1979)	H. Kubinyi
Klinisch-pharmakologische Kriterien in der Bewertung eines neuen Antibiotikums. Grundlagen und methodische Gesichtspunkte *23*, 327 (1978)	H. P. Kuemmerle
Adrenergic receptor research: Recent developments *33*, 151 (1989)	George Kunos
Über neue Arzneimittel *1*, 531 (1959), *2*, 251 (1960), *3*, 369 (1961), *6*, 347 (1963), *10*, 360 (1966)	W. Kunz
Die Anwendung von Psychopharmaka in der psychosomatischen Medizin *10*, 530 (1966)	F. Labhardt

Mechanism of drugs action on ion and water transport in renal tubular cells 26, 87 (1982)	Yu. V. Natochin
Progesterone receptor binding of steroidal and nonsteroidal compounds 30, 151 (1986)	Neelima M. Seth A. P. Bhaduri
Recent advances in drugs against hypertension 29, 215 (1985)	Neelima B. K. Bhat A. P. Bhaduri
High resolution nuclear magnetic resonance spectroscopy of biological samples as an aid to drug development 31, 427 (1987)	J. K. Nicholson Ian D. Wilson
Antibody response to two cholera vaccines in volunteers 19, 554 (1975)	Y. S. Nimbkar R. S. Karbhari S. Cherian N. G. Chanderkar R. P. Bhamaria P. S. Ranadive B. B. Gaitonde
Surface interaction between bacteria and phagocytic cells 32, 137 (1988)	L. Öhman G. Maluszynska K. E. Magnusson O. Stendahl
Die Chemotherapie der Wurmkrankheiten 1, 159 (1959)	H.-A. Oelkers
Structural modifications patterns from agonists to antagonists and their application to drug design – A new serotonin(5HT$_3$)antagonist series 41, 313 (1993)	Hiroshi Ohtaka Toshio Fujita
Serenics 42, 167 (1994)	Berend Olivier Jan Mos Maikel Raghoeba Paul de Koning Marianne Mak
GABA-Drug interactions 31, 223 (1987)	Richard W. Olsen
Drug research and human sleep 22, 355 (1978)	I. Oswald
Effects of drugs on calmodulin-mediated enzymatic actions 33, 353 (1989)	Judit Ovádi

An extensive community outbreak of acute diarrhoeal diseases in children *19*, 570 (1975)	S. C. Pal C. Koteswar Rao
Drug and its action according to Ayurveda *26*, 55 (1982)	Madhabendra Nath Pal
Oligosaccharide chains of glycoproteins *32*, 163 (1990)	Y. T. Pan Alan D. Elbein
Pharmacology of synthetic organic selenium compounds *36*, 9 (1991)	Michael J. Parnham Erich Graf
Moral challenges in the organisation and management of drug research *42*, 9 (1994)	Michael J. Parnham
3,4-Dihydroxyphenylalanine and related compounds *9*, 223 (1966)	A. R. Patel A. Burger
Mescaline and related compounds *11*, 11 (1968)	A. R. Patel
Experience with bitoscanate in adults *19*, 90 (1975)	A. H. Patricia U. Prabakar Rao R. Subramaniam N. Madanagopalan
The impact of state and society on medical research *35*, 9 (1990)	C. R. Pfaltz
Transfer factor in malignancy *42*, 401 (1994)	Giancarlo Pizza Caterina De Vinci H. Hugh Fudenberg
Monoaminoxydase-Hemmer *2*, 417 (1960)	A. Pletscher K. F. Gey P. Zeller
The oral antiarrhythmic drugs *35*, 151 (1990)	Lisa Mendes Scott L. Beau John S. Wilson Philip J. Podrid
Antifungal therapy: Are we winning? *37*, 183 (1991)	A. Polak P. G. Hartman

What makes a good pertussis vaccine? *19*, 341 (1975) Vaccine composition in relation to antigenic variation of the microbe: Is pertussis unique? *19*, 347 (1975) Some unsolved problems with vaccines *23*, 9 (1979) Eradication by vaccination: The memorial to smallpox could be surrounded by others *41*, 151 (1993)	N. W. Preston
Antibiotics in the chemotherapy of malaria *26*, 167 (1982)	S. K. Puri G. P. Dutta
Potassium channel openers: Airway pharmacology and clinical possibilities in asthma *37*, 161 (1991)	David Raeburn Jan-Anders Karlsson
Isozyme-selective cyclic nucleotide phosphodiesterase inhibitors: Biochemistry, pharmacology and therapeutic potential in asthma *40*, 9 (1993)	David Raeburn John E. Souness Adrian Tomkinson Jan-Anders Karlsson
Clinical study of diphtheria, tetanus and pertussis *19*, 356 (1975)	V. B. Raju V. R. Parvathi
Epidemiology of cholera in Hyderabad *19*, 578 (1975)	K. Rajyalakshmi P. V. Ramana Rao
Adenosine receptors: Clinical implications and biochemical mechanisms *32*, 195 (1988)	Vickram Ramkumar George Pierson Gary L. Stiles
New synthetic ligands for L-type voltage-gated calcium channels *40*, 191 (1993)	David Rampe David J. Triggle
Problems of malaria eradication in India *18*, 245 (1974)	V. N. Rao
Pharmacology of migraine *34*, 209 (1990)	Neil H. Raskin
The photochemistry of drugs and related substances *11*, 48 (1968)	S. T. Reid
Orale Antikoagulantien *11*, 226 (1968)	E. Renk W. G. Stoll

Mechanism-based inhibitors of monoamine oxidase *30*, 205 (1986)	Lauren E. Richards Alfred Burger
The hopanoids, bacterial triterpenoids, and the biosynthesis of isoprenic units in prokaryote *37*, 271 (1991)	Michael Rohner Philippe Bisseret Bertrand Sutter
Tetrahydroisoquinolines and β-carbolines: Putative natural substances in plants and animals *29*, 415 (1985)	H. Rommelspacher R. Susilo
Functional significance of the various components of the influenza virus *18*, 253 (1974)	R. Rott
Drug receptors and control of the cardiovascular system: Recent advances *36*, 117 (1991)	Robert R. Ruffolo Jr J. Paul Hieble David P. Brooks Giora Z. Feuerstein Andrew J. Nichols
Behavioral correlates of presynaptic events in the cholinergic neurotransmitter system *32*, 43 (1988)	Roger W. Russell
Epidemiology of pertussis *19*, 257 (1975)	J. A. Sa
Surgical amoebiasis *18*, 77 (1974)	A. E. de Sa
Role of beta-adrenergic blocking drug propranolol in severe tetanus *19*, 361 (1975)	G. S. Sainani K. L. Jain V. R. D. Deshpande A. B. Balsara S. A. Iyer
Studies on *Vibrio parahaemolyticus* in Bombay *19*, 586 (1975)	F. L. Saldanha A. K. Patil M. V. Sant
Leukotriene antagonists and inhibitors of leukotriene biosynthesis as potential therapeutic agents *37*, 9 (1991)	John A. Salmon Lawrence G. Garland
Pharmacology and toxicology of axoplasmic transport *28*, 53 (1984)	Fred Samson Ralph L. Smith J. Alejandro Donoso

Clinical experience with bitoscanate *19*, 96 (1975)	M. R. Samuel
Tetanus: Situational clinical trials and therapeutics *19*, 367 (1975)	R. K. M. Sanders M. L. Peacock B. Martyn B. D. Shende
Epidemiological studies on cholera in non-endemic regions with special reference to the problem of carrier state during epidemic and non-epidemic period *19*, 594 (1975)	M. V. Sant W. N. Gatlewar S. K. Bhindey
Epidemiological and biochemical studies in filariasis in four villages near Bombay *18*, 269 (1974)	M. V. Sant W. N. Gatlewar T. U. K. Menon
Hookworm anaemia and intestinal malabsorption associated with hookworm infestation *19*, 108 (1975)	A. K. Saraya B. N. Tandon
The effects of structural alteration on the anti-inflammatory properties of hydrocortisone *5*, 11 (1963)	L. H. Sarett A. A. Patchett S. Steelman
The impact of natural product research on drug discovery *23*, 51 (1979)	L. H. Sarett
Aldose reductase inhibitors: Recent developments *40*, 99 (1993)	Reinhard Sarges Peter J. Oates
Anti-filariasis campaign: Its history and future prospects *18*, 259 (1974)	M. Sasa
Barbiturates and the $GABA_A$ receptor complex *34*, 261 (1990)	Paul A. Saunders I. K. Ho
Platelets and atherosclerosis *29*, 49 (1985)	Robert N. Saunders
Advances in chemotherapy of malaria *30*, 221 (1986)	Anil K. Saxena Mridula Saxena
Developments in antihistamines (H_1) *39*, 35 (1992)	Anil K. Saxena Mridula Saxena
Pyrimidinones as biodynamic agents *31*, 127 (1987)	Anil K. Saxena Shradha Sinha

On conformation analysis, molecular graphics, fentanyl and its derivatives *30*, 91 (1986)	J. P. Tollenaere H. Moereels M. van Loon
Antibakterielle Chemotherapie der Tuberkulose *7*, 193 (1964)	F. Trendelenburg
Alternative approaches to the discovery of novel antipsychotic agents *38*, 299 (1992)	M. D. Tricklebank L. J. Bristow P. H. Hutson
Diphtheria *19*, 423 (1975)	P. M. Udani M. M. Kumbhat U. S. Bhat M. S. Nadkarni S. K. Bhave S. G. Ezuthachan B. Kamath
Biologische Oxydation und Reduktion am Stickstoff aromatischer Amino- und Nitroderivate und ihre Folgen für den Organismus *8*, 195 (1965) Stoffwechsel von Arzneimitteln als Ursache von Wirkungen, Nebenwirkungen und Toxizität *15*, 147 (1971)	H. Uehleke
Mode of death in tetanus *19*, 439 (1975)	H. Vaishnava C. Bhawal Y. P. Munjal
Comparative evaluation of amoebicidal drugs *18*, 353 (1974) Comparative efficacy of newer anthelmintics *19*, 166 (1975)	B. J. Vakil N. J. Dalal
Cephalic tetanus *19*, 443 (1975)	B. J. Vakil B. S. Singhal S. S. Pandya P. F. Irami
The effect and usefulness of early intravenous beta blockade in acute myocardial infarction *30*, 71 (1986)	Anders Vedin Claes Wilhelmsson

Methods of monitoring adverse reactions to drugs *21*, 231 (1977) Aspects of social pharmacology *22*, 9 (1978)	J. Venulet
The current status of cholera toxoid research in the United States *19*, 602 (1975)	W. F. Verwey J. C. Guckian J. Craig N. Pierce J. Peterson H. Williams Jr
Systemic cancer therapy: Four decades of progress and some personal perspectives *34*, 76 (1990)	Charles L. Vogel
Cell-kinetic and pharmacokinetic aspects in the use and further development of cancerostatic drugs *20*, 521 (1976)	M. von Ardenne
The problem of diphtheria as seen in Bombay *19*, 452 (1975)	M. M. Wagle R. R. Sanzgiri Y. K. Amdekar
Drug nephrotoxicity – The significance of cellular mechanisms *41*, 51 (1993)	Robert J. Walker J. Paul Fawcett
Nicotine: An addictive substance or a therapeutic agent? *33*, 9 (1989)	David M. Warburton
Cell-wall antigens of *Vibrio cholerae* and their implication in cholera immunity *19*, 612 (1975)	Y. Watanabe R. Ganguly
Steroidogenic capacity in the adrenal cortex and its regulation *34*, 359 (1990)	Michael R. Watermann Evan R. Simpson
Antigen-specific T-cell factors and drug research *32*, 9 (1988)	David R. Webb
Where is immunology taking us? *20*, 573 (1976) Immunology in drug research *28*, 233 (1984)	W. J. Wechter Barbara E. Loughman
Natriuretic hormones *34*, 231 (1990)	W. J. Wechter Elaine J. Benaksas

AGENTS AND ACTIONS SUPPLEMENTS

Edited by

K. Brune
University of Erlangen, Germany
M.J. Parnham
Bonn, Germany

Agents and Actions Supplements (AAS) is a series for rapid publication of the proceedings of symposia on topics of current interest in inflammation, allergy, related respiratory diseases, thrombosis and related fields. The series allows fast dissemination of surveys and specialized reports on, for example, research into the role of prostaglandins in inflammation and thrombosis, new trends in the treatment of rheumatoid arthritis, allergic reactions and asthma.

Variability in Response to Anti-Rheumatic Drugs

Edited by
P.M. Brooks / R.O. Day, *University of New South Wales, Sydney, Australia*
G.G. Graham, *University of New South Wales, Kensington, Australia*
K.M. Williams, *University of New South Wales, Sydney, Australia*

1993. 240 pages. Hardcover. ISBN 3-7643-2869-X (Agents and Actions Supplements 44)

Therapy of rheumatoid arthritis is undergoing dramatic changes. Greater appreciation of the long-term outcomes of this disease and the impacts of treatments has resulted in a more aggressive approach to therapy, especially in the early stages.

An increasingly diverse array of anti-rheumatic drugs with novel effects on inflammation and the immune system confronts us. One factor remains constant; individual response to anti-rheumatic therapy is highly variable, thus providing an important approach to under-standing the heterogeneity of the disease process, as well as the mechanisms of drug action.

Experts of international repute address in this volume relevant aspects of recent research into non-steroidal anti inflammatory drugs, stereo-chemistry, pharmacodynamics and pharmacokinetics, trials and trial design, combination therapy, new and old disease-modifying anti-rheumatic drugs, adverse reactions, and side effects. The result is a state-of-the-art review of anti-rheumatic drug therapy.

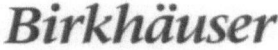

Birkhäuser

Birkhäuser Verlag AG
Basel · Boston · Berlin

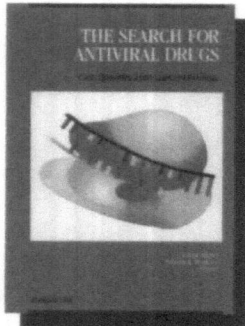

"The assembly in one volume of the contemporaneous views of the most active investigators in this field will probably come to be seen in the future as a landmark record..."

—from the Introductory Remarks by Herman N. Eisen

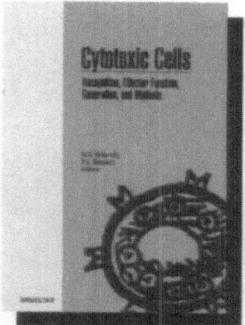

Cytotoxic Cells: Recognition, Effector Function, Generation, and Methods

Edited by
M. Sitkovsky and **P. Henkart**
National Institutes of Health, Bethesda, MD, USA

1993. 544 pages. Hardcover. ISBN 3-7643-3608-0

This collection of papers from the most important researches of cytoxic cells will make an excellent introduction to the study of cytotoxic T lymphocytes and other cytotoxic cells, including CTL, NK, LAK, TIL, ADCC, macrophages, mast cells, and platelets.

These topics are covered comprehensiviely, including generation, recognition, effector functions, and important methodologies. It will provide a state-of-the-art review of this important field. Special chapters cover the mechanisms of lethal hit delivery and immunopharmacological manipulations of cytotoxic cells which will be of interest to pharmacological researchers as well as cancer specialists. Adoptive immunotherapy is covered by experts in each field. The book is divided into brief, very readable chapters by experts in each field.

Leading the way as the first comprehensive work available in the field of Cytotoxic Cells and Cytotoxicity assays, this outstanding collection of papers by internationally renowned immunologists will serve as the reference source for immunology and cell biology laboratories, as well as allied fields of research.

Cytotoxic Cells provides an essential collection of methodologies, which are invaluable to every immunologist and cell biologist studying cellular regulation. The historical, molecular, cell biological, and clinical aspects of cell-mediated cytotoxicity are thoroughly covered by the leading researchers in their respective fields.

Over 50 chapters cover the following topics: • Introduction and Overview • Target Cell Recognition • Generation of Cytotoxic Cells • Molecular Mechanisms of Cellular Cytotoxicity • Granule Proteases • Alternate Mechanisms of Cytolysis • Biochemical and Immunopharmaceutical Manipulation of Cytotoxic Cells • Functions of Cytotoxic Cells In Vivo • Macrophage-Mediated Cytotoxicity • Methods

This is an invaluable introduction to the field for students, as well as a reference tool for practicing researchers, and a must for every laboratory bookshelf.

For more information on recent and forthcoming books and journals you can order the BIRKHÄUSER LIFE SCIENCES BULLETIN, published twice a year and free of charge.

Birkhäuser

Birkhäuser Verlag AG
Basel · Boston · Berlin

Fractals in Biology and Medicine

T.F. Nonnenmacher, *Mathematische Physik, Universität Ulm, Germany*
G.A. Losa, *Instituto Cantonale di Patologia, Locarno, Switzerland*
E.R. Weibel, *Anatomisches Institut Universität Bern, Switzerland*

1994. 397 pages. Hardcover. ISBN 3-7643-2989-0

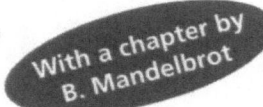

With a chapter by B. Mandelbrot

Fractals in Biology and Medicine explores the potential of fractal geometry for describing and understanding biological organisms, their development and growth as well as their structural design and functional properties. It extends these notions to assess changes associated with disease in the hope to contribute to the understanding of pathogenetic processes in medicine.

The book is the first comprehensive presentation of the importance of the new concept of fractal geometry for biological and medical sciences. It collates in a logical sequence extended papers based on invited lectures and free communications presented at a symposium in Ascona, Switzerland, attended by leading scientists in this field, among them the originator of fractal geometry, Benoît Mandelbrot.

Fractals in Biology and Medicine begins by asking how the theoretical construct of fractal geometry can be applied to biomedical sciences and then addresses the role of fractals in the design and morphogenesis of biological organisms as well as in molecular and cell biology. The consideration of fractal structure in understanding metabolic functions and pathological changes is a particularly promising avenue for future research.

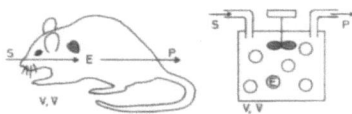

Please order through your bookseller
or directly from:
Birkhäuser Verlag AG, P.O. Box 133
CH-4010 Basel / Switzerland
Fax ++41 / 61 721 79 50
E-Mail: 100010.23@compuserve.com

Orders from the USA or Canada
should be sent to:
Birkhäuser Boston, 333 Meadowlands Parkway,
Secaucus, NJ 07094-2491 / USA
Call Toll-Free 1-800-777-4643

For more information on recent and forthcoming books and journals you can order the BIRKHÄUSER LIFE SCIENCES BULLETIN, published twice a year and free of charge.

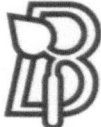

Birkhäuser Verlag • Basel • Boston • Berlin